"In *Five Spirits*, Lorie Dechar brings the long-forgotten tradition of the Mysterious Feminine back to the practice of acupuncture and Chinese medicine. She presents a compelling vision of the body as a vessel of spiritual transformation and provides life-changing, vivifying revelations about the true nature of health. This book offers a unique, invaluable approach to healing."—**Michael J. Gelb**, author, *How to Think Like Leonardo daVinci* and *BodyLearning: An Introduction to the Alexander Technique*

"A journey into Chinese medicine through a very personal vision. The author looks for a psychospiritual healing and development and presents it with her rich imagination and poetic language, inspired by Chinese characters and thinkers as well as by Western philosophers."—**Elisabeth Rochat de la Vallée**, sinologist; author, *Rooted in Spirit* and *The Seven Emotions*

"Dechar's book is admirable in its scope. . . . She strives not to translate Chinese medicine into a Western form of understanding but instead supports Western expansion of consciousness to allow for an understanding of this type of reality. Recommended for public libraries and alternative medicine collections and highly recommended for students in the field."—*Library Journal*

"An entirely original book. Dechar is in a unique position to address how classical acupuncture might be utilized to enable patients not only to transform their health concerns, but also to address their metaphysical and psycho-spiritual issues. While *Five Spirits* will be especially provocative for practitioners of acupuncture and Chinese medicine, it will also appeal to bodyworkers and psychotherapists, and their patients who are intrigued by Eastern perspectives on health and healing."—**Mark Seem**, director, Tri-State College of Acupuncture; author, *Acupuncture Energetics* and *New American Acupuncture*

"In *Five Spirits* Lorie Dechar has brought the depth of Chinese medicine into the present and opened the road ahead to a truly integrated vision for health."—**Nancy Rosanoff**, author, *Knowing When It's Right*; host, *The Listening Place*

"As a patient in Lorie's acupuncture practice, I have experienced profound physical, emotional and spiritual transformation; her work has helped me to find new faith in my fundamental ability to heal. *Five Spirits* has not only given me insight into the depths and directions of my own healing process, but also serves me as an essential text in learning how to assist others on their paths."—**Tom McCauley**, acupuncture student

師曰此經乃九天八會

道元始天尊昔經歷千

備生死五運遷變萬

唐景雲之上上清之境

祥生火□□不舍吾□

Five Spirits

Alchemical Acupuncture for Psychological
and Spiritual Healing

LORIE EVE DECHAR, M.AC.

CHIRON PUBLICATIONS / LANTERN BOOKS

NEW YORK

For Diane and Edouard
Who lit the fire
And Nina Shoshana
Who carries forth the flame.

2006
Lantern Books
One Union Square West, Suite 201
New York, NY 10003

Cover art © RubberBall / SuperStock
Cover calligraphy by David Shih
Interior calligraphy by David Shih, WeiChung Wayne Chen and Lorie Eve Dechar

The author gratefully acknowledges permission to reprint copyright material from the following:

Tao Te Ching: The Definitive Edition, by Lao Tzu, translated by Jonathan Star, copyright ©2001 by
    Jonathan Star. Used by permission of Jeremy P. Tarcher, an imprint of Penguin Group (USA) Inc.
The Secret of the Golden Flower, translated by Thomas Cleary, copyright ©1991 by Thomas Cleary.
    Reprinted by permission of HarperCollins Publishers.
The Heart: The Lingshu Chapter 8, by Claude Larre and Elisabeth Rochat de la Vallée. Reprinted by
    permission of Monkey Press.
Rooted in Spirit: The Heart of Chinese Medicine, by Claude Larre and Elisabeth Rochat de la Vallée,
    translated by Sarah Stang. Reprinted by permission of Station Hill Press.
Taoism: Growth of a Religion, by Isabelle Robinet, translated by Phyllis Brooks, copyright ©1997 by
    the Board of Trustees of the Leland Stanford Jr. University.
Wenlin® Software for Learning Chinese, Version 2.1 ©1987–2005 Wenlin Institute, Inc.

Printed in Canada

Library of Congress Cataloging-in-Publication Data

Dechar, Lorie.
    Five spirits : alchemical acupuncture for psychological and spiritual healing / Lorie Eve Dechar.
        p. cm.
    Includes bibliographical references and index.
    ISBN 1-59056-092-2 (alk. paper)
    1. Medicine, Chinese. 2. Hygiene, Taoist. 3. Mind and body therapies. I. Title.
R602.D34 2006
610'.951—dc22
                                                    2005022649

Acknowledgments

~

Just as a flower grows up from the soil that nourishes and supports it, this book has grown from the garden of my life, from the love, the challenges and the commitment of my friends, family, teachers, students and patients. Many people have played a role in the conception, gestation and creation of this book.

In particular, I want to express my heartfelt appreciation to Nathan Schwartz-Salant for seeing my strength as well as my vulnerability and for relentlessly calling me back to the Self. Gassho to Claude Anshin Thomas for opening me to the priceless treasure of my practice. And to Professor J. R. Worsley for giving me, from the very beginning of my career as an acupuncturist, permission to let nature be my master teacher.

Deep gratitude to Rudolph Ballentine for the years of intellectual partnership and mutual healing, Michael Gelb for the sheer joy of our unique and precious friendship, Ann Bingham for her clarity and dedication to this project, Patsy Roth for opening a space for my teaching and for being a source of inspiration in my life, and to Benjamin Fox for having the courage, eccentricity and devotion to be my partner on the journey.

In addition, I want to thank Sarah, Erin, Alyssa and Gene at Lantern Books for helping me to make the vision real. Noel Dechar and Laura Harmon for all the evenings by the fire. Peter and Natasha Dechar for bringing Tonya's radiant spirit into our lives. My mother, for reading the manuscript when it was still unreadable and believing in this project from beginning to end. My students at Tri-State College of Acupuncture, who continue to teach me how to learn and how to teach. My patients, who have revealed to me the mysterious alchemy of the healing process. And my daughter, Nina, for calling me down to earth and then flying with me to the stars.

Last but not least, I thank the waters, tides, winds, trees, light, earth, sky and people of East Blue Hill, Maine, who supported my spirits while I dreamed and wrote this book.

Table of Contents

∽

List of Figures

∽

As my inmost nature teaches me, whatever is necessary, as seen from the heights and in the sense of a great economy—is also the useful par excellence: one should not only bear it, one should *love* it. *Amor fati*: that is my inmost nature. And as for my long sickness, do I not owe it indescribably more than I owe to my health?

—Friedrich Nietzsche[1]

Author's Note

∽

As acupuncture becomes increasingly popular in the West, there is a tendency to view and practice it as if it were the product of our Western consciousness. We begin to think of it as a safe and economical alternative treatment for common problems such as headache, back pain, digestive disturbances and allergies. Although acupuncture is an effective treatment for many ordinary physical symptoms, this limited viewpoint does not open to us the richness of the tradition as it was originally taught and practiced in ancient China.

In this book, I am not offering proof of acupuncture's effectiveness or explanations of its methods from a Western perspective. Rather, I offer a view of the system from the inside out. Like a tour guide who speaks two languages, I hope to lead the reader on a journey into a foreign territory, the territory of ancient Chinese medicine. My goal is not to turn Chinese medicine and acupuncture into something Western consciousness can comprehend but rather to support the expansion of Western consciousness beyond its usual boundaries. Rather than fitting Chinese medicine into the box of Western rational thought, I hope to expand Western consciousness to contain this other way of organizing reality. To me, this is the only way we can be touched and changed by the transformational potential of traditional Chinese medicine, using it as a springboard to a new and more efficient system of emotional, psychosomatic, and psychospiritual healing.

In the following pages, I will use many Chinese words and key Chinese medical terms, along with some Western psychological terms, that are defined in the Glossary as well as in the body of the text. The reader is advised to note that certain English words are used to refer to Chinese concepts and may have a somewhat different meaning within the context of the book. For example, the English word "heart" is the commonly accepted translation of the Chinese word *xin*. However, the Western heart, which is thought of as a muscular organ that pumps blood through the body, is different from the Chinese *xin,* which is viewed not only as a physical organ but also as a complex of physical, emotional and psychospiritual functions.

The original Chinese characters for key Chinese medical and alchemical terms are included. From my own experience, the original characters provide the key to understanding ancient Chinese concepts and no translation can compare to studying the ancient graphics themselves. For etymological interpretation, I have relied on four main sources: *Chinese Characters*, by Dr. L. Wieger, S.J.; multiple texts and transcripts of talks by Claude Larre, S.J. and Elisabeth Rochat de la Vallée; *China: Empire of Living Symbols,* by Cecilia Lindqvist; and the Wenlin CD-ROM Software for Learning Chinese, version 2.1. In addition, I have amplified my interpretation of the characters through insights gleaned from studies of Buddhist and Taoist philosophy, archetypal psychology, and the symbolic language of dreams and the collective unconscious.

At the outset, I offer an explanation of four key concepts, followed by a note on Chinese characters, in order to facilitate the reader's entry into the terrain of the book:

Traditional Chinese Medicine. I use the term "traditional Chinese medicine" to refer to the original system of healing presented in Taoist alchemical texts and early classical Chinese medical texts—particularly the *Neijing Suwen,* or *The Yellow Emperor's Classic of Internal Medicine* (c. 350 BCE)—and practiced in ancient China. This original teaching includes Yin/Yang Theory, the Law of the Five Elements, the Five Spirits and other aspects of Taoist psychospiritual alchemy. While reading *Five Spirits,* distinguish my term "traditional Chinese medicine" from Traditional Chinese Medicine, or TCM, the term that is used to refer to the modern form of medical acupuncture and herbal pharmacology currently practiced in mainland China and taught in some acupuncture colleges in North America and Europe. Acupuncture is the cornerstone of traditional Chinese medicine; the system, however, also includes a variety of other treatment methods, such as massage, breath practices, moxibustion, herbal remedies, meditation, diet, and exercise.

Alchemy. Alchemy is an ancient spiritual discipline and natural philosophy that was practiced, in various forms, the world over for many centuries. Alchemy's main concern is the process of transformation and the attainment of immortality, in other words, the overcoming of entropy and death and the upgrading of material and psychic substances to form systems of ever-increasing complexity and value. The Taoist alchemical tradition can be viewed as the way Chinese people organized their understanding of the natural world after the waning of shamanism and before the emergence of modern science. It began around 350 BCE with the publication of Taoism's primary text, Lao Tzu's *Tao Teh Ching.* Although alchemical practices are currently outlawed in mainland China, they continue to play a part in Taoist ritual, Taoist and Buddhist meditation practices and Chinese martial arts. The development of Taoist alchemy in China parallels the development of Chinese medicine. It is the premise of this book that many of Chinese medicine's central principles derive from alchemical consciousness. The alchemical mystery at the heart of traditional Chinese medicine is the healing transformation of ordinary life experience—the lead weight of suffering, illness, loss and humiliation—into the golden light of wisdom, compassion and insight.

Taoist Psychology. The word "psychology" is not generally associated with Chinese medicine, since the system does not radically separate the healing of the spirit, mind and body. However, I believe that the term "psychology," in its classical sense, aptly describes an important part of the Taoist alchemical tradition and a crucial but overlooked aspect of traditional Chinese medicine. The English word "psychology" is derived from *psyche*, the Greek word for "soul." In Greek mythology, Psyche was a beautiful maiden who became a goddess. She is usually pictured with the wings of a butterfly and is emblematic of immortality. The word is related to the Greek word *pneuma*, which means "breath." The ancient Greeks viewed the breath as the connecting link between heaven and earth, divinity and humanity, between spiritual energies and the physical matrix of the body. They thought of the soul as a kind of breath body and likened it to a butterfly that flits between the air above and the world below. Like the breath itself, the soul was thought to move freely between spirit and matter, infusing one with the essence of the other as it brought animation and intention to living beings. The Taoists also had a very clear idea about a breath body. They believed that it came into being in the human embryo when the yin and yang essences of the parents joined at the moment of conception. Taoist sages spoke frequently of this breath body, diagrammed it and focused a great deal of attention on it in their alchemical and healing practices. Their understanding of the breath body led to the development of *wushen*, the Five Spirits, which we will see describes a complex breath body or *pneumatic* system that both lifts and stabilizes the human body, mind, and spirit. In this book, I use "psychology"not in its modern Western sense, to refer to the study of object relations, the traumas of early childhood and the development of individual personality, but in the classical sense, to refer to the study of the subtle breath body or what, in earlier eras, was spoken of as the soul.

The Five Spirits. The Five Spirits are the Taoist map of the human psyche. The system provides a mythical view of the nervous system and forms the basis of Chinese medical psychology. It also describes a precise and efficient technology for psychospiritual transformation. The Five Spirits can be understood as the Taoist version of the chakra system of Vedic India. Like the chakras, the spirits exist as centers of consciousness in the subtle body rather than as structures in the physical body. Just as each chakra relates to a particular level of consciousness, each spirit relates to a particular aspect of human awareness, a particular vibration or frequency of psychic energy. An understanding of the Five Spirits is the key that opens the doorway to the mysteries of Taoist psychospiritual alchemy. By taking advantage of the discoveries of Western archetypal psychology and new discoveries about the mind and nervous system, we can decipher the Five Spirits and reorganize the system in a way that has proven to be clinically invaluable in treating psychosomatic, emotional and psychospiritual distress.

The Structure of Chinese Characters

While English words are made up of letters which are abstract phonetic symbols, Chinese words or "characters" are concrete visual images, pictures that are grounded in direct somatic experience of the world. For example, the charcter *ri*, which means "sun," is a circle with a dot at the center, much like a picture drawn by a young child. It is easy to see how this round circle represents the round sun in the sky.

Most characters, however, are not simple figures such as the character for "sun." Rather, they are compound figures formed by combining two or more graphic elements. The elements or components may themselves be simple characters with their own meaning, or they may be phonetic components that indicate the pronunciation of the word but do not add to the logic or meaning of the character.

Western scholars of the Chinese language, known as sinologists, refer to the meaning part of the character as the "radical." They refer to the part that does not give meaning but indicates pronunciation as the "phonetic." While more modern students of the Chinese language now use the terms "signific component" and "phonetic component," in this book I have chosen to use the more classical term, "radical," when referring to a meaning component of a character. For the purposes of this book, the pronunciation of Chinese words is not relevant, so I will not make reference to phonetic components.

Caveat

The therapeutic strategies presented in this book are meant as general guidelines that should be tailored to the reader's level of expertise. These strategies are drawn from standard Chinese medical texts, from Western psychology and from my own experience working with patients.

Acupuncture is powerful medicine, and it takes years to learn to practice it safely. Only licensed acupuncturists should use needles or moxa on any of the acupuncture points mentioned in this book. However, there are safe methods that make it possible for nonprofessionals to benefit from the healing effects of Chinese medicine. Acupressure, using touch to stimulate the acupuncture points and meridians, has proven to be a safe and effective treatment for many common physical ailments as well as for emotional distress. Gentle touch exchanged in an atmosphere of acceptance and trust can go a long way toward shifting a person's state of being. Sensitive touch and the use of intention to move and tonify qi (as described in this book) can be safely exchanged between family members and friends and practiced professionally by licensed massage therapists and other trained body workers. Charts showing the exact location of points are not included in this book but are readily available in standard Chinese medical textbooks.

The flower essences cited can also be safely used by trained practitioners as well as general readers. They are readily available in most health food stores, although they too should be used with respect for the potent energies that accompany psychological healing processes. Chinese herbs, however, are complex medicines and should not be prescribed, even in low doses, except by trained practitioners and herbalists.

Preface

By Rudolph Ballentine, M.D.

∽

Let's imagine for a moment that Mao Tse Tung's mission on Planet Earth was to repackage Chinese culture so that it could enter the West—especially its healing traditions—so as to provide help for the desperately neurotic, suffering denizens of the "developed" world. So he snipped off the offending features of acupuncture (its "Eastern" spirituality, for example) and packed it off, freshly shorn and almost passably "scientific," to the Western hemisphere. And there it was gradually accepted.

Then, surprise! Like a Trojan horse, it opened and out poured a richly complex, spiritual approach to healing that was totally different from—and a much-needed antidote to—the prevailing technological medicine of the day.

There may be more truth to our little fantasy than is apparent at first glance. Indeed, Mao did strip Chinese medicine of its deeper psychological and spiritual aspects. And indeed it did, largely as a result of that, slip adroitly into Western clinics and hospitals. And now, after it has indisputably arrived, the time is ripe for its belly to open and for the warriors of transformation to charge forth.

And that's where this book, with its magician of an author, enters the scene. Lorie Eve Dechar brings forth the spiritual heart of Chinese medicine, hidden within the materialistic version that was rolled into the West. She reveals to us an authoritative, profoundly authentic portrait of the subtle, multileveled healing system of Taoist alchemy—the tradition that was obscured and even outlawed during the "modernization" of Mao's Cultural Revolution and its purges.

Uncovering the lost essence of the Chinese healing tradition has been a collaborative effort, and many scholars have made their contributions. But Lorie's clinical work, which employs acupuncture to trigger psychospiritual transformation, brings a special flavor to her research. I had the privilege of teaching with her during many of the years she sifted and searched through Taoist philosophy texts, pored over calligraphy and attuned herself to the guidance of the Taoist alchemists. Lorie's perspective is uniquely grounded in her embodied feeling experience as a woman as well as in her firm commitment to the value of rigorous research.

Her evolving understanding of the transformational essence of healing and its resonance with the ebb and flow of nature's changes helped me deepen my own grasp of the healing process. The colloquium that we co-led on comparative alchemy (Taoist, European and Tantric) opened doors for both of us and for those who participated. We lived what we taught, and as Lorie needled me, I prescribed homeopathic remedies for her—each administered to move the alchemical process along.

Lorie has dug deeply and lifted from the shadows of history powerful insights and approaches that have much potential for treating the mind/body ailments that plague the growing population of human beings who live alienated from nature and suffer for it. I know that the vision this book represents—reconnection between the spirit and embodied life, recovery of the knowledge of how to work skillfully with the five spirits of Taoist Chinese medicine, and recognition of the role of healing in the emergence of a new, more viable consciousness—will strike a deep chord in this new century and help catalyze the momentous planetary shift that is now underway across the globe.

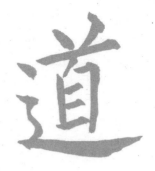

Introduction

Beginning the Journey

BEGINNING

In the wild, unpopulated mountains of China, beyond the Western gateway of the state of Chou, a man ground a lump of dark pigment with a gray stone. He mixed the pigment with water and stirred until the ink was smooth enough to mirror the sky. He picked up a brush and painted a series of black lines on a white scroll. His lines formed pictures, shaping thoughts into words on a page. With these words, the man gave rise to a philosophy that for centuries influenced an entire culture's religion, art, literature, and medicine.

The man wrote a simple question, something like

How do I know the way of things at the beginning?[1]

The man was wondering about the beginning of the world, a time of Origin, a time that had always been and would be forever. He was wondering about his own beginning, how it was he could be at all. He was wondering about how nothing becomes something and how something returns to nothing and then what happens in between.

Was it one man or many? Was the man old or young? Was he an ordinary man or a sage? We do not know the answers to these questions. We do know, however, that a man named Lao Tzu—the Old Young Master of ancient China—is said to have asked and answered this question:

> How have I come to know the way of all things in their beginning?
> I know by what is within me. I know by the Name, Tao, the Name
> that is sounding right here, right now, at this place where I am, at
> this point where my foot stands, at the ending and beginning of the
> world.[2]

Two thousand years later, more or less, on a day in late September in a sunlit room on the eastern end of Long Island, a woman picked up a hair-thin silver needle and inserted it into a point on the instep of my left foot.

As the needle penetrated my skin and sank into the hollow between the bones, I felt a powerful surge of energy rush through me and then, deep relaxation. A breeze stirred the curtains at the open window and suddenly the scent of green apples poured into the room from a gnarled tree in the garden. A veil that had been covering my senses lifted. Skin, sky, warmth, breeze, green, apples: The world cracked open and light rained like water through my body.

This was my first experience with acupuncture. It was not what I had expected. Rather than discovering a way to get rid of the persistent headaches and fatigue that had bothered me for over a year, I discovered something that transformed the way I experienced being in my body, something that changed my perception of the world and supported me in living my life differently. After the first few treatments, my headaches were gone and my energy had returned. But, much more importantly, those early treatments were the beginning of my journey into the territory of Taoist philosophy, Eastern spirituality, alchemy and Chinese medicine. They were the first steps in a journey that has led me away from the person I thought I was and back to myself, many times over, a journey that endlessly begins again each time I insert a needle into an acupuncture point or read a verse of a Taoist text or wonder about the meaning of an ancient Chinese character.

Five years after my first treatment, I graduated from acupuncture school and became a practitioner of traditional Chinese medicine. Over the twenty years I have been in practice, I have worked to integrate this medicine and philosophy into my being—and yet, the truth is that Chinese medicine is as changed by me as I am by it. The needle I hold between my fingers is not the same as the needle held between the fingers of an acupuncturist living half a world away in China, five hundred, a thousand or fifteen hundred years ago.

WHAT IS TRADITIONAL CHINESE MEDICINE?

As an American acupuncturist, the first question I am usually asked is, "Does acupuncture work?"

To this question, my answer is, "Yes . . . and no." Yes, acupuncture works, but it does not work in the way that Western medicine does. Acupuncture emerges from a four-thousand-year-old Eastern worldview, a pre-rational perspective radically different from our own. So although acupuncture is effective for a wide range of physical, emotional, and psychosomatic symptoms and is now practiced in modern hospitals and clinics all over America and the world, its effectiveness cannot be explained by the rational mind alone or proven through the exclusive use of modern Western scientific methods. The key to a more complete understanding of acupuncture, as well as other aspects of Chinese medicine, is found in the ancient art of Taoist alchemy, and an even earlier tradition, the tradition of the Neolithic healer priests, known as the *wu*.

The wu are the spiritual ancestors of Taoism, which along with

Buddhism and Confucianism is one of the three great religions of China. The wu were also the first acupuncturists, the first to insert bits of sharpened jade and bone under the skin in order to heal sickness and shift psychological states. Through their dedicated and precise observations of the natural world, these shamanic healers developed many of the concepts that later became the foundation of the Taoist alchemical tradition.

Taoist alchemy is an ancient spiritual discipline that was practiced in China for thousands of years. Unlike Western science, which is based on technical experimentation and the objective measurement of quantities, alchemy is based on personal observation and the subjective experience of qualities. When viewed from the perspective of modern rational thought, the wisdom of alchemy is easily overlooked or mistaken for superstition and fantasy. Its goal has been misunderstood and trivialized into an attempt to turn base metal into gold, but if we look more carefully, we discover that the authentic alchemical quest was for the spiritual mystery at the heart of the material universe, the source of life itself. The gold the alchemists were searching for was not only material. Their *true* gold was the golden light of the divine; their *true* work was the fixing or crystallizing of the golden light of the soul. Through alchemy, they sought to overcome the forces of decline and death and to transform an ordinary human being into an immortal or sage.[3]

The wisdom of the Taoist alchemists and the insights of the wu combine to create the seminal theories of traditional Chinese medicine. This aspect of Chinese medicine goes beyond the healing of pain and disease, beyond the maintenance and repair of the physical body. Its goal is transformation—the reorganization and spiritual upgrading of organic life.

BASIC CONCEPTS OF TAOIST PSYCHOSPIRITUAL ALCHEMY

Tao

The system we now know as Chinese medicine was influenced by each of the three main spiritual and philosophic traditions of China: Buddhism, Taoism and Confucianism. Most of the psychological theories that we will examine in this book—and many of Chinese medicine's core ideas—are based on the principles of Taoism and in particular Taoist alchemy.

There is no precise date set for the beginning of Taoism. Unlike Confucianism, Taoism does not have a political, social status. It does not have a specific historic figure recognized as its originator. Some contend that Taoism is not a religion at all but rather a loose combination of teachings and philosophies based on the revelations of mystics, priests and sages over time. According to Thomas Cleary, one of the West's most renowned Taoist scholars, "the basis of Taoism may be thought of as the primary body of knowledge underlying original Chinese culture. Its legends and traditions reach back to prehistory, preserving within themselves memories of an earlier matriarchal tradition preceding the historical emergence of patriarchal Chinese civilization."[4]

The word *Tao* has no exact English translation, but it relates most closely to the Western idea of wholeness, to the unknowable unity of the divine. When used by the Taoist philosophers, Tao became the Way, the path or cosmic law that directs the unfolding of every aspect of the universe. So Tao is the wisdom of the divine made manifest in nature and in my individual life.

The Chinese word Tao has an etymological relationship to the Sanskrit root sound "da," which means "to divide something whole into parts." The ancient Sanskrit word dharma is also related to this root. In the Buddhist tradition, dharma means "that which is to be held fast, kept, an ordinance or law . . . the absolute, the real."[5] So, both dharma and Tao refer to the way that the One, the unfathomable unity of the divine, divides into parts and manifests in the world of form.

Tao is not an answer to the question "What should I do?" but a response to the question "How do I do it?" This knowing how—how to heal, how to grow, how to live, how to rediscover my self and my origin—is an ongoing process, a way to walk through our lives rather than a static thing or way to be. It is a stone rolling down a hill, a leaf falling from a tree, light replacing shadow as the sun rises above the tops of the trees. Tao makes a space in the known where the unknown can happen. Poised right here, right now, at the place where I stand, Tao is the ongoing ever-imminent, ever-astonishing arising of the possible.

"Something invisibly formed," writes Lao Tzu, "born before heaven and earth. In the silence and the void, standing alone and unchanging . . . perhaps it is the mother of ten thousand things. I do not know its name. Call it Tao."[6]

The Mysterious Feminine

Tao, although ever hidden, can be seen in the movements of the clouds, in the twisting of the pine trees on the windswept ocean cliffs, in the shifting tides and the great cycles of the seasons. Tao is the unknowable Origin of being and non-being, nothingness and form. But there is a way that Tao can be perceived. Tao is perceptible through its reflection in the "Ten Thousand Things," the infinite diversity of life and form in the natural world. In the very first chapter of the Tao Teh Ching, the principal text of the Taoist tradition, we read,

> Tao is both Named and Nameless
> As Nameless, it is the origin of all things
> As Named, it is the mother of all things[7]

Tao is both the wholeness and the parts. But since the divine wholeness is not accessible to human consciousness, Taoists focused on how the integrity of Tao was reflected within us and all around us in the natural world. Their primary interest was not in the ascension of human spirit to the heavenly realms but in the descent of spirit into our lives, and their focus was on the yin, the "Mysterious Feminine," which through its potent receptivity and miraculous productivity could make manifest the mystery of Tao.

Through meditation, ritual and other spiritual practices, the Taoist sought to align and harmonize the various aspects of his inner being so that he could become like a mountain, a conduit between above and below. The energies of heaven swept down and manifested on earth through his spontaneous actions, much as the wind sweeps down and moves the leaves and branches of the trees. In this way he became impregnated by spirit and could give birth to his true nature, his divine mandate, his destiny or Tao.

Thus the brush stroke of the master calligrapher brought the breath of heaven down to earth as a line of black ink on a white page. The tai ch'i master manifested the divine through the gestures of his body as he practiced his form. The Taoist practitioner brought his awareness to the breath and the breath down to the belly so that spiritual embryo of the sage could come into being in his womb. And the master acupuncturist became like a mountain, a connecting link between heaven and earth, through the effortless yet absolutely precise placement of the acupuncture needle—a celestial lancet—in the point on his patient's body.

Qi

At the center of Chinese medicine is an alchemical mystery, the insubstantial substance known as qi or ch'i (pronounced "chee"). Qi is the breath, the vital force of life. It is the wind that comes from the whirling vortex of Tao.

Qi streams through the body along a complex system of invisible conduits known as meridians. The ancient Chinese mapped and identified the places on the meridians where qi accumulates or comes close to the skin. According to the classic Chinese medical texts, the body has over 365 of these accumulations, which are known as points and are the places where the qi is most easily accessed, where it can be regulated, balanced, toni-fied, or sedated through skillful use of the acupuncture needle.

Like quicksilver, qi is ungraspable and ever changing. It cannot be seen with the physical eye or measured with scientific instruments. Qi is devoid of mass or velocity, yet it exists in space and time as a quality of being, as vitality, mood, presence or animating life force. The eye of the heart and the ear of the soul can recognize its presence. We experience its effects in the liveliness of a young child, the luster of a fresh-picked apple or the rich fragrance of a pine forest. And the more deeply we immerse ourselves in the world of the ancient Chinese, the more the mys-tery of qi becomes a subtle, ever-present influence in our daily lives.

Yin and Yang

Yin and yang have become a part of American culture. The taiji or yin/yang symbol, the interconnected swirling of dark and light, turns up in the oddest places. People wear it on T-shirts, earrings and necklaces. It shows up in advertising logos and in works of art. We feel an irresistible affinity with this symbol even if we have no more than a vague conscious understanding of its meaning, because it represents a truth about the cre-ative power of opposites that we know in the deepest parts of our being.

Yin/yang symbols are found on bronze vases that date from the sec-ond millennium BCE. The terms "yin" and "yang" were initially descrip-tions of topography. They were used to designate the shady and the sunny slope of a mountain, the northern and southern banks of a river, the dark and the sunny seasons, and so on. Eventually, they came to also imply the masculine and feminine aspects of life.

When the heavy qi falls and the light qi rises, yin and yang are born. Yang relates to heaven, to spirit and to the mind, while yin relates to mat-ter and to the body. Yin is related to the moon, cold, dark, water, moisture, quiescence and night. Yin is reflective; it receives and brings into form the impulses of the yang. Yang is related to the sun, heat, light, fire, dryness, activity and day. Yang initiates possibility while yin manifests form.

Yang qi is the ephemeral, formless, initiating, spirit-polarized psychic energies of breath, consciousness, mind and imagination. Yin qi is the substantiated, formal, manifesting, matter-polarized energies of flesh, embodied awareness, body and instinct.

"When the absolute (Tao) goes into motion," writes the Taoist alchemist Yu Yuwu, "it produces yin and yang. When motion culminates, it reverses to stillness and in stillness produces yin. When stillness culminates, it returns to movement. Movement and stillness in alternation constitute bases for each other. This is the wonder of Creation, the natural course of the Way."[8]

CHALLENGES AND OPPORTUNITIES

Mythical versus Modern Consciousness

Both Chinese shamanism and Taoist alchemy are based on pre-scientific forms of logic, which is nonlinear and integrative, as opposed to Western logic, which is linear and analytic. It focuses on relationships between objects, events and experiences, not distinctions between them. Its conclusions emerge from the coincidence of connections and impressions, not as the result of linear deduction.

The Chinese tend to look at the totality of a situation. Their fundamental belief is that no single part can be understood except in its relationship to a whole complex pattern or process. In Chinese thought, it is the overall pattern rather than the linear relationship of cause and effect that is the significant factor in understanding. This difference in logic is mirrored in the metaphysical system that arose in each culture. The Western Judeo-Christian tradition has a fundamental belief in a divine Being, a God who created or caused the manifest universe. The Chinese Buddhist or Taoist tradition has no such creator. Creation is always and forever manifest in the patterns and cycles of the world around us, which is, in the words of Ted Kaptchuk, "a web that has no weaver."[9]

Modern scientists and philosophers sometimes refer to this kind of logic as primitive, which implies that it is not only older but also less elegant and efficient than modern logic. But I propose that this older logic is simply different from modern logic. It organizes information differently, asks different questions and is useful for solving different kinds of problems. It allows us to notice different aspects of experience and to play different games with the world.

This other logic is less effective than modern logic in predicting the behavior of mechanical systems. Through my own clinical and personal experience, however, I have found that it far surpasses linear, scientific thought when it comes to understanding the psychological and spiritual dimensions of human beings as well as the instinctual language of the body. An understanding of this level of consciousness is crucial for healing symptoms that are rooted in distresses of the emotional, instinctual, or spiritual life.

I use the term "mythical"[10] to describe this nonlinear way of organizing reality. This term expresses the poetry, sacredness and symbolic wisdom that we experience as we open to this other way of organizing the world. The word also reminds us that this other logic is not an outmoded organizational structure but one that is operating in us right now, functioning alongside our modern, linear consciousness. Although inaccessible to our thinking mind, this realm is readily accessible to us through the experiential knowing of our bodies, our imagination, our emotions, our creativity and our dreams.

Directed Thought

Modern logic gives us access to one of the most powerful tools that human beings have ever discovered: directed thought. Directed thought allows us to determine what is and is not relevant to a given purpose. It allows us to focus the power of the mind on a single objective and to throw out information that is not directly useful in the achievement of a specific goal. Directed thought goes beyond the present and forges ahead into the future. In Western medicine, directed thinking has allowed scientists to isolate disease-causing entities such as microbes and viruses and find ways to destroy them. It has led to the synthesis of powerful pharmaceuticals that can reverse the effects of life-threatening illnesses. And it has led to a highly developed understanding of anatomy and physiology that has opened the doorway to nearly miraculous surgical procedures, including the repair and replacement of internal organs of the body.

However, the strength of directed thought is also its weakness. Because its focus is so pinpointed, it often misses subtle but crucial parts of a problem, just as a high-powered focusing lens enhances the minute details of the foreground object while it dims or renders invisible details of the background. Directed thought isolates one thing after another but loses out on the relationships that connect things into the matrix of an integrated whole. It focuses on quantities of objects but has a tendency to ignore their quality or *essential nature*.

Directed thought discards aspects of reality that oppose or contradict its position. It allows us to focus the power of the mind on a single objective and to throw out information that is not directly useful in the achievement of a specific goal. Without the creative tension of contradiction, no new possibility is born of the relationship between two opposites. So directed thought eliminates the possibility of an integrating third, a mediating substance that can reintegrate the severed parts of a shattered or analyzed wholeness. It eliminates the healing and integrating influences of paradox and ambiguity. In its zeal to exclude anything not central to its immediate goal, directed thought has lost the capacity to see, speak about or work with what pre-scientific Western consciousness recognized as the integrating threads of the soul or subtle body or the insubstantial substance that the Chinese call qi.

When we want to know how many apples there are on the apple tree or to analyze the chemical composition of the apple seed, we need the modern analytical mind. But when we want to understand how a ripe apple tastes on the first cool morning in September or how the atmosphere in the orchard feels when the tree is struck with blight, we must turn to mythical consciousness, to what the ancient Chinese referred to as *xin*, the heartmind.

When we want to repair a broken bone in a person's arm, we need the directive, goal-oriented clarity of modern Western surgery. Likewise, for a patient presenting with a simple case of muscular pain due to overuse, the linear, medically oriented strategies of modern acupuncture may work best. But when we need to unravel some long-forgotten trauma lodged in the frozen muscles of a patient's upper back, to heal at the level of what Western psychologists refer to as the body unconscious, we must turn to the fluid, nonlinear logic of mythic consciousness.

The Mythical Nature of the Chinese Language

According to Chinese mythology, language came to human beings as a gift of the gods. Spirits from heaven handed down the characters that form the Chinese language during prehistoric times. The characters were referred to as "cloud scrolls," "breaths of the Gods," heavenly vapors. Language was honored as a form of communion with the divine. Like the incense and smoke sent up to heaven during ritual, words formed a bridge between the physical and psychological, the body and mind, the earthly and heavenly realms. The characters were regarded as nets or fish-traps in which the light of spirit could be gathered.

The earliest signs of the use of graphic symbols are found at Bampo, an archeological site on the bank of the Yellow River. Here, primitive symbols were discovered etched onto pottery shards carbon dated at 4800 BCE. The earliest actual writing discovered by archeologists can be traced back to the Xia (2100–1600 BCE) and Shang (1600–1066 BCE) dynasties. This writing comes to us in two forms: as characters carved onto ceremonial bronze vases and as inscriptions carved onto the backs of tortoise shells and ox bones for divination purposes. The archeological fragments include over 1,098 characters with over 4,000 variations. In the third century BCE, the First Emperor of Quin codified the wide variations of bronze and bone graphic into a unified written language called the Small Seal Script.

Unlike our own string- or sentence-based language, the language of the ancient Chinese is pictographic. The characters are multidimensional gestalts, immediately perceived wholes that integrate and unify a host of related multisensory impressions and ideas. Sinologist Claude Larre says, "The Chinese text is an expression of something we already know from our own personal, bodily conscience."[11] In other words, the characters are symbols, universal graphic images that arise from the sensory images of the human body.

FIGURE 1: SENTENCE STRING VERSUS CHARACTER

The sun shines
subject   verb

uni-directional sentence string—linear "analytic" logic
reflects the chronological analytic logic of modern Western
consciousness

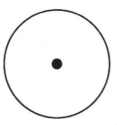

Chinese character for sun, *ri*
reflects the global synchronous logic of mythical consciousness—
it is a symbol that gathers together multiple impressions of the sun
including roundness, centrality and mystery

Like dream symbols, the Chinese character condenses many layers of meaning and interrelated experiences into a unified image or group of images. Like dreams, the characters are governed by an associational, non-linear logic that reflects the synesthetic montage of sensory experience. The images contained in the characters are rooted in organic truths that transcend culture and time. They bring us back to deeply felt, embodied understandings about our selves and the natural world. Because they evolved slowly over thousands of years, Chinese characters graphically synthesize centuries of human experience and wisdom. They arise from the collective unconscious of humanity and reflect universal archetypes that can in fact be said to relate to the transpersonal or the divine. Attempting to directly translate a character into English cannot convey the complex layer of meaning woven into the symbol.

Although the designs of the words have mutated through time, when we look at the patterns of a Chinese character, we catch a glimpse of how human beings related to the world over forty centuries ago. The lines are the tracings of the consciousness of an ancient civilization. Spending time contemplating a character is like lifting the lid of an alchemical vessel in which human ideas and experiences have been simmering for thousands of years. In addition, spending time with the characters opens us to forgotten parts of our own being. Psychiatrist Fritz Perls believed that most of our mentality consists of pictures and words—the unconscious having a greater affinity to pictures, the conscious mind to words.[12] Meditating on the characters can open us to our unconscious, especially our *body unconscious*, the memories and messages hidden in our nervous system and neuromuscular holding patterns. In this way, the characters can be used as powerful tools in the healing process.

Just as much as any drug, herb or acupuncture needle, words can have a powerful effect, a resonance that vibrates through space and time to shift our physical as well as psychological experience.

The characters contain the energies of mythical consciousness and, like any ancient symbol, they affect us on subtle levels. For this reason, many ancient characters are included in this book, and readers are encouraged to regard them as potent catalysts that can transform the way they see the world.

The Psychology of Traditional Chinese Medicine

Traditional Chinese medicine is now accepted in the West as a viable cure for chronic pain and functional diseases. It is less widely known that Chinese medicine is also a powerful psychological healing modality that can be used to promote emotional healing and psychological and spiritual transformation. In fact, it is the premise of this book that the Taoist system of the Five Spirits presents us with a symbolic map of the human psyche and nervous system and that this system forms the basis of traditional Chinese medical psychology. There are two main reasons that this important aspect of Chinese medicine has been overlooked.

The first is that when the People's Republic of China reinstated Chinese medicine in the 1960s (after outlawing it for over a decade), the psychospiritual dimension of the tradition was mostly left aside. The form of acupuncture and Chinese pharmacology developed in mainland China in the 1960s is a highly effective system of medicine, but its chief concern is bringing economical health care to large numbers of people. It does not focus on the psychosomatic or psychospiritual causes of disease but rather on eliminating physical suffering as quickly and economically as possible.

In this "modern" form, acupuncture is a viable treatment for symptoms that are rooted in the physical structure of the body. It is highly successful in the treatment of acute physical pain, muscle spasm and superficial structural imbalances. It is a safe, economically sound treatment option for internal diseases such as digestive disturbances, sinusitis and endocrine disturbances. And, in cases where long-standing emotional and psychological distress is not a factor, this modern style of acupuncture is an effective treatment for headaches, allergies, asthma and gynecological problems.

In the mid 1960s and early 1970s, groups of pioneering Western scholars and doctors went to China to study traditional Chinese medicine. As China was still under the sway of communism with its strong anti-spiritual bias, this first wave of students learned a Maoist style of modern, materialistic acupuncture that had been stripped of its spiritual and psychological insights. This was the kind of acupuncture that was first brought back to Europe and America. It was only later, through the emergence of original texts preserved and translated by missionaries before the Communist takeover and through teachings preserved in Japan, Korea and Vietnam, and by master practitioners from the mainland, that the deeper transformational aspects of the tradition began to come to light.

The second reason that the psychology of Chinese medicine has been overlooked is that the Chinese approach is fundamentally psychosomatic. Chinese medicine views the human bodymind as a unified system with no distinct line drawn between physical, emotional, psychological and spiritual experience. For this reason, it has been difficult to tease apart the pieces and easy to overlook the sophisticated psychological understanding and spiritual wisdom embedded in the tradition.

The ancient Chinese regarded physical, emotional, psychological and spiritual experiences as an expression of qi, the life force. The qi that relates to the psychological level of experience is more ephemeral, less physically structured than the qi that relates to the blood, bones and muscles of the physical body, but qi is "all one thing." Whether it is manifesting at a more ephemeral or more material level, qi continues to obey the same laws and behave in similar ways. Nevertheless, qi exists in a state of perpetual transformation. Just as water is constantly changing from solid to liquid to vapor yet always remaining essentially the same substance, qi is constantly shifting between physical, psychic and spiritual states.

From the perspective of Taoist philosophy, it is not only logically impossible to radically separate and isolate the various states of qi, it is a threat to the integrity of life and of living organisms to try. To impede or block the intermingling of yin qi and yang qi, form and animation, body and mind, is to impede the dance of life itself.

The Dilemma: The Body/Mind Split

When we try to isolate the various states of qi, we obstruct the movement of the life force and eventually come to an impasse. Without the intermingling of yin qi and yang qi, there can be no creativity, no new life, and eventually the system runs down. Similarly, when we separate the terrain of body and mind and segregate the treatment of physical, psychological and spiritual distress into specialized disciplines, we often find ourselves stuck in devitalized impasses, endless circles that produce no new possibilities.

Humanist psychologist and philosopher Eugene Gendlin presents what he calls the "dead end problem" in his book *Focusing-Oriented Psychotherapy*. Gendlin approaches the dead end from the perspective of psychotherapy—from the mind side of the bodymind continuum. He describes the dead end as a situation in which a process gets stuck on a mental level. According to Gendlin, this kind of dead end appears quite often in talk therapy and psychoanalysis. An example would be attempting to ease the discomfort of stomach cramps by discussing why we get them. The discussion may be very interesting, but it usually does nothing to relax the cramps. Our vocabulary and logic may make perfect sense, but the intellectual understanding does nothing to change our experience. Such discussions lead nowhere because they do not bridge the gap between the mind and the body. The mental insights are not grounded in an embodied, experiential process that goes to the level of the autonomic nervous system. There is no marriage between yin and yang, so nothing new can come to life.

Bodyworkers such as massage therapists, physical therapists and acupuncturists commonly encounter another kind of dead end. Here the process bogs down on the body side of the bodymind continuum. Stress-related shoulder tension, for example, might improve after a session but returns the next day when the person goes to work. In this case, the best, most relaxing physical treatment goes nowhere. The patient could be treated every day, but the symptom would return because the therapy does not bridge the gap between the body and the mind. The physical experience is not lifted to the level of conscious insight and imaginative vision that could change the way this person is relating to the world.

The split between body and mind is the cause of both dead ends. Yang and yin have separated. Yang qi—the ephemeral, formless, initiating, spirit-polarized, vital energies of breath, consciousness, mind and imagination—does not mix with yin qi—the substantiated, formal, manifesting, matter-polarized energies of flesh, embodied awareness, body and instinct. From a Taoist alchemical perspective, the body/mind split is a pathological state because there is blockage when the qi cannot transform freely from yin form to yang formlessness, from yang formlessness to yin form. An excess accumulates on one side, bringing deficiency and exhaustion on the other. When yin and yang separate, we head away from movement toward impasse, away from life toward death. Unless there is a mingling of yin and yang, life processes are arrested and there can be no transformation.

Traditional Chinese medicine regards these splits and blockages as the cause of all disease and pain. Disease is the inevitable outcome when there is a lack of communication between the yin and yang aspects of an organism and the free-flowing transformations of qi are impeded. This is expressed in the Chinese medical principle that states:

> *tong zhi butong/ butong zhi tong*
> If there is pain, there is no free flow.
> If there is no free flow, there is pain.

By re-enlivening acupuncture and Chinese medicine with the ancient alchemical consciousness at its heart and integrating it with the insights of depth psychology and modern understanding of the nervous system, I have found that I am able to help my patients bridge the gap that modern Western consciousness has placed between body and mind. I call this integrated way of practicing acupuncture Alchemical Acupuncture because its principles are based on Taoist alchemical ideas. The process is also alchemical because it reunites yang and yin, spirit and matter, mind and body and reorganizes these split parts to form a new, more complex and efficient whole. By illuminating the somatic experience initiated by the insertion of the acupuncture needle with the light of the imagination and the insights of the conscious mind, something new comes to life in the treatment room.

The goal of this method of treatment is to restore communication between mind and body and thus to bring a person closer to the experience of his or her own wholeness and connection to Tao. Treatment is a way to bring movement and consciousness to deadened, unconscious parts of our being buried in the matrix of the physical body. It is also a way to call back parts of our being that have flown off and disassociated from sensory, embodied experience. We restore communication by fostering an "alchemical" or transformational relationship between the mind, the imagination and the vital functions of the body. Our tools include needles, moxa and touch as well as conscious awareness and imagination.

In order to communicate with the body, the mind must learn to understand its language. The body speaks through sensations, symptoms, longings, symbols, poetic images and dreams. As opposed to mental cognition, which is analytic and mediated by thought, cognition at the body level is synthetic and unmediated. While the conscious mind can only process one thought at a time, the body takes in hundreds of pieces of information at once and organizes them into patterns below the level of conscious awareness.

Chinese medicine can be a great help to Westerners working with psychosomatic distress because its synthetic nature—looking for connections and relationships instead of causes and effects—is compatible with somatic awareness. Healing happens at the sensory level, directly on the body. Symbols, patterns and poetry play a large role in its theoretical organization. By incorporating Chinese medicine with modern tools of somatic psychology, we can enhance the depth and potency of treatment.

If we are willing to move beyond the limitations of linear logic and integrate the ancient principles of acupuncture into our current way of looking at the world, we can take the practice of acupuncture to a new level and be able not only to heal acute physical pain and chronic internal diseases but also to address symptoms arising from the ephemeral myth-making faculties of the psyche, the invisible light of the spirit and the primal, non-rational, instinctual forces of the body. We will be able to tap acupuncture's greatest potential: its use as a tool for transformation, a permanent change in the quality, complexity, and creativity of our being, life and consciousness.

I have found Alchemical Acupuncture particularly well suited to my Western patients. It allows me to guide people beyond the thinking mind and through various levels of the psyche without abandoning the organizing capacities of the ego. The wisdom of the body is brought to the level of awareness in the form of conscious insight, and it becomes possible to heal challenging, multifaceted symptoms that cannot be sharply defined as physical or psychological. It is only through this descent into the fertile, chaotic waters of the deep unconscious that permanent changes at the level of behavior, identity and vision can occur.

This way of practicing acupuncture is not for every patient or every acupuncture practitioner. It is difficult. It challenges our accepted ideas about reality and does not offer any quick fixes. I do believe, however, that it is the way we can fully realize the healing potential of acupuncture and Chinese medicine, especially its ability to heal painful splits in the modern human psyche, such as the splits between spirit and matter, mind and body, and individual identity and the cosmos.

Many of the principles and tools of Alchemical Acupuncture can be used not only by trained acupuncturists but by all who are willing to tune in to their own body, their qi, and the natural world. These are tools that have been used by healers for thousands of years. Today these alchemical tools can help us to heal ourselves and each other, to problem-solve, to move through seemingly impossible impasses and to transform our lives. In this kind of acupuncture, it is not only the needle that facilitates the healing process. Meditation, visualization, breathing, touch and psychological insight—in fact, anything that stirs the life force—can be used as a tool of healing.

ALCHEMICAL ACUPUNCTURE

- Is a system of psychological and psychosomatic healing organized around the Five Spirits of traditional Chinese medicine, the Taoist alchemical map of the human psyche

- Follows the Tao of each patient individually, avoids expectations, views chaos and surprise as openings through which new possibilities emerge

- Combines traditional Chinese medicine, Taoist alchemical principles and insights drawn with modern Western depth psychology and somatic psychotherapy

- Is especially effective for the psychosomatic and psychospiritual problems of modern Western patients

- Does not fix something broken or find something lost but supports transformation, the constellation of a completely new integrity made up of the disintegrated fragments of the old

- Leaves nothing out, treasures irritating symptoms, contradictory signs, chronic pains, obsessions and compulsions as the raw material of transformational processes, i.e., the trash that is really the treasure
- Is based on mythical rather than rational logic
- Uses the tools of traditional Chinese medicine as well as active imagination, meditation, visualization and archetypal amplification to move qi and support transformational processes
- Is a creative process in which both practitioner and patient are actively engaged—healing is more like a work of art than a work of nature or science
- Uses skillful means, follows the flow of the life force using the Five Elements and Five Spirits of Chinese medicine as guides

THE FIVE SPIRITS

The Five Spirits are the finest, most ephemeral aspect of qi. An understanding of the Five Spirits is the key that opens the doorway to the mystery of Taoist psychospiritual alchemy and the art of Alchemical Acupuncture. At the grossest level, the Five Spirits can be understood as a symbolic description of the human nervous system, the frontal lobe, the spinal column, the peripheral nerves and the autonomic nervous system, with its sympathetic and parasympathetic expressions. At a subtler level, the spirits can be conceptualized as divine animating and vitalizing forces, the Taoist version of the Western soul or psyche.

As a precise and efficient technology for psychospiritual development, the Five Spirits can be understood as the Taoist version of the chakra system of Vedic India. Like the chakras, the spirits function to balance the yang and yin aspects of our being. Like the Indian chakra system, the Taoist concept of the Five Spirits is based on the recognition of the inherent divinity of both feminine and masculine, earth and heaven. Just as each chakra relates to a particular level of consciousness, each spirit relates to a particular aspect of human awareness, a particular vibration or frequency of psychic energy. Like the chakras, the spirits exist in the subtle body or breath body, an invisible yet vital structure that forms a kind of pneumatic link between the realms of spirit and matter. Like the chakras, the spirits relate to the vertical axis of the human body, the spinal column, and the endocrine, nervous and functional organ systems that constellate around the center pole of the spine. However, unlike the chakras, which are visualized as abstract wheels of swirling energy fields, the Five Spirits are thought of as soulful psychic entities, each with its own nature, preferences, tendencies, needs, organic magnetism, emotional resonance and psychospiritual function.

Many modern acupuncturists regard the Five Spirits as a quaint but obsolete superstition; hence the wisdom contained in this theory has been largely ignored by modern acupuncture both in China and the West. However, through the investigation of Chinese characters and the reading of alchemical texts, we discover that the theory of the Five Spirits is much more than an intriguing story or beautiful fantasy; it is the core of an ancient spiritual psychology. By taking advantage of the discoveries of Western archetypal psychology, we can decipher the ancient symbols and their obscure references and reorganize them in a way that has proven to be clinically invaluable in treating psychosomatic, emotional and psychospiritual distress.

As we delve into this system, our modern Western ideas about the nature of spirit and consciousness are called into question. From a Taoist perspective we see that spirit exists not only in the distant heights of heaven but also as an ever-present phenomenon that illuminates the stars and penetrates to the darkest depths of matter. Similarly, consciousness is transformed from an abstraction into real and tangible light, an illuminating spark of spirit that rests in our hearts and guides us through our lives.

This vision of the Five Spirits allows us to view the psyche as a unity. The line between body, mind and spirit blurs, and psyche emerges not as a noun but as a verb, a process, an ongoing dance of transformation. From this perspective, we see that conscious and unconscious processes emerge from an organic, visceral matrix animated by the Five Spirits—by the energies of the divine.

The most important stories of ancient civilizations contain encoded information about priestcraft, astrology and social custom as well as information about psychological, astronomical, agricultural, temporal and geological occurrences.[13] The Five Spirits present an encoded description of ancient Taoist healers' observations of psychic and neurological phenomena in the human organism. The spirits illuminate the aspect of our being that in earlier times was referred to as the soul. This is the aspect of our being that allows us to transform our lives from the monotony of day-to-day survival into an intentional creation, a psychospiritual event.

The Five Spirits—the *shen, hun, po, yi,* and *zhi*—are the resident deities of the Taoist psyche or subtle breath body. Together they form a complex pneumatic system that both lifts and stabilizes the psychic and vital processes of the human organism. The Five Spirits give us a vocabulary to speak about the behavior and function of psychic phenomena that exist at the far edges of Western conscious awareness—fluid, ungraspable animating psychic energies such as inspiration, insight, imagination, mood, perceptions, intention, instinct and will. This vocabulary allows us to intentionally work with these subtle yet potent psychic energies in a precise and effective manner. Later in this book, the Five Spirits will be introduced in detail and we will look at ways these soul entities can be used to support integrated healing of the body, mind and spirit.

Although modern acupuncture practice is strongly influenced by the linear logic of Confucianism and modern scientific thought, acupuncture's seminal theories and practices—especially those pertaining to psychological healing and psychospiritual transformation—arise from mythical consciousness. In order for us, as modern Westerners, to come to an authentic understanding of these ancient theories and to use them most efficiently, we must move beyond the limitations of linear logic and directed thought and rediscover the mythical world within us.

From the point of view of modern linear logic, it is impossible for human beings of the present time to ever really know how the ancient Chinese experienced the world around them. Our modern intellect cannot begin to grasp the atmosphere and wisdom of this distant era. Yet, when we open ourselves to aspects of awareness that are often ignored by rational Western consciousness, we enter a dimension of embodied emotional awareness that transcends linguistic, cultural and historical contexts. This level of awareness lives in us alongside the logic of our modern mind. It lives in our dreams, bodies, instincts, symbols, archetypes, mythologies and fantasies as well as in many of our most irritating, peculiar, chronic somatic and psychological symptoms. And it is this level of knowing that leads us not only to the mysteries of acupuncture and Chinese medicine but back to our own bodies and our own souls.

In this book, I am not proposing a regressive return to earlier ways of being and organizing the world. I do not believe that this kind of sentimental turning backward will help us heal the complex psychological and psychosomatic problems that afflict us today. Rather, I am suggesting a conscious illumination of the past, a turning backward that is simultaneously a moving forward to the future. Earlier forms of consciousness remain active even if we are not consciously aware of them. By shining the light of our awareness onto these "deeper" levels, we can intentionally make use of the insights and capabilities that are waiting there in a dormant state.

An Awareness of Tao

In my practice, I try to remain open to all possibilities. Body, mind, soul or spirit? On what level does a patient's problem need to be addressed? Is a pain in the shoulder due to a repetitive sports injury or a chronic muscle tightness that shields a wounded heart? Is elbow pain simply elbow pain or is it a symbolic message from the body that is calling out to be interpreted? Although it sometimes takes time to know which way to go, I trust the qi to lead me in the right direction.

In the background of every treatment, I hold an awareness of Tao, that sacred presence that cannot be spoken or rationally understood. I try to remember that on the other side of the needle is the breathing of the infinite. Acupuncture is, at its Taoist core, a transformational form of healing. From its origins in the shamanic rituals of aboriginal Chinese tribes along the Yellow River, acupuncture's primary function was the realigning of the cosmos. Chinese medicine's original concern was facilitating the unfolding of the Tao in our lives here on earth. Unfortunately, it has lost much of its power in the necessary but limited service of pain relief for a slew of modern ailments. Yet these very symptoms are actually the expression of the deep distress of the modern Western soul and are indicative of how far we have strayed from our alignment with the Tao, our connection to the wisdom of nature and our own bodies.

It is not easy to allow ourselves to be touched and changed by the world of Chinese medicine. It takes time and patience as well as a willingness to be temporarily disoriented and confused. Chinese medicine, when practiced from an alchemical orientation, dares us to explore maligned and forgotten parts of ourselves in order to rediscover our own wholeness. It dares us to let go of old, outmoded ways of being and to open to new, more authentic possibilities. This kind of healing takes courage, insight, trust, sweat and tears.

But only in this way can we fully benefit from the wisdom of the ancient Chinese. And only in this way can we discover the doorway to a lost part of our own selves, a part that I believe is vital to our personal and collective healing as well as to the future of our planet.

During the thousands of years of Chinese medicine's evolution, language, symbols, visions, dreams and intuitions have combined with unrelenting empirical observations of nature to form a healing system that has the unity and perfection of poetic genius. This ancient, intricately woven tapestry of healing may at first seem impossible for the modern Western mind to penetrate. Yet in the following pages we will discover a path to the heart of traditional Chinese medicine, a path that leads us back to a distant past and at the same time guides us forward to the future. By pulling gently yet persistently on the thread of our own experience, by following the thread of our own insights and understanding, we discover an opening, no bigger than the point of a needle, through which we can enter the vast majesty of the world of Tao—the world of Chinese medicine that lies not only in the ancient past but here and now, in the world outside as well as within us.

道

This book is written for professional acupuncturists, shiatsu and acupressure practitioners, counselors and psychotherapists, as well as lay readers interested in healing themselves, their friends, and their families. Clinical cases and suggestions, including specific points and strategies, are scattered throughout the text of the book. At the end of each chapter in Part II is a related case study and a description of points and treatment strategies for each of the Spirits.

In this book, I show how the mythical language, concepts, theories, and practices of acupuncture can be integrated into our current way of looking at the world to create a new kind of healing process.

- In Part I, we "Explore the Territory." Here the reader is introduced to the main theories of Taoist psychospiritual alchemy and the concepts that form the philosophical ground of Chinese medicine: the heartmind, *wuwei*, alchemy, lead, gold and transformation, entropy and negetropy, the Five Elements and the Five Spirits.

- In Part II, we "Descend the Mountain" as we follow the path of the Five Spirits from heaven to earth and back again. In Part II, we explore each of the Five Spirits in depth as the reader is guided on a journey through the various levels of the psyche and nervous system. Beginning at the level of the shen spirit, the yang, "sunlit" regions of the mind, we descend to the deepest realms of the zhi spirit, the watery, yin instinctual knowing of embodied life.

- In Part III, we enter the timeless, spaceless mystery of "Transformation" and then "Return" with new vision and new possibilities. Here, the *huntun*—the whirlwind of chaos—is introduced as a tool of healing and transformation, and the Mysterious Feminine—the visible face of Tao—is revealed. Then lead—the paradoxical yet crucial energy of the ego's resistance to the chaos of transformation—is explored. And finally we encounter the Golden Flower, the concretized light that is the key to hua, Taoist alchemy and psychospiritual transformation.

Part I:

Exploring the Territory

師曰此經乃九天八會

道元始天尊昔經歷于

備生死五運遷變萬豪

唐景雲之上上清之境

聲生火慾不舍吾

Introduction to Part I

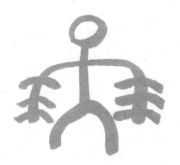

First take Heaven and Earth for the cauldron,
then make a ball of yin and yang and cook it up.

—ALCHEMICAL TEXT[1]

In order to gain the know-how to effectively use alchemical healing methods and tools presented in this book, one must first be familiar with the culture of Taoist alchemy and the vocabulary of Chinese medicine. So, in Part I we begin by looking at the central principles of Taoist psychospiritual alchemy and the alchemical aspects of traditional Chinese medicine. The chapters in Part I include:

- an overview of general philosophical concepts
- an introduction to the principles of Taoist psychology and Chinese medical theory
- a practical guide to methods and techniques
- an in-depth case study that demonstrates how the theories and tools can be used effectively in healing
- an analysis of key Chinese characters and detailed explanations of how to turn abstract concepts into effective clinical strategies

The ancient Chinese placed great emphasis on the symbolic function of numbers. We follow their lead as we progress through the five chapters that make up the first part of the book—beginning at zero, the place of origin. Chapter One addresses the concept of the empty center, the place where Taoist alchemy begins and ends. Several key ideas that relate to this core concept are introduced, including the heartmind, *wuwei*, the empty center and the miraculous pivot. We explore how the idea of emptiness informs the theory and practice of Chinese medicine and how this idea can transform our Western ideas about the psychology of the self.

Alchemy is the subject of Chapter Two, "Lead Into Gold." The central concern of alchemy is how Tao, the unbroken unity of the divine, polarizes into yin and yang, two opposites that reunite to create a child or new possibility. In this chapter, we look at the ancient art and science of alchemy, examining the points that distinguish alchemical consciousness from modern scientific thought and exploring why and when an alchemical attitude may facilitate healing more effectively than scientific logic.

In Chapter Three, "The Axle and the Wheel," we explore how qi—the alchemical third—unfolds into the "ten thousand things," the multitude of forms and energies that make up the living world. We discuss *wuxing*, which are the Five Elements—the yin, sustaining and structured aspect of qi. We also discuss *wushen*, the Five Spirits—the yang, ephemeral, motive aspect of qi—and examine the relationship between these two systems and their clinical usefulness in working with emotional and psychosomatic issues.

For Taoists, the number four is the number of the earth. It represents the way that the divine extends outward horizontally to create the four directions—the compass rose of life on earth. So, in Chapter Four, "Tao Lost and Rediscovered," we look at how the unknowable Tao extends itself into an individual healing process. This chapter presents a case study that demonstrates how the previously introduced concepts can be successfully integrated into actual treatment and how Chinese medicine can support a person in redis-covering his or her Way.

Five is the child of one. It is the place where the four directions cross to form a new center point. For Taoists, Kunlun Mountain is the mythical center pole of the cosmos. It is a symbolic expression of the spinal column that is the vertical center pole of a human being and the core of the human nervous system. In Chapter Five, "The Mountain," we begin the inner alchemical journey as we descend Kunlun Mountain from heaven to the underworld. The Five Spirits are the resident deities of this inner mountain, and, like the nature deities that preside over the woods, winds and waters of the natural world, these spirits preside over the psychic energies that animate the bodymind.

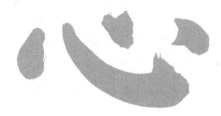

Chapter One

The Empty Center

Wu

The sage considered his situation. "Who is this 'I' who is wondering about the Way? This I is me," he thought, pointing to his nose. "This me is my breath streaming in and out through my nostrils."

Lao Tzu picked up a cup of tea and looked down at his face. He took a sip and swallowed. He thought about wu—emptiness or non-existence. Picking up a brush, he painted some lines on a white scroll. "It is only the empty space," he wrote, "that makes the cup useful. It is only the hole at the center that allows the wheel to spin. It is only the doors and windows, the empty spaces in the walls that make the room a place to live."

He wrote:

Thus, when a thing has existence alone
    it is mere dead-weight
Only when it has *wu*, does it have life[1]

Why Does Wu Matter?

Wu, emptiness, is a question that can never be answered, a mystery that can never be solved. Yet, just as spirit brings meaning and vitality to the material world, wu brings coherence to Taoist philosophy and effectiveness to Chinese medicine's most important treatment strategies.

Wu is not simply an abstract theory or a neat philosophical construct. Although it cannot be measured, touched or seen, wu is real. Without wu, our earthly life is dead weight. Without wu, things have no quality, usefulness or value. Without wu, the Way cannot wander and Tao will not be found.

Wu as a philosophical idea translates seamlessly into wu as psychological insight. We discover wu at the core of the Taoist understanding of self. It is the original nature of the heart, the organ responsible for organizing and maintaining individual identity.

In practical terms, wu, the emptiness at the center, is a principle that is used in acupuncture and Chinese herbal medicine, especially as it pertains to emotional and psychospiritual healing. Emptiness and fullness are principles that have a direct impact on diagnosis and treatment planning. Obstruction, stagnation and accumulation cause emotional problems, and, as acupuncturist and author Giovanni Maciocia reminds us, "Obstruction of the Mind causes mental confusion because the obstructing factor impairs the Mind's activity."[2] The treatment principle in obstruction of the mind is to open the mind's orifices, in other words to clear the way for the life force and make a space so that spirit can move freely into matter.

Even the acupuncture point is a kind of wu. The Chinese word is *xue,* which refers to a cave, a hole or hollow space. So the acupuncture point is viewed as a doorway, a nothingness, an opening in the material matrix of the body. The point's effectiveness lies in its emptiness, the space it opens for the spinning pivot of the acupuncture needle.

A Look at the Chinese Character

The ancient Chinese character for *wu* is a picture of a dancing shaman in fancy sleeves or tassels. The character gives us insight into the word's meaning.

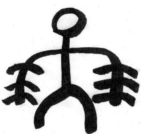 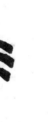 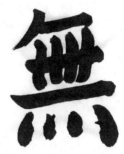

Wu, emptiness (ancient)   Wu, emptiness (modern)

The shaman played a central role in the life of the ancient Chinese. Shamans had mysterious powers and were able to effect changes beyond the capacities of ordinary human beings. Shamans cured diseases, ended droughts, managed floods, controlled evil spirits and invoked the gods. In their role as tribal leader, healer and priest, shamans mediated between the everyday world and the spirit world beyond. The shaman was the go-between, the free and easy wanderer who roamed the Cloud Realms between heaven and earth. Through ritual chanting, incense burning, drumming and incantations, shamans opened passageways between the human and divine realms. Through their ritual practices, shamans penetrated the Great Mystery, entered the ineffable and gained access to Tao.

Dancing was an important part of shamanic practice. It was the Hidden Way, the secret path that led them from one world to the next. The ritual dances of the shamans were based on complex combinations of steps and long periods of rapid spinning. The dances altered consciousness and induced states of ecstatic trance in which the shamans sprouted wings, rode through the empty vastness of space and traveled to the bright stars of the Milky Way and to the dark labyrinths beneath the earth. During these journeys they contacted the spirits of above and below who guided their healing work and gave them supernatural powers.[3] Through dancing, the shaman entered wu, the empty vortex, the whirlwind of the Tao.

In describing the nature of the wu shaman, Ge Hong, a third-century Taoist alchemist, wrote,

> He is so high that no one can reach him,
> so deep that no one can penetrate to his depth;
> he rides the fluid light,
> he whips space in the six directions . . .
> he emerges beyond height,
> he penetrates below depths . . .
> he sails to the point of the indefinite . . .
> he absorbs the nine efflorescences at the edge of the clouds . . .
> he goes here and there in the shadowy darkness . . .[4]

The meaning of the wu character is found in the center of the shaman's spinning, a vortex that is the pathway between above and below. It is wu, the empty center, that makes the dance useful. Ge Hong described this vortex as "so wide, it encompasses the eight cardinal points . . . it surges up like a whirlwind and streaks away like a comet. . . ." Like a funnel, this emptiness gathers the light of the divine, which it sends as sparks of spirit into the world.

The spinning emptiness at the center of the dance creates a magnetic field, a receptive yin hollow that draws the yang initiating spirits down into the realm of matter. The spinning is the circulation that continually infuses divine radiance into the world. According to Taoist philosophy, the spirits are drawn irresistibly to wu—to the whirling emptiness at the heart of matter. And once the spirits arrive at the center, matter changes from dead weight into something that has life, something that has purpose, something that evolves, something that has Tao.

The concept of the empty center is at the core of Taoist philosophy. But it also informs the basic principles of traditional Chinese medicine and is a crucial part of the Taoist ideas about psychological healing and the self.

FIVE

The number five is related to the empty center. Five is the child of one. It is the embodied reflection of divine unity. After Tao divides into the opposites of earth and heaven, yin and yang, matter and spirit, it further divides and manifests as the four directions, the cardinal points of the compass wheel. At the center of the four, at the meeting point of space and time, here and now, is five. Five is the centered four, the unknowable Tao made manifest as individual being.

According to sinologist and Jesuit priest Claude Larre, five represents organization, the constellating of cosmic vitality into discreet units of organic function. Five is the "dimension where the permutations of time and space have an action . . . the way in which the spirits govern my life at the deepest level."[5] In *Number and Time,* Marie Louise von Franz says that five "represents the alchemical idea of the *quinta essentia,* the most refined, spiritually imaginable unity of the four elements. It is either initially present in and extracted from them or produced by the circulation of these elements among one another."[6] C. G. Jung also relates the number five to the unknowable quincunx or quintessence, the ungraspable mystery of life. "By unfolding into four," Jung wrote, "the one, accentuated as the center, acquires distinct characteristics and can therefore be known."[7]

The Chinese word for "five" is also pronounced "wu." The word sounds similar to the word for "emptiness"; however, the Chinese character is different. On early ceremonial bronze vases, five is represented by X, two crossed lines that symbolize the meeting point of earth and heaven, yin and yang, the inhalation and exhalation of the breath. Later, two parallel strokes were added above and below the crossed lines to represent heaven and earth, between which constellated qi, the field of life. At the crossing point of two lines, at the midpoint of the four directions, is five, the center point or "knot of life."[8]

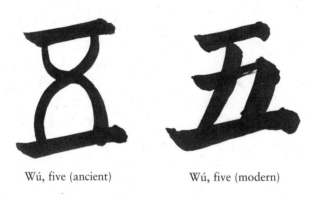

Wú, five (ancient)   Wú, five (modern)

According to the ancient Chinese, all of life is a manifestation of the number five: the Five Elements, the five yin viscera, the Five Spirits. X, the cross point of the inhalation and exhalation of heaven and earth, marks the spot where life begins and ends. X marks the spot: me, the empty center, the point where something and nothing meet to manifest as my particular life. X also represents the entire field of life that forms at the interface of opposite polarities. Much as modern science locates electromagnetic fields between opposite polarities, the ancient Chinese located the field of life at the crisscross point where the opposite breaths of yin and yang meet.

Five is the return to origin where one meets itself again. Five is where the great mystery of Tao meets itself in the little mystery of me, where Tao meets tao at the crossing point of my life, here and now, this very place where my foot stands.

THE HEART

How can a person know Tao? By the Heart.

How can the Heart know? By emptiness, the pure attention that unifies being and quietude.

The Heart is never without treasure, yet it is called empty. . . .

The Heart is alive and it possesses knowledge, it knows, and from knowing makes distinctions. To make distinctions is to know all parts of the whole at once.

—Chuang Tzu[9]

The Chinese word for "heart" is *xin*. The Chinese word refers to the organ Western medicine recognizes as the heart as well as what is sometimes referred to as the heartmind, the central organizing principle or processing unit of individual life. For the ancient Chinese, xin was much more than a muscular blood pump. It was the residence of the spirit, the center of psychological life and function. In philosopher and sinologist Chad Hansen's words, "We understand the faculty of xin best as the faculty that guides the body's behavior."[10] Hansen compares xin to a black box, an emptiness in which all the opposites of sensory life, the likes and dislikes, the thises and thats, are gathered, evaluated, and then reintegrated into a single appropriate and effective action.

In traditional Chinese medicine and ancient Taoist thought, the heart is likened to the ruler of a kingdom. Like an emperor, the heart is the organizing principle of a person's being, the regulating principle of the body and the mind. It is found at the crossing point of the upper and lower body, at the X point of the arms and the legs. The ancient Chinese character for the heart is a primitive rendering of the actual organ; it shows the hollow vessel of the organ itself as well as the main arteries leading to and away from it.

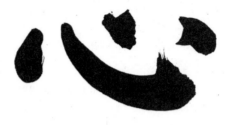

Xin, heart

In addition to being a rudimentary picture of the heart, the graphic can be viewed as a picture of an empty bowl that is open at the top. The emptiness at the center of the heart makes it useful. This emptiness creates a space for the shen—the fiery sparks of spirit that, according to Taoist mythology, come to us at the moment of conception, directly from the stars. This fiery cosmic light illuminates our capacity for consciousness and self-awareness. It is the spark that ignites all other aspects of personal awareness, represented by the spirits of the hun, yi, po and zhi. Look at the small brush stroke at the center of the heart as representing the shen, the tiny spark of divine fire that resides in the heart space and radiates out into the world as the light of individual awareness and identity.

Taoist psychology places special emphasis on the heart, whose rhythms are closely related to a human being's mental and emotional life. Classical Chinese medical texts say that the heart is the residence of the mind. Even today, the character *xin*, heart, is used to refer to the mind. This does not mean that the ancient Chinese were unaware of the brain but that they did not associate the faculties of the mind—awareness, perception, feeling, imagination, thought, intention, sensation, desire and will—with that particular organ.

THE SELF: EAST MEETS WEST

Most classical Western philosophies and religions begin with the premise that at the center of being, there is something rather than nothing.[11] According to the Western view, at the center of a person, there is some unique structure or principle that endures throughout life and possibly even after death. At my core, there is a self that is separate from other selves as well as from the material world around me (including my own body). It is likewise separate from the divine world that lies beyond the world I know with my ordinary senses. The edges of the self are defined by the boundary of the physical skin, and its scope is limited by the constraints of time, space and cultural context.

Taoist philosophy, on the other hand, is grounded in the concept of wu, the unknowable emptiness at the center of being. The Taoist alchemists, who were the original psychologists of traditional Chinese medicine, had no conception of a self as an enduring, unchanging entity at the center of a human being. For them, the individual self—if it existed at all—was not limited and defined by the boundary of the skin but rather existed in a continuum with the cosmos. Like other cosmological phenomena, the self was seen as the meeting point of external and internal conditions, a fleeting event, a moment in time. Like a drop of dew, a snowflake or a morning breeze, the self was ungraspable, a momentary manifestation of the continually changing interplay of cosmic forces and circumstances. The boundary between "me" and the world around me was barely recognized. From a Taoist perspective, "I" am the cosmos in miniature. There is no distinct line between me and the visible natural world or the invisible world of the divine.

The Chinese word that comes closest to our word *self* is *zi*. The character is a picture of a nose. In China, one points to one's nose to indicate "me," "myself." The nose is a passageway through which the breath travels in order to mingle with the blood and animate the body, and then returns on its way back to the ether. Zi, the self, is a conduit, a breathing space, an empty center where outer and inner meet face to face, where something and nothing mingle to create my life.

From the perspective of Taoist psychology, there is no self at the center of me, nothing that is graspable or nameable or permanent. Rather, there is a process of ongoing transformation, a whirlwind of qi that spins from the most yin, material vibrations of my existence—the bones, organs, muscles and blood—to the most yang vibrations—the visions, desires and inspirations of the mind and the spirit. At the far limits of this whirlwind, the vortex extends from my being outwards to the ineffable and infinite, to the whirling chaotic unity that is the origin and goal of my life, where self and no-self, being and non-being mingle in the endless cosmic dance of Tao.

From this perspective, nothingness is not an abstraction. It is not far away and beyond being. Rather, nothingness informs and breathes life into being. Although it cannot be known by the conscious mind, under special circumstances wu may be experienced directly. Through the heightened awareness produced by meditation, ritual, shamanic dance and the esoteric practices of inner alchemy, as well as the transcendent states of consciousness that are sometimes entered during times of illness and overwhelming suffering, the boundaries of the identity dissolve and self meets no-self, being meets non-being.

From a Taoist perspective, it is only through this encounter with wu, the emptiness at the center, that human beings come to know their own true nature. As something and nothing collide in the direct encounter with wu, we are returned to the ever-present mystery of our original wholeness, to the tiny but perfect reflection of the Tao that lies within us—the unified chaos where opposites unite and polarities mingle, the vortex that whirls like the shaman's dance at the center of our lives.

Closer to the Taoist vision of the unknowable mystery at the center of being than many other traditional Western approaches—but also, in some ways, essentially different—is the psychological perspective of C. G. Jung. In 1928, Richard Wilhelm sent Jung the translation of a Taoist alchemical text, *The Secret of the Golden Flower.*[12] In *jin hua*—the golden flower—Jung recognized a parallel to the circular mandala drawings of blossoming flowers painted by his patients. For Jung, the golden flower—like the flower that unfurls from the seed point at the center of the mandala circle—came to symbolize the mystery at the center of being. Jung referred to this mystery at the center as the self.

As Jung delved into the writings of the Taoist alchemists as well as the esoteric writings and mythologies of other ancient wisdom traditions, he recognized relationships between the images and symbols of the texts and the contents of his modern patients' unconscious. Although his patients had no previous knowledge of Chinese mythology, Taoist philosophy or alchemy, there appeared to be an overlap between their unconscious fantasies and dream images and the visions and symbols expressed in the ancient texts. In addition, Jung discovered that the process of psychospiritual development outlined in *The Golden Flower* closely paralleled processes of psychic development followed by patients in his practice. This led him to infer that these images, symbols and psychic growth patterns transcended time, geographical locale and culture, that they must be an innate part of the human psyche. He concluded that human beings, through their long process of evolution, had developed certain basic ways of mentally organizing and grasping the phenomenal world that were somehow "hard-wired" into the brain and nervous system. He referred to these organizing patterns as archetypes and believed that they were the psychic equivalent of the innate instinctual impulses that arise from our physical being. He believed that the archetypes, like the instinctual behavior of animals, were universal and highly resistant to change. In his Commentary to *The Secret of the Golden Flower,* he wrote,

> . . . just as the human body shows a common anatomy over and above all racial differences, so too, does the psyche possess a common substratum. I have called the latter the collective unconscious. As a common human heritage it transcends all differences of culture and consciousness . . .[13]

As Jung continued his exploration of the collective unconscious, his view of the self expanded beyond the skin boundary and the confines of personal identity. He began to view the self as a mystery that transcended time, space, individual identity and the limitations of culture and history.

In several significant ways, Jung's view of the self parallels the Taoist view of Tao. Jung regarded the self—as the Taoists regarded Tao—as a divine wholeness that transcends ordinary human experience, a wholeness that could never be known with ordinary consciousness or spoken of using ordinary language. Like Tao, the self exists as the ever-present ground of being. Even when we are completely unaware of its presence, this vast mystery pervades every aspect of our lives.

Taoists spoke of a connection between the great cosmic Tao, which lies far beyond human experience, and tao, the tiny but perfect reflection that lies within each individual being. Similarly, Jung recognized a uniquely personal self that incarnates in an individual through a process of inner work. This small self within reflects in miniature the wholeness of the great self, which Jung sometimes referred to as the Self. Just as Taoists looked to the tao within as the

"Way," the path that leads a person back to her own true nature, Jung looked to the incarnate self as a mysterious organizing principle, a speck of crystallized spirit or embodied divinity at the center of being, that could bring integrity, meaning and purpose to the seemingly random experiences of life.

Like the small tao within, the inner self exists as an ever-present potentiality in every human being. The seed of the self is planted within us at the moment of birth, and the infant lives in a state of unconscious connection to this divine wholeness. But as consciousness develops in the growing child, the connection to the self is eclipsed by the power of the developing ego and individual will. According to both the Taoist and the Jungian perspective, the recovery of connection to our original inner wholeness is the ultimate goal of every human life.

Yet for Jung, anything beyond the consciously conceivable remained beyond human experience. It was something "about which nothing can be determined."[14] He did not deny that phenomena existed that were beyond the scope of the conscious mind, but as a scientist, he was determined to refrain from speculation and to speak only about what he had directly observed or experienced. So, unlike the Taoists, who contended that the wholeness of Tao could be experienced by human beings through the relinquishing of individual consciousness to wu through an encounter between being and non-being, self and no-self, Jung believed that the wholeness of the self could only be approached through a conscious process, a gradual deepening and broadening of ego awareness. For Jung, this broadening of ego awareness occurred through the assimilation of the contents of the collective and personal unconscious into consciousness.

Through his work with patients and his explorations of his own psyche, Jung came to believe that modern Westerners (unlike people of ancient Eastern traditions, who were less invested in their own individual identities) needed to approach the experience of inner wholeness through the conscious integration of unconscious contents, especially the rejected parts of their own nature. Jung believed that the contents of the collective unconscious of humanity could be approached and known by the ego through an exploration of dream images, symbols, active imagination and projected fantasy. As the ego expands its range through the assimilation of our desires, instinctual drives, and especially the shadowy, hidden parts of our personality that are at odds with civilized collective values, we come closer to a state of inner wholeness and the Self is gradually incarnated as self. Through this process, a felt sense of inner richness, integrity and multidimensionality emerges in the psyche. The Self is no longer experienced as something outside and beyond human life, but rather is incarnated in the psyche as a stable inner center, a spacious container for the conscious ego. The ultimate goal of this integration process is a shift in emphasis from the one-sided, limited viewpoint of the ego to the expansive, multifaceted totality of the self.

Jung referred to the encounter between the conscious ego and the archetypal images of the collective unconscious as "conscious life."[15] For him, this conscious life, making the unconscious conscious, was the ultimate goal of psychological development and the closest a human being could come to wholeness. He referred to this process as individuation and believed that it began at mid-life when the ego had reached the limits of its own potency and the individual made a conscious decision to follow the "backward-flowing path,"[16] turning away from the endless distractions and desires of the outer world toward the inner realms of the psyche.

While Jung's view of the self overlaps in important ways with the Taoist view, the ultimate goal of Jungian archetypal psychology differs from that of Taoist psychology. The process of individuation that Jung held as the ultimate goal of human development was an earth-bound, psychic experience. It was an experience that could be talked about and known. Consciousness was not obliterated in the swirling vortex of nothingness but rather, carefully cultivated and protected as a hard-won treasure. The expansion of consciousness and the strengthening of relationship between the conscious ego and the self was a clearly stated goal of the work.

The Taoist process of enlightenment, on the other hand, regarded consciousness as a useful but expendable tool that could be discarded once the inner alchemical process was underway. For the Taoist, consciousness was the spark that ignited the engine of inner work but was not regarded as the illumination itself. The adept's task was to sacrifice the spark to a much greater light as he was lifted out of time and space, off the three-dimensional plane of the earth toward a direct encounter with the divine.

According to Jung, the self incarnates at the center of a human being through the integration of the shadow parts of the personality and the archetypal energies from the unconscious into consciousness. The Taoists, on the other hand, begin the process by emptying the center so that something much greater than individual consciousness can come to life in the void. Jung's process of individuation and conscious life opens a doorway to the transpersonal—to realms of experience that extend horizontally beyond the limits of individual identity. Taoists worked to open a vertical conduit that led the adept directly to the absolute—to the realms of the transcendent.

Ken Wilber defines the transpersonal as a realm of experiences that takes us beyond individual identity. In his book *No Boundary*, he writes, "in transpersonal experiences, the person's identity does not quite expand to the Whole, but it does expand or at least extend beyond the skin boundary of the organism."[17] Transpersonal experiences extend the range of the psyche so that the sense of self grows horizontally in emotional scope, psychological depth and wisdom. But, as Wilber states, transpersonal experience does not bring us into direct contact with the Whole, the divine unity at the core of being. For this, we must turn to transcendent states, experiences that allow us to extend the self along the vertical axis of spirit, to climb the spinning ladder of light that leads us away from our selves, that leads us to wu, to the realms of the dancing Taoist shamans.

At the present time on our planet, as the cultures of East and West collide, as the Western tradition of rational thought and the Eastern tradition of mystical experience mingle, it may be that the way back to our own center, to our own experience of inner wholeness, will be found through the integration of these two viewpoints. In order to accomplish this integration, we must create healing modalities and practices that allow us to expand our experience of the self beyond our current notions of spatial and temporal reality. We must develop horizontally along Jung's transpersonal line and vertically along the Taoist line of transcendent experience. We must reconsider our notions of inner and outer, spiritual and material, vertical and horizontal, personal, transpersonal and transcendent as we develop a new, more integrated kind of embodied spiritual awareness.

For us, it may not be not enough to directly encounter the divine through the relinquishing of identity in the experience of wu. Perhaps we must find a way to enter into the encounter while remaining conscious of our somethingness, of our own individual identity. In other words, for human beings at the current time, the return to wholeness may require that we come into conscious relationship with the self, to the spark of divinity that illuminates the entire spectrum of our being—from the brightest peaks of the mind to the darkest labyrinths of the body. This is the hidden potential of the newly emerging embodied energetic systems of healing. Although acupuncture—when practiced from an alchemical perspective—is only one of many such systems, it is one that has stood the test of time and proved effective for human beings all over the world. As we explore the world of Chinese medicine through the lens of archetypal psychology and Taoist alchemy, we discover a way to not only deepen the practice of healing but also reinvent our notion of the self.

Ancient Understandings and Recent Trends:
The Return to Origin

In ancient times, every individual Chinese person saw himself as a miniature reflection of the cosmos. In Asian art historian Stephen Little's words, for them "the structure of the human body mirrors the universal order inherent in the Tao. This system of divine correspondence between human microcosm and celestial macrocosm is a fundamental and continuous element in the tradition of religious Taoism."[18] The organizing principle of this cosmos, Tao, was reflected in the rhythms and movements of the natural world and the unfolding destiny of each individual human life. Despite the seemingly random effects of chance and fate, life had an integrity and harmony that sprang directly from Tao. A human being's essential task was to know his or her place in the cosmos and to cultivate a life that was an expression of the effortless elegance and essential wisdom of the natural world.[19] From the perspective of the ancient Chinese, all disease was caused by a loss of Tao. The central concern of traditional Chinese medicine was the restoration and maintenance of Tao and the ongoing cultivation of a harmonious relationship between human beings and the natural world.

Today, the unities once possessed by human beings—the unity of life and nature, mind and body, action and instinct—are shattered beyond repair. The health and psychological well-being that the ancient Chinese derived from their trust in nature and the integrity of the cosmos are not available to us. In modern American culture, we do not have the grace of confidence in the wisdom of nature and the integrity of the cosmos. We live in a world that has fragmented into a dot matrix of TV images and syncopated sound bites. Our minds, emotions and bodies are divided; our heads, hearts and feet move in different directions. We have lost touch with the Mysterious Feminine, the receptive yin wisdom of the earth and the body that supports and nourishes the arising of life.

In his Commentary on *The Secret of the Golden Flower*, Jung began to explore how ancient Taoist and alchemical concepts could be used to resolve the problem of the modern psyche's fragmentation, the splits between conscious and unconscious, mind and body, individual will and destiny, matter and spirit, mundane and divine, self and cosmos. He believed that this fragmentation, which had served an important purpose as part of the development of rational, analytic thought and the individuated ego, had gone far beyond what was healthy for human beings and was causing tremendous psychological distress among his patients. Alienation, psychosomatic disturbances, addiction, anxiety and depression were only a few of the symptoms caused by the shattering of the psyche. In the Commentary, he wrote,

> The unity once possessed has been lost and must be found again. Tao is the method or conscious way by which to unite what is separated. . . . There can be no doubt that the realization of the opposite hidden in the unconscious signifies reunion with the unconscious laws of our being, and the purpose of this reunion is the attainment of conscious life or, expressed in Chinese terms, the realization of the Tao.[20]

For Jung, Tao was a doorway into the fluid, synchronous consciousness of the East. The ideas of Taoism gave him images and a language with which he could express not only his developing theories but also less familiar parts of his own psyche. Jung felt that Eastern consciousness mirrored many aspects of the Western unconscious and that an understanding of Eastern thought offered crucial insights into hidden parts of the Western mind. It was a way to bring the ego-awareness of Western consciousness into relationship with the instincts, dream symbols and creative potentialities of the deep unconscious.

Through the restoration of communication between ego consciousness and the deep psyche, Jung felt that a new, more complex psychic wholeness could come to life. This new wholeness would preserve individual identity while reconnecting modern man to the revitalizing energies of nature, the unconscious and the cosmos. His investigations in this area eventually became a significant part of modern depth psychology.

But Jung failed to recognize crucial aspects of Taoist philosophy that were expressed in the text of *The Secret of the Golden Flower*. Although he went beyond the bounds of Western rational consciousness when he entered the transpersonal realm of archetypal images, myths and symbols, he hesitated at the edge of a full, transcendent illumination experience. He did not yet have the tools that later somatic therapies could provide to move the archetypal energies of the unconscious through the nervous system of the body—nor did he have a full, embodied understanding of Eastern yogic practices.

Even more significant was a basic theoretical misunderstanding that Jung expressed in his Commentary on *The Secret of the Golden Flower*. Here, Jung equated shen, the "light of heaven," which Taoists regarded as the quintessential alchemical mystery, with consciousness. He further stated that to follow the way of Tao meant to go consciously, or, to follow "the conscious way." Thus he missed the crucial underlying message of the text, which urges the spiritual seeker to use consciousness and individual will only as the spark to fuel the descent into wu and then to surrender the light of individual consciousness to the dark, chaotic waters of transformation. In the text, the adept is urged to "use action to achieve non-action" and is told that "the awakening of spirit is accomplished because the heart has died first." Further, we read that "when no idea arises, the right ideas come." Taoist alchemists viewed consciousness not as a goal but as a tool that allows us to initiate the inner alchemical opus. But, once the opus is undertaken, the goal is to surrender the will and to release the grip of consciousness so that a new form of awareness, a new illumination, can come to life from "down below." The light of consciousness that allows us to initiate the process must be sacrificed to the emptiness and darkness of the Void so that it can be reborn in a new and more precious form, a completely new, multi-dimensional form of awareness, a new flesh that is a body of crystallized light.

Jung's "conscious life" did not include an essential aspect of Eastern religious experience: the direct encounter with the unknowable, unnamable mystery of the Tao. While this "conscious life" took into account the conscious and unconscious aspects of the self, it did not attempt to deal directly with the transcendent aspect of human experience, the aspect that Taoists and Chan Buddhists refer to as no-self, the Great Void, the Nameless Mystery, the Formless Form of Nonbeing.

For Jung, this transcendent aspect of Tao was beyond human experience. In the *Commentary*, he writes,

> The fact that I restrict myself to what can be psychically experienced, and repudiate the metaphysical, does not mean, as anyone with insight can understand, a gesture of skepticism or agnosticism pointed against faith or trust in higher powers, but what I intend to say is approximately the same thing Kant meant when he called *das Ding an sich* (the thing in itself), a "purely negative, borderline" concept. Every statement about the transcendental ought to be avoided because it is invariably a laughable presumption on the part of the human mind, unconscious of its limitations. Therefore, when God or Tao is spoken of as a stirring of, or a condition of, the soul, something has been said about the knowable only but nothing about the unknowable. Of the latter, nothing can be determined.[21]

But, for the ancient Taoists as well as the Zen Buddhist practitioners who followed in their footsteps, the purely negative quality of the "thing in itself" is precisely the goal of the work. For them, focusing on the image or attempting to use consciousness to achieve wholeness is a case of "confusing the finger with which one points to the moon with the moon itself."[22] For them, the unknowable is not something far away and beyond our experience. Rather, it is the medium and ground of being. Like fish who swim in water yet never know the sea, we live in the swirling current of Tao and do not realize it. This unknowable mystery permeates the entire universe and a tiny speck of it is in each and every one of us, waiting to be recognized.

The Taoist practitioner's ultimate goal is not conscious understanding but the embodied experience of transcendent light, illumination as an actual presence of being. In order to arrive at this experience of illumination, he must first encounter wu—the absolute negation of his individual being. This means that he has transcended the limitations of form, that his awareness is no longer limited to his five senses and the boundaries of his individual, physical self or even of the temporal and spatial constraints of the earth plane. He has been "reborn" through a descent into darkness and illuminated by the divine light that waits, in seed form, in the depths of his own being. This rebirth into the realm of incarnate light is not an experience of consciousness but rather a direct experience of wholeness. It is the crystallization of the golden light of the divine into material form.

> The light is not in the body alone, neither is it only outside the body. Mountains and rivers and the great Earth are lit by sun and moon; all that is this Light. Therefore it is not only within the body. Understanding and clarity, knowing and enlightenment, and all motion (of the spirit) are likewise this Light; therefore it is not just something outside the body. The Light-flower of Heaven and Earth fills all thousand spaces. But also the Light-flower of one body passes through heaven and covers the Earth. Therefore, just as the Light is circulating, so Heaven and Earth, mountains and rivers, are all rotating with it at the same time. To concentrate the seed-flower of the human body above in the eyes, that is the great key of the human body.[23]

During the healing process or the journey of spiritual transformation, the encounter with wu marks a turning point. This encounter happens without warning and immediately extinguishes our capacity to "know" in any traditional sense of the word. It is an encounter that turns us upside down and inside out. Old patterns and ways of being disintegrate and new possibilities spontaneously emerge. If we survive the encounter at all, we survive through a rebirth that fundamentally reorganizes our entire being.

At these moments, Tao can be felt as a vast mystery, a blue wind at twilight, a flickering light barely discernible . . . seen and not seen . . . something known as it remains, forever, unknowable. And it is this night wind, this invisible light, this luminous darkness, the unknowable mystery of the Tao, that is at the core of all truly transformational healing.

Modern Western depth psychologists speak of the emergence of inner integrity as the individuation process. They view it as a spontaneous reconstellation of psychic order, a new level of structure and organization. The new wholeness that constellates through this process is referred to as the Self. It is a unique expression of the person's essential nature and a reflection in miniature of the unknowable integrity of the divine.

The Taoist alchemists recognized a similar phenomenon in their own work with psychospiritual development. When I turn inward and encounter the unknowable nothingness at the center of me, something meets nothing and a reorganization of my entire being occurs. The outcome of this is a new integrity: I know myself as something beyond knowing, a minute but perfect expression of divine wholeness, a miniature version of Tao—not a what but a how, not a something but an ever-unfolding way of being. In alchemical texts, this miniature Tao is pictured as an embryo or small child curled in the belly or floating above the head of the meditating sage.

Taoist alchemists regarded this reorganization as the ultimate goal of a human being's psychospiritual journey, the end and the beginning of the quest. They referred to it as the "return to original nature," "the birth of the sage," or the "return to the wholeness of Tao."[24] They referred to the individuals who had endured the ardu-

Embryo in Belly of Meditating Sage

要兒現形圖

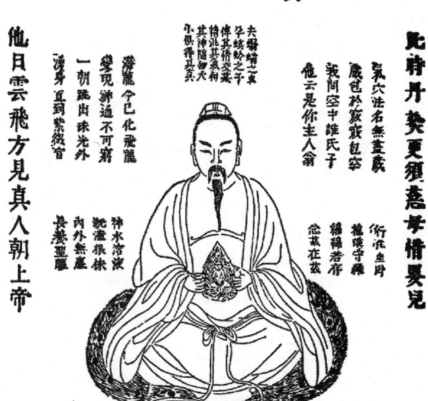

他日雲飛方見真人朝上帝

潛龍令已化飛龍
變現神通不可窮
一朝踴出珠光外
渾身直到紫微宮

長養聖胎
內外無塵
玩漾狠休
神水溶溶

夫欲嬰兒真
孕嬰始之子
傳其情交媾
媾泥其氣相
其神隨如火
小焰得其真

氣穴法名無盡藏
歲包於寂寂包空
我聞空中誰氏子
他云是你主人翁

銜准坐臥
攝懷守雌
綿綿若存
念茲在茲

此身丹藥更須慈孝悌要兒

ous experience of return as sages or masters. The Chinese character for the word *tzu*, master or sage, is a picture of a dancing child. The character reinforces the idea that the master is one who has returned to origin, someone who is capable of combining the wisdom of experience with the unbroken spontaneous innocence of a child. Thus the sage, who grows younger as he ages, achieves immortality!

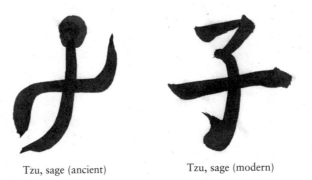

Tzu, sage (ancient)   Tzu, sage (modern)

The character for *tzu* also alludes to the Taoist idea that this return is a new birth or rebirth that happens in the middle of a person's life. The ancient Taoists viewed the return to original nature as the sprouting of a seed, the unfolding of an embryonic wholeness that was already waiting in a person's being. The sage was a child of Tao, a five that is born from one, a reflection in miniature of the integrity of the divine. The conditions that support this special birth could be cultivated, but the actual emergence of wholeness could never be forced or willed. It was a miraculous but natural event, like the sprouting of a flower or the crystallizing of a precious gem.

But for modern Westerners, the return to wholeness may require an attitude different from that of the ancient Taoist sage. Unlike the Taoists, whose seamless connection with the natural world allowed them to easily slip beyond the boundary of their own skin, modern Westerners have a sophisticated and highly developed sense of their own unique identity. The complete surrendering of identity to the energies of nature and the cosmos may not be enough to bring about the constellation of the new integrity. Jung warns that "It is not for us to imitate what is organically foreign. . . . [I]t is our task to build up our own Western culture. This has to be done on the spot, and into the work must be drawn the real European as he is in his Western commonplaces, with his marriage problems, his neurosis, his social and political illusions and his philosophical disorientation."[25]

Before we can climb the ladder toward transcendent states, we must first deal with our suffering at the relational, personal and transpersonal level. Through conscious, active work with the less conscious parts of our selves—our bodies, our dreams, our longings, our fantasies—we can actively begin to create a wholeness that is made up of our broken parts. Until this wholeness is constellated at the transpersonal level, it cannot be sacrificed in service to the transcendent.

In Lao Tzu's words, Tao is found *within us,* but for modern Westerners, this finding is not the result of a restoration of something lost or the fixing of something broken. Wholeness capable of reintegrating the fragments of the modern Western psyche must include all the weird, paradoxical, messy, irritating annoyances of our individual and hard-won identities. Such a new wholeness can only constellate through the suffering, longing and determination of single individuals striving to discover their own authentic nature.

CLINICAL IMPLICATIONS: SHOCK, TRAUMA AND THE EMPTY CENTER

Chinese medicine often uses mythical language and metaphor to express its meaning. The beauty and the poetry of the language is in itself a part of the healing process. The symbolic images of Chinese medicine and Taoist psychology describe actual phenomena that we can see every day. These images give us a way to bring dignity and meaning to seemingly random psychological symptoms. This poetic language is unerringly accurate in its description of physical and psychological phenomena that are routinely encountered, not only in the acupuncturist's treatment room but in daily life. The philosophical ideas and poetic images we have explored in the preceding pages form the basis of many of Chinese medicine's most important theories and practices.

From a Taoist perspective, the process of psychospiritual development begins with a shock, a lightning bolt, a shattering that opens the way for the influx of light into unconscious matter. It begins at the moment of conception, when the phallus of the father penetrates the body of the mother and the essences of the parents meet in the yin darkness of the womb. Then the light of the stars pours down into the heart of the embryo. Thus, when the baby is born, it comes into the phenomenal world trailing vapors of cosmic fire and divine light.

The staggering loss of light that the infant experiences at the moment of birth is partially made up for by the light of the shen that pours down in the form of love from her mother's and father's eyes. In order for this light to flow freely from mother to child, the mother's heart must be empty and tranquil so that the light of the shen has a place to rest. As long as this light is present, the child will move along into the unfolding experiences of life and weather the shattering pain of incarnation and the suffering of embodiment, until she eventually finds her way back to the wholeness of her original nature. However, when the mother has lost touch with her own divinity and her heart is filled with depression, worry, anger or despair, then her shen will not be present to entice the newborn infant into the world. The child then turns back to the womb or clings regressively to the mother's subtle body, a cold, wet, lifeless web of psychic flesh that cannot truly nurture or support her. Now, according to the Taoist vision, the self is possessed by *gui*—disembodied hungry ghosts with swollen heads, shrunken bodies and necks too thin to permit the passage of food. In this case, emptiness is a pathological state. This kind of nothingness is not a conduit for spirit and light but rather a clogged and stagnant void.

The image of the hungry ghosts aptly captures the current atmosphere of the modern Western psyche. Without the light of spirit to guide us out of the morass of the material world, we wander in a haze of endless desire and hunger that can never be satisfied. In order to transcend this condition, we must open not only to the transpersonal energies of the self but to the shen light that courses through the material world and through our own flesh.

As we have seen, from a Taoist mythological perspective, the light of the shen or spirit comes to us directly from the stars, directly from the divine, and resides, during our lives, in the empty space at the center of the heart. The shen is the illuminating spark of personal awareness, the source of the radiance of individual presence that streams from a person's being. The shen controls and directs the movements of the qi on a physical, mental and emotional level. Thus, all bodily and psychic functions are organized by the shen. The Five Spirits are the expression of the shen as it extends itself outward from the heart to function as discrete, increasingly embodied forms of awareness, i.e. intuition, vision, imagination, intention, sensing, somatic reactivity and instinctual knowing.

In order to maintain a suitable resting place for the shen, the heart must remain in a state that is close to its original nature. This is a state of *wuwei*—being by not being, doing by not doing, a state of serenity, acceptance and active receptivity. The light of the shen effortlessly radiates from such a tranquil heart to illuminate the lives of all those it touches.

According to Chinese medical theory, early maternal deprivation, parental neglect and unrelatedness, emotional and physical shock and trauma all directly impact the heart and spirits. In the poetic language of the ancient Chinese, the violent emotions that arise as a result of such experiences cause the heart to shake and tremble like a tree in a storm wind. Thus, the shen no longer rests tranquilly in the heart space. The spirits scatter, and their light no longer guides the movements of qi through the body and the mind. All bearings lost, the qi becomes chaotic and the light of the heart grows dim. In modern psychological terminology, the departure of the spirits is equivalent to the numbness, emotional paralysis, disassociation and mania that are the common sequelae of long-standing emotional neglect, shock and trauma.

Similarly, prolonged emotional strain and unresolved psychological issues impact the heart's ability to maintain its empty center. When a person is overwhelmed with worry, resentment, craving, or other intense emotions, there is no longer room in the heart for the shen. The spirits fly away and the radiance of present awareness no longer illuminates the person's life. When the shen have departed, signs that indicate psychological well-being are absent. The light in the eyes, the quality of presence and appropriate emotional responsiveness—all the signs of healthy spirits—are gone. We see instead the vacant stare, the unpredictable emotions, erratic reactions, absence of affect and disassociation that are common results of shock, trauma and overwhelming emotional experiences. From a Taoist perspective, healing entails finding a way to clear the heart of the negative emotions and to entice the spirits back to their nest. Once this is accomplished, the illumination of the shen—the light of awareness—can effortlessly guide a person back to the authentic wholeness of Tao.

Both patient and practitioner recognize the moment when the spirits return to the heart space. Sometimes it comes after months or years of treatment, sometimes during a first or second visit. It comes when the spirits are seen and touched, revived and called back to the heart, which may be the needle penetrating the empty center of the acupuncture point, clearing the way for wu, or a word or touch that hits the point, making contact with the spirits of the patient. In all cases, however, an opening is followed by a return of radiance that brings light to the eyes, color to the cheeks, and an overall return of animation and relatedness that the Chinese would refer to as the returning of the shen.

Case Study: Calling Back the Shen

Ten days after two planes crashed into the twin towers of the World Trade Center, I was back at work, teaching at the Tri-State College of Acupuncture on Fourteenth Street in downtown Manhattan. From the open windows of the classroom, we could still smell the ash and fire in the air, and fire trucks and police cars still raced down the avenue.

At the break, a young woman came up to me shaking and crying. For the past ten days, she said, she had been unable to sleep. She was disoriented and terrified. Although most New Yorkers were in shock that month (as are many human beings all over the planet on any given day following any given terrorist assault or other disorienting trauma), this was the one person in shock who stood in front of me at that very moment. I pulled myself together to bring my focus onto her distress. What I saw was that her eyes were moving rapidly back and forth and that she didn't make contact with me as she spoke. She was talking rapidly but to the air, as if she didn't really see me. The best way to describe it was that there seemed to be no one at home inside her. After talking with her for a few minutes, I suggested that she come to my office the next day for a treatment.

When she arrived, she was in the same state as she had been the day before. She still had not slept and was shaking and crying almost continuously. The first thing I did was give her a few drops of Bach Flower Rescue Remedy, a homeopathic mixture of flower essences that I have found to be remarkably effective for shock.[26] The Rescue Remedy calmed her down a bit, and as I sat with her and listened to her story, I felt the shen begin to gather back around her like bits of light—an awareness, hovering in her field, but not yet venturing back into her body.

I had her lie down on the treatment table and took her pulses.[27] All were chaotic, but the pulse that related to the heart was especially troubled. I decided first to do a treatment that would clear away pernicious qi, a treatment called "Aggressive Energy Clearing" that was developed by Dr. J. R. Worsely.[28] After I cleared the meridians, my patient was calmer but her eyes were still vacant.

Rather than going directly to a needling point on the Heart meridian, I decided instead to use the powerful tools of imagery and poetry to entice the shen back to their nest in the heart. I began by describing the shen spirits, explaining how the Taoists viewed the energies of the spirit as tiny wild birds and how these birds could get very frightened and scatter after severe trauma. As I spoke, I saw her eyes come into focus. She was really looking at me for the first time. When I explained how the heart can become filled with fear or other kinds of distress and leave no room for the spirits to rest, a look of understanding came to her face.

"That's exactly how I felt," she said, "as if my chest was filled up. I couldn't breathe. And it was like a part of me was just gone . . . just gone and I couldn't find myself."

With each small insight, a bit more of her came back. Her eyes stopped flickering, and color began to come into her cheeks. When I felt the moment was right, I asked her to turn her palm up and I needled Heart 7, Spirit Path. The name of this point tells us its function. The path is an emptiness, a conduit that opens the way for the shen to come back to their home in the Heart. I inserted the needle into the point and turned it a half-turn to the right to gently open the doorway for the qi.

That was all I needed to do. She looked at me and said, "I feel like I'm back." And we both knew that she was.

Reinventing the Self and the Practice of Alchemical Acupuncture

Alchemical Acupuncture invites us to reconsider our Western concept of the self as a fixed identifiable "something" that exists solely in the material realm of three-dimensional space and linear time and begins and ends at the boundary of the physical skin. Although from the perspective of the rational mind a needle is a needle and a point is a point, it becomes clear in the treatment room that the quality of the hands that hold the needle is as important as the quality of the needle itself. When the needle penetrates the boundary of the skin, it is not only the physical flesh of the patient that is touched, not only the metal of the needle that touches. There is an exchange of qi, a joining of energies, a mingling of soul and spirit that defies our traditional Western concept of limited individual identity.

In the words of the *Lingshu,* the primary classical Chinese acupuncture text, in order for a practitioner to bring acupuncture to its fullest potential, "the method is above all not to miss the rooting in the Spirits."[29] Claude Larre, in his book *Rooted in Spirit*, amplifies this citation by saying that the text "reminds us that pricking with a needle is effective only when accomplished by the hand of an acupuncturist whose Spirit can go all the way to the heart of animation, to the Spirits of the patient."[30] In order to heal not only the body but the psyche and the spirit, the soul and the spirits must be seen and related to. This means that the practitioner's vision must be able to penetrate beyond the material. She must be able to extend her self beyond the limits of her own skin, to feel into the felt sense of another. She must consciously stand in the emptiness at the center of her own being so that her eyes can see the unseeable, her ears can hear the unhearable and her hands can touch the most untouchable places in the patient's heart. In order to work at this level, a practitioner must surrender her individual will to the power of wuwei so that the needle can be guided not by her but by Tao.

Through the practitioner's vision, the patient also learns to experience the unity between spirit and matter, body and mind. The patient learns to experience the qi—the ungraspable life force that flows like a stream of light through his entire being. In this way, he comes to know himself as more than matter, to truly know himself as flesh—a living, breathing emptiness that both contains and is contained by spirit.

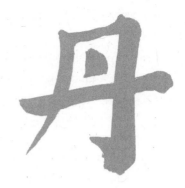

Chapter Two

Lead into Gold

Lao Tzu sat still and silent on a rock by a stream. He watched the water as it flowed downhill, leaving a trail of silt behind.

After rain, the water was cloudy.

But some hours later, the water cleared and he could see the pebbles and stones at the bottom.

Things change, he thought.

Then he picked up his brush and wrote:

Through the course of Nature
    muddy water becomes clear
Through the unfolding of life
    man reaches perfection
Through sustained activity
    that supreme rest is naturally found

Those who have Tao want nothing else
Though seemingly empty
    they are ever full.
Though seemingly old
    they are beyond the reach of birth and death.[1]

Taoist alchemy's central concern was the process of transformation—how something whole can be broken into parts and then reorganized to form a new wholeness of greater value and complexity than the preceding one. The alchemical opus can be summarized as an attempt to reverse the process of entropy, the running down and degradation of energetic systems with the passage of time. This focus is symbolically epitomized in the alchemical project of transforming base lead into gold. But, although the alchemists were passionately involved with the transformational properties of matter, their true quest was immortality—the transformation of an ordinary human being into a sage, one who had returned to the unbroken wholeness of Tao by reintegrating the opposites of life on earth. Through this reintegration, the sage became immortal and, rather than deteriorating with the passage of the years, grew increasingly infused with vitality and illumination. In Lao Tzu's words, such a being "though seeming old [was] beyond the reach of birth and death."

To the modern Western mind, the Taoist alchemical quest seems like a naïve fantasy. Through the influence of modern science and rational logic, as a culture we have come to accept that the parameters of linear time and three-dimensional space mark the boundaries of human experience, that life runs in one direction—from birth to death—and that the physical body defines the scope of a person's being. Yet even scientists admit that there is more going on in the universe than the rational mind can understand, and in fact the connection of events other than by cause and effect is an important exploration of modern physics. In the words of the scientist Enrico Fermi, "It does not say in the Bible that all laws are expressible linearly!"[2]

Western depth psychology has demonstrated that in the realm of the psyche and deep unconscious, events occur that defy rational understanding and the limitations of ordinary time and space. At the level of the psyche, synchronicity—the law of meaningful coincidences and acausal relationships—rules human experience, rather than the law of linear cause and effect. At the unconscious level, the reversals of time and the inversions of space that we discover in alchemical thought, like the strange reversals of the dream world, are commonplace occurrences. The inner life of subjective experience—and, more particularly, the inner activity of creating identity, inner wholeness, and a self—occurs in a different dimension than events in our outer life. In the words of psychoanalyst Nathan Schwartz-Salant,

> When we come to the problem of how a sense of identity comes into existence, we touch upon the boundaries of our understanding of the nature of the psyche. At bottom, what we call identity is a name for a fluid process which depends upon both [past history] and another, acausal dynamic. The latter is the basis for the mystery that surrounds the idea of identity. It is the process by which archetypal reality incarnates in historical time.[3]

Once we leave the materialistic world of modern Western rationalism and enter the deeper realm of the human psyche, we discover that the mythical viewpoint of the alchemists comes closer to the "truth" than our own mental, analytic worldview. In fact, when we dip beneath the conscious thinking mind, we discover that at the level of psychic and somatic awareness, the level of the soul, alchemical consciousness makes perfect sense. This ancient, seemingly antiquated system actually offers us indispensable tools for organizing and manipulating psychic reality.

Alchemical concepts are at the core of Chinese medicine. The movements of qi, the interplay of yin and yang, and the cyclical transformations of the Five Elements and the Five Spirits are all firmly rooted in the ground of alchemical consciousness. Many important Chinese medical terms and practices still in use today derive from Taoist alchemical ideas.

There are four main ways that the alchemical approach differs from the approach of Western science, and these differences directly influence the practice of Alchemical Acupuncture.

Cleaving versus Mingling

The first difference relates to basic strategies of investigation. While science is analytic, alchemy is synthesizing. While science focuses on discreet events and outcomes, alchemy focuses on relationships and processes. The word "science" comes from the Latin *scire,* meaning "to distinguish, to separate, to cut apart." It is related to *scindere,* "to cleave." The nature of modern science, by definition, is analytic. It seeks to cut apart the world in order to know it. In fact, we find this root, scire, again in our word con*scious*ness. The underlying assumption embedded in this term is that, in order to be aware of something, we must be able to recognize it as distinct from something else. Conversely, the word "alchemy" comes from the Greek *chemeia,* which means "a mingling or infusion." The nature of alchemy, by definition, is synthetic. It seeks to discover the underlying wholeness, the ways that the parts of the world mingle and unite.

In medicine, the cleaving strategy shows up in the radically separate specializations of Western doctors. It can be seen in Western medicine's focus on eradicating specific symptoms and identifying specific pathogens as opposed to focusing on the terrain of the whole person. It reaches its pinnacle in the practice of surgery, the cutting out of diseased portions of the whole, which is one of the great achievements of modern medicine.

The mingling strategy shows up in the Chinese physician's focus on the whole person, the view that physical, mental and spiritual symptoms are related, and the resonance that is recognized between the microcosm of human life and the macrocosm of the planet. It reaches its pinnacle in the endless web of interconnecting links made by the acupuncture meridians where, for example, a point on the left little toe is used to relieve pain in the right eye.

Yang versus Yin

From a Taoist perspective Western science would be considered the product of yang or masculine consciousness. It is active, penetrating and guided by the values of a basically patriarchal culture. Western science has a definite bias toward the active, sunlit mental realms of the yang as opposed to the receptive, shadowy, embodied, feeling realms of the yin. Western medicine works with what can be seen in the light of pure reason as opposed to what can be felt or intuited in the moonlit awareness of the soul.

In opposition to modern Western science, the primacy of the yin is explicitly stated and implicitly felt in every aspect of Taoist alchemy. Alchemists honored all aspects of the feminine, including the female body, genitalia, sexual fluids and reproductive organs. They viewed the uterus, with its empty center, as a sacred vessel where the mystery of creation occurred. The female body became symbolic of the cauldron in which matter could be alchemically renewed and transformed. "[N]ever lose sight of the Mother," writes Lao Tzu, "for the Mother brings the harvest, she alone causes all things to endure."[4]

Like the empty space at the center of the heart, the empty space at the center of the alchemical cauldron provides a nest for the speck of fiery spirit. It is analogous to the uterus that makes a space for the initiating spirit of the male essences and for the possibility of new life. Thus the heart, the hollow alchemical cauldron, the pelvic bowl and the uterus are all alchemical "burning spaces" where transformation can occur.

Alchemists recognized the divine preciousness of matter as well as spirit. They treasured the yin energies (the organic, earthbound, downward-magnetizing energies of disintegration and dissolution) as well as yang energies (the spiritual, lifting, upward-magnetizing energies of growth, diversity and complexity). This treasuring of the yin underlies the principle of wuwei—action through non-action, doing by not doing—that is central to Taoist psychospiritual alchemy. Silence, receptivity, patience, mystery and introspection are yin attitudes highly valued by Taoist alchemy. They are also attitudes that are indispensable to the practice of Alchemical Acupuncture, for it is in the silences, in the empty spaces in between the words, in the vast unknown that lies beyond our rational knowing, that the potent new possibility waits like a seed in the dark fertility of the yin.

Analytic versus Synthetic: Parts versus Whole

Modern scientific logic is analytic. It breaks things down in order to understand them better. It focuses on the parts of a system rather than the relationships that support and sustain wholeness. In contrast, the ancient logic of alchemy is synthetic. It focuses on the way severed parts combine to form new forms of wholeness.

The authentic practitioner of alchemy was committed to wholeness, to leaving nothing out of the system. He valued the transformational potency of the seemingly unimportant dregs of life, the bits of unintegrated stuff left over from creative processes. The old adage that "the treasure is found in the trash" comes directly from this ancient alchemical wisdom. In alchemy, every part of the whole is meaningful and valuable. Nothing is thrown out. Broken pieces are recombined to form new patterns of wholeness. What is more, the new wholeness is not something that has been planned and systematically worked toward in an intentional, directed way. It comes as a surprise that emerges as a kind of revelation. Like a kaleidoscopic image, the new wholeness appears suddenly as the bits and pieces of our lives reorganize to form a completely new pattern.

The integrating capacity of alchemical consciousness is beautifully expressed in the Zen Buddhist parable of the *tenzo* or Zen cook. The modern chef is a scientist who chooses a specific recipe, makes a list of ingredients, purchases what he needs and then puts the new pieces together in a directed way to create his intended dish. However, the tenzo works with what he finds, with the ingredients that are already in the cupboard. The true tenzo regards the lowliest dry clove of garlic with the same reverence as the most precious saffron threads or exotic mushrooms. The Zen cook throws absolutely nothing out! Everything finds its way into the cooking pot. Yet his work is effortless. The final dish is an expression of Tao, the vast organizing principle of the cosmos that transcends the dualities and limitations of directive thought and the modern scientific mind.[5]

Physical versus Psychic

Modern Western science is based on the idea that the natural world (including the human body) is a physical phenomenon, devoid of spirit and made up of unconscious matter that can be objectively observed and definitively measured. Since spiritual and psychic phenomena are timeless, weightless and spaceless, Western medicine places them outside of its domain and at times even denies their existence. Alchemists, however, were concerned with not only the quantities but also the qualities and qualitative effects of the observable world. For them, matter was filled with psychic energies or soul. The world was alive and vibrated with wisdom, intention and spirit.

While the materialistic, linear focus of Western science has given us the ability to make huge advances in the realm of technology as well as in the physical realms of medicine, it has proved less effective when it comes to working with the subtle, non-physical realms of the soul. In addition, Western science does not recognize the negentropic effects of spiritual and psychic energies on the physical world. This purely materialistic perspective has left us deadlocked in irreversible entropy, the physical universe's one-way ride downhill toward degradation and decay. As scientist and author James Lovelock puts it, the laws of entropy "read like the notice at the gate of Dante's Hell."[6]

Alchemy's capacity to recognize and work with psychic as well as physical phenomena gives us a way to begin to question the absolute inevitability of entropy. The very nature of psychic phenomenon is that they are pneumatic—that is to say, breathy, light, lifting, animating, energizing and negentropic! It is the breathy quality of the qi that gives it the capacity to animate and lift things up, to bring vitality to inert matter. And it is the breathy quality of the Five Spirits that allows them to function as a kind of pneumatic tube or pump that can renew vitality and empower transformation.

The clinical value of alchemical principles will be described in the case studies presented in this book. Next, however we turn to the central problem that alchemy is attempting to resolve.

ALCHEMY AND THE LOSS OF TAO

The alchemical story begins when the perfect reciprocity between human beings and the Tao was disrupted. According to myth, the earliest humans lived in absolute alignment with the Tao. Their universe was timeless, a closed energy circuit that went round and round in perfect harmony, without change. But at a certain moment in mythological time, as a natural part of the unfolding growth of the cosmos, the unity of Tao shattered and polarized. This rupture caused human beings to lose their alignment with Tao. Once this perfect alignment was lost, they began to live recklessly, out of accord with the laws of nature and the cosmos.

This problem is articulated in the first chapter of the *Neijing Suwen*, or *The Yellow Emperor's Classic of Internal Medicine*—the first and most famous acupuncture text. On the first page, the legendary Yellow Emperor, the first emperor of China and the inventor of the Chinese language and acupuncture, presents the central problem that traditional Chinese medicine was attempting to resolve when he asks his teacher the following question:

I have heard that in ancient times the people lived to be over a hundred years old and yet they remained active and did not become decrepit in their activities. But nowadays people reach only half that age and yet become decrepit and failing. Is it because the world changes from generation to generation? Or is it that mankind is becoming negligent of the laws of nature?[7]

The Yellow Emperor's teacher, Ch'i Po, responds to his question by saying that the people of old lived in harmony with cosmic energies and patterned themselves on yin and yang and the designs of nature. They were "tranquilly content in nothingness and the true vital forces followed them everywhere."[8]

"How could such people become ill?" Ch'i Po asks.

These mythic people who lived in ancient times had not yet separated from the natural world. They had no consciousness of self or other. Thus they lived in a state of wholeness and unity with Tao. They were tranquilly content and had no capacity to imagine or desire anything beyond what was. For these people, change was impossible because past and future did not yet exist. All that was and ever would be was present in the very moment. According to the text of the *Neijing*, these people of old lived in states of unbroken perfection. Order and disorder, life and death—these opposites had not yet entered human awareness. Consciousness that could desire something different from what was given, *a priori*, by nature had not yet arisen in human beings.

But by the time of the writing of the *Neijing* (approximately 400 BCE), human consciousness had begun to develop beyond this primal state of unbroken unity and harmony with nature. "Nowadays," says Ch'i Po, "people are not like (these people of ancient times). They do not know how to find contentment in themselves."

By the time of the writing of the text, human civilization had left behind the simple lifestyles of tribal people. People no longer went to bed when darkness fell or rose with the morning sun. They no longer lived in harmony with the rhythms and cycles of nature. They made their own rules and lived by their own inclinations and desires. In addition, shamans no longer made the sacrifices or correctly performed the rituals that could deal with leftover chaos and restore the lost harmony between human beings and the natural world.

The central dilemma of the text of the *Neijing*, as well as of acupuncture and traditional Chinese medicine, is whether it is better for the healer to try to restore the harmony that is inevitably lost when human consciousness develops beyond instinctual life, or to face the unknown and move forward toward some completely new possibility. The decision not to restore but to move forward toward an unknown possibility was the beginning of Taoist alchemy. The conscious choice to endure the pain, suffering, and breakdowns that accompany the birth of a completely new possibility from the disintegrated parts of a previous wholeness is the first step in the process of alchemical transformation.

THE PROBLEM OF ENTROPY

The central problem of the loss of Tao described by the ancient Chinese is related to the modern problem of entropy. The ancient Chinese were concerned with a break in reciprocity between human beings and the Tao and the subsequent deterioration of life. The modern scientist is concerned with the nature of energetic systems and the inevitable deterioration of their quality and potency.

The Law of Entropy is presented in the First and Second Laws of Thermodynamics, which assure us that while the energy in a system can never be lost, it will irreversibly degrade in quality and complexity as energetic processes occur in time.[9] The First Law states that the total amount of energy—comprised of any of its forms—cannot be destroyed. However, the Second Law qualifies the First by stating that while the quantity of energy in a closed system is conserved, the quality or energy value—the potency and vitality of the energy—will inevitably decrease. Another way of stating the Second Law is that the disorder, randomness and inefficiency of a closed system can never decrease with the passage of time or work. While quantity is conserved through the course of energetic processes, qualities such as potency, differentiation, order and complexity always degrade.

As systems move towards states of uniformity, the polarizing tension of discreet opposites is lost and the available functional energy decreases. So, after a taut spring discharges its force, the spring will lie inert unless recharged by a force outside the system. The electromagnetic energy that arises from the tension of opposite polarities will inevitably run down as positive and negative lose their polarization and merge. And the potency and vitality of the human organism will inevitably decrease with aging and the passage of time. While Taoist alchemists understood that the quality of energy systems has a tendency to degrade with the passage of time, they did not believe that degeneration is the inevitable end point of all organic and psychic processes. They knew that there were ways to conserve and nurture the quality of an organic system through the renewing effects of psychic and spiritual energies. But beyond this, alchemists believed that it was possible to promote change that resulted in the upgraded energy value of systems. They sought to discover ways to actually reverse entropy and to support change in time that resulted in states of being of higher value, complexity and potency. The specific goal of alchemical transformation was to resolve the paradox of how something whole can break down and shatter, endure its own destruction, and reorganize to form a more efficient and complex wholeness.

The capacity to at once shatter and sustain under the pressure of the tension of opposite polarities was the secret of alchemical transformation. Taoist alchemists referred to this secret in various ways, using symbolic language and poetic terminology. At the core of all these symbols and metaphorical descriptions was the understanding that alchemical transformation can only occur when there is a mingling of opposites, in particular the mingling of the negentropic energies of the upper spirits, the shen and hun, and the entropic energies of the lower spirits, the po and zhi, in the cauldron of matter. In psychological terms, this means that there is a conscious decision made to endure the energies of entropy, the energies of disintegration and decay—to sacrifice yang activity, to do nothing but wait—until a creative reversal, a new possibility, emerges spontaneously from the yin depths of the body and the unconscious.

This alchemical process can only occur in a container that is strong enough to withstand the powerful energies of its own shattering. Taoist alchemists found the prototype for this kind of special container in the female body, the womb that can be broken open by the stormy energies of the birthing process and yet maintain its own integrity. This is what Lao Tzu's describes as the "[e]ndlessly creating, endlessly pulsating . . . Spirit of the Valley,"[10] the hidden creator who never dies. But to the synthesizing, metaphorical mind of the alchemist, just as the heart is related to the emperor, to light and to spirit, the womb is related to the empress, to darkness and to matter. So all transformation must happen in the womb of the goddess, in the darkness of matter, in the underworld beneath the surface of the earth, in the deepest, most hidden places of the body and the unconscious.

TRANSFORMING WILL INTO WISDOM

A central principle of alchemy is that the yang contains a speck of yin and the yin contains a speck of yang. The yang speck hidden in the yin is the basis of the potency of the . It is a fiery spark that fuels her endless pulsating creativity, which never dies. This yang within yin is a magical negentropic potency that comes from down below, from the lower spirits. It is a high-grade energy that like uranium or oil is buried deep in the darkness of matter. At the moment of conception, every living being is endowed with a drop of this precious essence. The ancient Chinese called this high-grade energy *jing*.

Every human being comes into the world with his or her own maximum allotment of jing. We receive this jing from the essences of our two parents, but indirectly jing comes to us from earth, from the source of life, the Dark Goddess, the underworld deity known by the Taoists as Xi Wang Mu, the Queen Mother of the West. It is from the body of this Dark Goddess that the jing or juices of life flow.

Our jing is our instinctual will to live. It is the spark of our life force. It is the same vital energy that causes the seed to sprout, the leaf to unfurl, the flower to blossom. Jing endows us with the potency of our sexuality, the vitality of our reproductive organs. It is that most powerful drive, the will to be and manifest the self as it emerges from origin.

In the first stages of life, the jing is like a tightly coiled spring, full of potential energy and force. Like the coiled spring, the organic system as it emerges from the source is filled with potent vitality. It uses the jing to power its movement against entropy, upward towards the sunlit realms of the spirit, as it grows toward higher states of organization and complexity. It is the compressed jing of a rice kernel that causes the tiny first leaf to sprout or the dicotyledon to burst through the seed's hard casing and push upward through the dark soil toward the light.

But as ordinary organic systems reach the fullest, most complex expression of their natures, their jing begins to lose its potency. As the jing is depleted, the organism can no longer counteract the forces of entropy. Instead of the organic system continuing to move upward toward spirit and growth, its structure begins to deteriorate. Eventually the organism dies and returns to the underworld realm, where it disintegrates completely and can no longer be distinguished as an independent form. In mythological language, we would say that the organism has been torn apart and devoured by the Dark Goddess. It returns to a state of chaos and its dismembered parts lie in the belly of the Goddess, waiting to be digested, revitalized and reintegrated into the life cycle.

In natural, ordinary circumstances, the cycle is repetitive rather than transformational—it does not produce some completely new form. Under ordinary circumstances, depleted jing cannot be replaced, just as under ordinary circumstances we cannot turn back time. Organic systems come into life with their maximum allotment of jing, and the jing runs down as the organism moves from birth toward death. Taoist alchemists were passionate in their search for immortality, for ways to reverse entropy and replenish the value and potency of organic systems. They developed many esoteric practices that included breathing exercises, visualizations, meditation and the channeling and transmitting of sexual energies. They also experimented with herbs and acupuncture in an attempt to reinvigorate and upgrade the jing. The greatest sages, however, did not focus their efforts on renewing the potency of the jing with exercise, breath, or herbs but rather on transforming it internally as it degraded.

Taoist alchemists saw that under normal circumstances, energy value deteriorates from the high-grade vitality of youth, from infinite possibility and vast curiosity, to the low-grade sluggishness and rigidity of old age, to impotence, finite certainty and lack of curiosity. But they also saw that this process was not inevitable. Within the closed system of the human body, the process of entropy could be reversed. They discovered that they could actually use entropy, the energies of gravity, matter and the yin—the energies of stillness, receptivity and surrender—as a way to gain rather than deplete energy value. The secret of this alchemical reversal was to surrender the natural strivings of the will and to align one's life and one's actions with Tao. Just as a swimmer moves more quickly when she swims with the current rather than against it, alchemists found that they could gain potency by going with the tide of natural flow rather than trying to impose their individual will on the world around them. Two thousand years later, Friedrich Nietzsche came to the same realization when he discovered the redeeming power of *amor fati*: to love your fate rather than wasting energy raging against it.

Taoist sages saw that, paradoxically, the more they followed the way of the receptive yin, the more they surrendered the potent yang striving of their will to the infinitely more potent will of Tao, the more vitality, spontaneity, compassion and joy they attained. As they surrendered their limited personal will to the greater will of the divine, their capacity to do, to be, to illuminate and to manifest increased rather than decreased as they aged. In the life of the sage, energy value increased as will transformed to an even more potent substance called wisdom. Thus, "though seeming old, they were beyond the reach of birth and death."[11]

FIGURE 2: ALCHEMICAL TRANSFORMATION OF JING FROM WILL INTO WISDOM

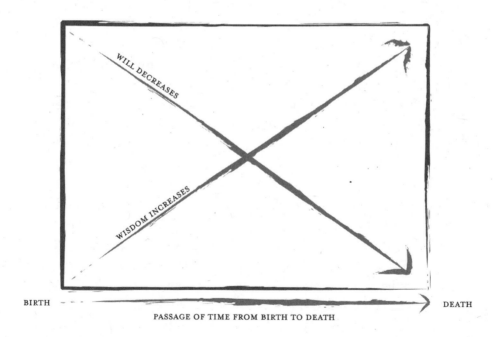

CHILD— ORIGIN

SAGE— RETURN TO ORIGIN

How the Giant Pan Gu Created the Universe

The problem of the loss of Tao and the recovery of wholeness through the creative use of fragmentation and disintegration is told in the Chinese creation myth of Pan Gu. This story defines the elements and stages of transformation, whether on a physical, psychological or cosmic level.

According to the story, the universe was once a swirling mass of chaos encased in a huge egg. At the center of the egg, sleeping and growing for eighteen thousand years, was the giant Pan Gu. When at last the egg became too small for him, the giant became uncomfortable. He needed room to move. He raged and flailed, ranted and raved until his hand came upon a huge axe.

Pan Gu grabbed the axe and swung it wildly from side to side until suddenly, with a huge crash, the egg cracked open. Then, all that was light rose up to form the heavens and all that was heavy dropped down to form the earth. And since Pan Gu did not want heaven and earth to close up again around him, he stood up to support the heavens with his head and to hold down the earth with his feet. He held up the heavens and held down the earth for eighteen thousand years until they were finally fixed in place. Then he lay down to die.

As Pan Gu was dying, his body began to shift, to sink and to rise until it became the parts of the earth we live on. His breath became the winds and the clouds, and his voice became the thunder. His left eye became the sun, his right eye the moon. His legs became the mountains, his blood the rivers, and his muscles the rich soil. Pan Gu's hair turned into pearls, and his teeth became the precious gems beneath the ground. His sweat and tears became the rain and mists that moisten the fields. And after all this, the human race was born from the tiny insects that crawled on Pan Gu's body and the lice that swarmed in his hair.

The Myth of Creation and the Alchemical Healing Process

The legend of Pan Gu can be interpreted in many ways. Like any myth, it exists outside of ordinary space and time and so can be used to help us understand the ancient past as well as the present and the future. This myth describes not only the creation of the cosmos but also the evolution of human consciousness and the development of a human being from embryonic beginning to death.

The elements of this story apply universally whenever creative and transformative processes are activated. For this reason, it can be used as a template for the transformational healing process, the process through which a particular way of being, a psychological state or energetic system, dissolves and reorganizes in a new energetic system of higher quality and complexity. While every individual transformation is different, there are certain steps and stages that are necessary and universal. The stages may backtrack and overlap,

FIGURE 3: THE PROCESS OF TRANSFORMATION

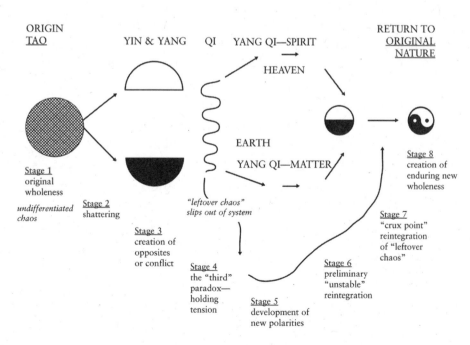

but ultimately transformational healing follows the same pattern as the process of creation outlined in the myth. See figure 3 for a graphic description of the process of transformation.

The Chinese character *pan* means "vessel, tray, or disk." The character *gu* means "ancient, original." So the giant Pan Gu represents the original alchemical vessel. But a tray or disk is also round, and roundness in mythological language means unbroken wholeness. So Pan Gu also represents our original wholeness, our identity with Tao. He is the beginning and the end, the fullness and the emptiness, the contained and the container.

The transformation process begins when this original wholeness becomes self-aware and two parts, a self and another, are created from one. The initiating spark for the transformation process is the spark of consciousness, implicit at origin but not activated until the wholeness becomes self-aware through the experience of discomfort or suffering. Through the ignition of self-awareness, the original wholeness shatters into parts and movement begins. In the myth, the giant's awareness that his "egg has become too small" is the beginning of his transformation.

The possibility of self-awareness is a seed that lies dormant in every human being. It is the conscious spirit or shen, the tiny spark discussed in the previous chapter, that has the power to ignite the alchemical fire of transformation. The ignition of consciousness is symbolically represented by Pan Gu's discovery of the axe. The axe, like consciousness, gives the giant the capacity to cut the world into pieces. As we see in the myth, once the spark of self-awareness ignites, transformation can begin. But this is only the first step in a long and difficult process.

The separation of wholeness into opposites—in the myth, "the rising of the light and the descent of the heavy"—is felt as a conflict. This stage is the equivalent of the biblical fall, the loss of the paradise of unified, unconscious bliss. It also represents the emergence of the law of entropy in the universe, the tendency for the energy of orderly systems to degrade back towards chaos. Entropy is introduced symbolically in the myth by the danger of heaven and Earth collapsing and once again enveloping Pan Gu. In the healing process, it shows up in our regressive wishes to "just get back to the way things used to be," to take the easy way out, or to compulsively act out or fall into a frozen state of depression.

Not giving in to the forces of entropy, not collapsing or rushing into premature action, marks the third stage of the process. Like Pan Gu, at this stage, we must "bear the weight" of the creative process until a new set of polarized opposites can form.

This third stage paves the way for the fourth, in which the new polarization crystallizes and the structure of Pan Gu's body dissolves to create a new wholeness or "cosmos." In the healing process, it is the time when a person is strong enough to let go of old behaviors and attitudes so that new possibilities can emerge.

But between the third and fourth stages, a crucial event occurs. At the moment of his dissolution, Pan Gu must make a choice. When the forces of entropy finally overtake him, Pan Gu could either choose to return to the bliss of primal chaos or sacrifice his own being so that some new organization of higher complexity can come to life. Pan Gu, like an alchemist, gave himself up to the process of transformation. His body was dismembered and the parts were used to create a new pattern. Every single part of Pan Gu's body was used to form a new, more complex order.

The Leftover Chaos

Once the world was created, there was a new problem. After Pan Gu's body dissolved and reformed, the order and disorder that had been perfectly blended in the original chaos of Pan Gu's egg was not restored. When the new cosmos formed from the parts of Pan Gu's disintegrating body, a bit of extra chaos was left over. In the myth, this leftover chaos is represented by the insects and lice that crawl on the giant's body. The insects are, and yet are not, part of the wholeness.

The leftover chaos that hangs around as the by-product of creative processes is like the sludge that accumulates at the bottom of an engine or the dregs at the bottom of the soup pot that no one wants to eat. In the story of the Zen cook, or tenzo, the leftover chaos takes the form of a tiny roach that falls into the soup pot that the head monk or *sensei* deliberately places in his bowl. The Zen master understands that even this part of the soup is necessary. Unless it is somehow dealt with, the sludge will eventually muck up the engine and the roach will spoil the soup.

In practice, the dregs are the irritating symptoms we want to get rid of. They are the personality traits and negative emotions we do not want to face. They are the bugs in the system, the things that wake us up at night, alerting us to the fact that the healing process is not complete. From this vantage point, our obsessions, desires, instinctual cravings, pet peeves and fantasies are the precious raw material of personal transformation! Chronic pain, itches, depression, tics, gas, eczema, tightness around the left shoulder blade . . . when viewed as manifestations of disorder that have been left out of the dynamic equation of a person's life, these irritating symptoms begin to reveal themselves as valuable.

The myth tells us that the return to Tao or final healing cannot take place until this leftover chaos is somehow integrated. And the myth reminds us in no uncertain terms that this leftover chaos is a particularly human problem that only human beings can resolve. In fact, it is the very stuff that we are made of.

To the Taoist alchemists, the chaotic dregs left over after the creation of the cosmos were a divine legacy that came directly to human beings from the unfathomable perfect chaos of Tao. So, to the Taoist alchemist, the leftover chaos is the most precious substance of all. It is the treasure in the trash, the precious junk that fools pass by without noticing on the street. The annoying, seemingly meaningless bugs, dust balls and sludge piles of life are, in fact, the secret treasure of the alchemist. The leftover chaos is the *prima materia*, the stuff of transformation. Through the magical reversal of alchemy, this leftover chaos is not a problem but rather our most valuable treasures. It is the fabled lead the alchemist transforms into gold.

AN ALCHEMICAL VIEW OF THE PSYCHE

Although the ancient Greeks used the word *psyche* to refer to the soul, today it most often refers specifically to the mental as distinct from the physical aspects of a human being. Webster's defines "psyche" as the "spiritual being as distinct from the body," also "the mind, the mental life of an individual comprising intellect, emotion and the activities and predispositions of the self." The dualism of rational thought has divorced the psyche and its energies from the body, and the psyche or soul has been reduced to an abstraction that, in modern Western culture, has very little real significance.

One of the notable exceptions to this practice of abstracting psychic energy is found in the work of C. G. Jung, who spent most of his adult lifetime exploring the nature of psychological experience. Much of his work took him into the realms of spiritual and mystical phenomena, and rather than approaching the psyche as an abstraction, he regarded it as a very real energetic system that could be studied and analyzed.

In his writing, Jung described the psyche as a bipolar spectrum of energy that extends from a red instinctual pole to a violet or spiritual pole. Toward the middle range of the spectrum, psychic phenomenon enters the realm of human life. But at both ends, individual psychic energy dissolves into transpersonal realms where it becomes inaccessible to ordinary consciousness. At the red, instinctual side of the middle range, the psyche is experienced physiologically through body symptoms, instinctual impulses, perceptions and desires. At the violet, spiritual side of the middle range, the psyche is experienced psychologically as ideas, dreams, images and fantasies.

Jung's view of the psyche comes very close to the Taoist alchemical system of the Five Spirits, which provides us with a symbolic map of the psyche that extends, like Jung's spectrum model, from material to spiritual—or, in Taoist terminology, from earth to heaven. At the yin, vital, instinctual pole, the lower spirits represent the autonomic nervous system, primitive brain and lower spine as well as the reproductive, digestive and basic survival functions. At the yang, psychic, spiritual pole, the upper spirits represent the frontal lobe and cerebral cortex as well as the thinking, planning and visioning functions of the mind and imagination. From a Taoist alchemical perspective, the upper and lower spirits, the yin and yang aspects of this system, must be in balance and communication. Their separation, disharmony and lack of communication lead to pathology and ultimately to death.

Both the Jungian and alchemical systems emphasize that the psyche is not an abstraction, not simply a mental and spiritual idea but a polarized energetic system that is grounded in the matrix of physical being. The vitality of the system is dependent on its bipolarity and the free flow of energy between the poles. When an excess of psychic energy accumulates at one end of the system, the other end becomes depleted and eventually manifests its depletion negatively in the form of disease—psychological symptoms on the psychic end or somatic symptoms on the vital end.

From an alchemical perspective, in order for healing to occur, it is not enough to simply focus on the end of the spectrum where the symptom is manifesting. Increasing order at one end will only increase disorder at the other. So, for example, focusing only on the psychological aspect of a problem, analyzing it intellectually or talking about its causes, may increase order at the mental end, but it will usually not result in a change at the level of the body, at the level of behavior, desire, or physical symptoms. Conversely, focusing only on the body may temporarily relieve a symptom but will not result in change at the level of insight or cognitive understanding. As order increases at one end, the real, transformational energy—the true gold—is found in the disorder at the other end of the spectrum. Work that happens at only one side of the spectrum usually leads to a dead end. There may be restoration or temporary change, but there can be no real transformation, no new possibility, unless there is a reintegration of opposites. In order for change to occur, a connection must be made between the two poles—or, in Taoist terms, there must be a marriage of the upper and lower spirits.

The following case studies explore the difference between the restorative and alchemical approaches. Both forms of treatment have their merits and usefulness, but they are not interchangeable. When a physical problem is complex and rooted in emotional or psychological issues, or when a psychological problem is long-standing and has taken hold at the level of muscle armor and autonomic nervous responses, then a deeper, alchemical approach is needed. In these cases, restorative treatment will usually produce unsatisfactory results for both practitioner and patient.

Two Approaches to Acupuncture

The Restorative Approach

As currently practiced, many of the theories and techniques of acupuncture and Chinese medicine are restorative. From this perspective illness is viewed as a problem to be gotten rid of rather than a treasure to be consciously worked with. In restorative acupuncture, the practitioner's job is to detoxify pathogenic factors, to rebalance yin and yang, to tonify deficiencies and reduce excesses. This allows the flow of the energies of the patient's body to resynchronize with Tao and retores the natural flow of organic rhythms and cycles.

When I practice this form of acupuncture, I feel that I am a magician. I take on the role of the "organizing principle" of a chaotic cosmos. The needle is a magical tool that I use to restore harmony and balance to the patient's organic processes. No conscious participation or even any cognitive understanding is necessary on the part of the patient. The process unfolds like a ritual. . . .

I stand beside the treatment table, a hair-thin, shining needle poised between my fingers.

"Take a breath," I say to the patient on the table.

I watch as he inhales, the palace of his rib cage expanding to receive more air.

I center myself. Feet planted firmly on the floor. Neck and back relaxed. Every nerve attuned to the faint vibrations of qi. I empty my mind and focus my attention on this moment. I invite the energies of earth and sky to flow freely through my body.

The tips of my fingers begin to tingle. I palpate the point. I feel its magnetism drawing down the needle.

I stand still. I do nothing. I become a conduit for the qi. I feel the needle vibrate with energy as a pathway clears between my patient and myself. I prepare for the moment when the needle between my fingers will break the boundary of his skin, penetrating the interface between spirit and matter.

"And breathe out," I say.

My patient exhales. The needle, like a silver bird, dives below the surface of his body. I feel the familiar tug of the qi on the needle, like the tug of a fish on a fishing line. He grimaces, then laughs. His face floods with color.

"You got it," he says. "I felt that all the way down to my feet."

I pick up his wrist and place my fingers lightly above his radial artery in order to take his pulses. Pulse taking plays a crucial role in Chinese medical diagnosis, and after many years of practice, I am now able to read the pulses in order to diagnose pathology as well as to determine whether or not a treatment has been successful.

From my patient's pulses, I can tell that the point I have just needled has had the desired effect of rebalancing his qi and releasing his abdominal muscles.[12]

"It's starting to ease up now," he says. "Yeah, it's already much better." He continues to relax. His breathing softens.

With that, he closes his eyes. A moment later, he is sound asleep, the healing qi coursing through his body.

Studies have shown that acupuncture treatment results in shifts in the body's biochemistry. In particular, cerebrospinal fluid levels of enkephalins and endorphins, the body's natural opiates, rise during and after treatment. In my clinical experience, most patients report feelings of deep relaxation and mild euphoria after acupuncture. More than half fall asleep or drift into a relaxed meditational state after treatment, which I believe is extremely beneficial and actually functions as part of the healing process, allowing body chemistry to reset, brain and neurological impulses to reorganize. This kind of acupuncture is a powerful tool in the healing of physical level problems. It also has effects on a psychological level, as it often restores balance and tranquility to the emotions. When acupuncture is practiced this way, its results are often very good, but they rarely last long.

The problem with the restorative approach is that human beings have strayed way too far from the cycles of cosmic energies to be able to permanently sustain the effects of restorative acupuncture. The return to a state of primal unity with the rhythms of the natural world lasts for a brief time but quickly recedes under the barrage of tensions and disharmonies of modern life. Unless the effects of treatment penetrate to the deepest layers of the nervous system and effect change at that level of behavior and character, the organism surrenders to the forces of entropy and returns to its habitual state of imbalance. Then the original symptoms quickly return or are replaced by others.

The Alchemical Approach

When we approach physical and emotional distress not only as a symptom of a loss of integrity but also as a kind of chaos that can be used to create a new kind of wholeness, then we open to the possibility of a more long-lasting and alchemical kind of healing. I have found that this kind of healing is much more challenging than healing that is restorative or compensatory. It requires a willingness of the patient to engage in the healing process, to face the unknown and to consciously endure painful states of being. It also requires a willingness of the practitioner to be in a relationship with the patient that goes beyond the hierarchical relationship of doctor or magician. The patient and practitioner work together to build a bridge between the body and the mind, the vital energies of the body and the psychological energies of the soul.

Let's return to the restorative treatment example described above and see how it would look from an alchemical orientation.

"And breathe out, I say.

My patient exhales. The needle, like a silver bird, dives below the surface of his body. I feel the familiar tug of the qi on the needle, like the tug of a fish on a fishing line. He grimaces, then laughs. His face floods with color.

"You got it," he says. "I felt that all the way down to my feet."

I pick up his wrist and place my fingers lightly above his radial artery in order to take his pulses.

"It's starting to ease up now," he says. "Yeah, it's already much better." He continues to relax. His breathing softens. His eyes close.

As his body relaxes, rather than stepping away and letting him drift off into sleep, I ignite the alchemical process by using a technique from Five Element Acupuncture known as the Spirit of the Point. Here I use the information and poetry that is embedded in the name of every acupuncture point to deepen the treatment.

I begin by telling him the name of the point. "Zhong Wan—Middle Hollow," I say.

I pause for a moment. In the silence that follows, the healing power embedded in the name of the point begins to work. He's alert, listening in an easy, relaxed way. I see he's digesting the point, taking in the name, letting the words combine with the sensation of the needle in his stomach so that they become part of his inner experience.

"Middle Hollow. This point is related to the earth element. It's on the Stomach Meridian. It's in the center of the solar plexus, the power center. It's all about the center, the stomach. You always say that's where your problems tend to show up."

"Hmmm . . ." I see he's traveling around inside his body, checking his body sensation for connections to this point that is gradually becoming his own special point. Then, he opens his eyes and looks at me.

"That's just the spot where the knot is. I always feel it in my stomach. Like a rock, a frozen block of ice, always there, always telling me to do more, do more. It's never enough. It's all on me. I'm the center of the family, the center at work. Then the indigestion starts and I feel lousy."

I see by the light of recognition in his eyes that his upper spirits are engaged in the process. He's thinking about the feelings and connecting them to images. But I also know he tends to go off into his head, to leave his body when he gets wrapped up in ideas so, I invite him to bring the spirits down to the level of physical sensation.

"So maybe just take a minute to be with that," I say. "What's it like to just be with the knot, right where that needle is? Take a breath in there and see if you can get a look at it."

He takes a breath. He closes his eyes again and his breathing becomes more even. There is a silence and I am not sure if he has fallen asleep. I just stand there and do nothing. I trust that the needle is continuing to affect his nervous system.

A few moments later, he opens his eyes again. "The truth is, I can't do it all," he says. "I have to let some of it go."

He takes a long, deep breath. I see the tension in his jaw relax as his psychological insight combines with the movement of qi to affect a small transformation at the level of the spirits.

"I like that," he says. "I like the idea of letting it go." And then he adds,

"This needle is really working. I actually can feel the ice starting to melt." He closes his eyes. A moment later, he is sound asleep, the healing power of qi coursing through his body.

This is a simple example of how an alchemical approach that connects mental and physical experience can help a person heal on multiple levels. Unlike Western psychotherapy, where the therapist might delve into the question of why this patient manifested his feelings of hyper-responsibility through his digestive problems, focusing on past history and parental insufficiencies, Chinese medicine focuses on the immediate moment, the climate of this person's life right now and how it may be out of rhythm with Tao. Rather than offering personal support or sympathy for his early suffering, the symbols and concepts of Chinese medical theory give the patient a way to find a path that might work better for him now.

The language and ideas of Chinese medicine are rooted in mythical consciousness and can be intentionally used to create healing images and symbols in the imagination. This supports a person in bringing the mind and imagination—the fiery energies of the yang upper spirits—down into the alchemical cauldron of the body where they can mingle with the watery essences of the lower spirits—the energies of the nervous system, muscle tissue and instincts. In this way an alchemical transformation can occur, an insight or "Aha!" that leads to an upgrade in a person's way of being. Through this descent of spirit into matter, a truly new possibility emerges and one begins to see one's life differently.

When I practice this kind of Alchemical Acupuncture, I think of the altered state induced by the acupuncture needle not only as a respite for the patient from the stresses of life but as a way to open the door to deeper layers of the nervous system, the imagination and the body unconscious. I support the patient so the relaxation of the body initiates a descent into mythical consciousness. As the nervous system reorganizes, the thinking mind recedes to the background and body awareness becomes more acute.

At this "in between" moment, as the shock of the needle dissolves rigid holding patterns that have been embedded in the muscles and nervous system, an image or a symbol (in this case, the name of the point) can be used as a kind of organizing principle, a tiny grain of sand, around which the pearl of a new possibility can form. The subtle shifts of sensation and nervous responses that occur as a result of the needle are leftover chaos that can be reorganized and fixed into the matrix of the psyche through the use of the images and metaphors of Taoist alchemy.

The needle produces a shock to the system that is the first stage of transformation, the moment when the egg is cracked by self-awareness. Like lightning the needle initiates a process of change that includes both shattering and reorganization. If both patient and practitioner are able to withstand the powerful energies unleashed during the process, the end result is transformational. Even in the simple case described above, we see that reinforcing the systemic shock of the needle with imagery and conscious insight can bring about the creation of a new possibility, a new organization of higher quality, efficiency and complexity.

In Chinese medicine, the basic law of free flow holds true on every level of the being, the physical as well as the psychological. When the qi in the area of a block becomes congested and stagnant, the qi in other areas becomes undercharged. This situation results in physical pain, illness, emotional upsets and psychospiritual distress. The basic technique of the restorative approach involves locating the block and releasing the stuck qi so that the system can be restored to its former organization, the life force can once again flow freely, and the person can return to the full expression of his or her original nature. In the example, I was able to release the qi stuck in my patient's abdomen by needling an acupuncture point on the Stomach Meridian that was related to digestive function. Unless my patient's relationship to his inner and outer life changed, however, the forces of entropy will almost certainly result in the dissolution of this new order. Most likely, he will return to his old pattern of overworking and holding stress in his abdominal muscles. Sooner or later the qi will once again become blocked. The treatment will have to be repeated and nothing essentially new will have come to life.

But when I approach the case from an alchemical perspective, I view my patient's stuck qi as an indispensable component of the transformation process, the lead without which there can be no gold. The pain, malaise, discontent, chronic indigestion and depression that arise from the patient's block are the base material out of which something new and precious can be made. In this case, unblocking on a vital or lower spirit level at the point of stuck tightness in the belly, released qi that was gathered up by the psyche and incorporated into a conscious insight. The stuck abdominal tension was the "lead," the primary material to be used in the work of transformation. Rather than simply needling the qi and releasing it back into the life cycle, I supported my patient in treasuring the stuck qi and working with it in various ways. The goal in this kind of treatment is to use the needle to dissolve the qi, which is stuck at the physical level. As order and efficiency is restored at the level of the vital energies of the autonomic nervous system, the disorder at the level of the cerebral energies of the psyche becomes apparent.

The tendency at this point is for the patient to drift off to sleep while the nervous system reorganizes. However, if we encourage a patient to stay aware of the reorganizing process, it is possible to work with the new disorder and use it to create a new, more enduring integrity. In this way, when the system reorganizes it forms a new, more stable wholeness that is far less likely to deteriorate.

These dark areas or blockages of qi coagulate in the tissues of the body as chronic pain, lumps and tumors. They accumulate in the psyche as obsessions and depression and can be seen in regressive, repetitive behavior patterns that do not support the arising of life. In the ancient alchemical text *The Secret of the Golden Flower*, Master Lu Tung Ping describes this place as the abysmal, the "place where the sun sinks into the Great Water . . . when the thunder [the creative force] is in the middle of the Earth quite hidden and covered up."[13]

In Taoist alchemical texts, work at the level of the stuck qi was spoken of as a crucial stage of the process of transformation. It is the hard, boring, seemingly meaningless work, the surrendering of the will and the enduring of uncertainty, that precedes and precipitates the *weiji* or crux point—the moment of the spontaneous "Aha!" when the split realms of body and spirit reorganize to form a new integrity.

ACUPUNCTURE AS AN ALCHEMICAL ART

The goal of alchemy is transformation, change that results in an increase, a reinvigoration, or a rebirth. The alchemist's ultimate quest is the transformation of a human being from an ordinary person into a spiritually enlightened or "illuminated" sage. The goal of Alchemical Acupuncture is to facilitate this kind of transformation through the healing process.

After twenty years of working with Taoist alchemical principles and inserting acupuncture needles into the human body, I am convinced that acupuncture *is* an alchemical art and that it has the capacity to reverse entropy. Sometimes this reversal is so slight and short-lived that it is barely noticeable beyond a brief surge of energy or relaxation of muscle tension. But in other cases, if the patient is committed and willing to withstand the challenges of an authentic transformational process and the acupuncturist is willing to work at an alchemical level, the reversal of the forces of entropy results in a permanent upgrade in the organization of a patient's being. In these cases, acupuncture supports psychospiritual changes that alter the course of a person's life and destiny.

As an acupuncturist, I have seen vitality return to devitalized patients through the insertion of the acupuncture needle. I have seen qi stuck in the physical body in the form of chronic pain or stagnation dissolve into freely moving, vitalizing emotion. And I have watched as destructive behavior patterns shatter and transform into the pure light of spiritual insight and wisdom. The energy that has fueled these transformational processes has come not from outside the patient but from within. No medicine or electro-stimulation has been injected or added to the closed system of the patient's bodymind, yet vitality, potency, curiosity, animation and wisdom have increased.

Through my years of observing patients in the treatment room, I have come to believe that the energy that fuels this seemingly miraculous reversal of entropy results from acupuncture's ability to re-polarize yin and yang energies of the qi, specifically the energies of the upper and lower spirits. Through this repolarization, the qi oscillates more quickly and intensely between the realms of psyche and body, spirit and matter. As entropy and negentropy increase at opposite poles, the overall tension of the system also increases and vitality is restored to the body and the mind. If a patient stays with the process long enough, the new organization of the qi can be fixed at the level of the spirits or autonomic nervous system and permanent transformational upgrades can occur.

Western scientists have attempted to explain this phenomenon by saying that acupuncture affects the electromagnetic field of the body. But to me, this attempt to study one system using the logic of another is counterproductive. Studies and tests have successfully proved that acupuncture works by measuring its effects. However, so far there have been no Western scientific theories, tests, or experiments that have successfully explained how it works. I believe that Western tests have been unable to prove the validity of the electromagnetic theory, the Gate Theory,[14] or any other modern scientific explanation because acupuncture is alchemical. Its logic is mythical. It works in a non-linear realm that exists between matter and spirit, at the level of the subtle body. The energies that are activated by the acupuncture needle cannot be quantitatively measured because they exist in a dimension that transcends the temporal, spatial and causal limitations of Western science. Yet they can be qualitatively experienced as real changes that can be seen and felt in the patient's body, emotions, spirit and daily life.

The physiological system that most closely correlates to the terrain of the acupuncture meridians is the nervous system, but the nervous system alone is not enough. It is only when we restore the autonomously animating energies of the divine to the fleshy structures that sustain organic processes that we begin to get a picture of the territory where acupuncture happens. This mysterious realm of alchemical transformation is what we in the West describe as the soul.

Tan: A Look at the Chinese Character

The Chinese character for "alchemy" is *tan*, the same character used to refer to cinnabar, the prized mineral of Taoist alchemists as well as the color red. *Tan* is sometimes said to represent a fragment of red cinnabar buried in an underground mine. Other interpretations of the character describe the speck of cinnabar as enclosed in a crucible or alchemical cooking vessel.

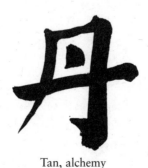

Tan, alchemy

Cinnabar has a long and complex history in Taoist alchemy and Chinese medicine. In *waidan*, or outer alchemy, the primary concern was the decomposing and recomposing of this bright red mineral to form medicines, tinctures, pigments, works of art and jewelry. In *neidan*, or inner alchemy, the focus was on the inner nature of cinnabar and its parallels to the inner nature of human beings and the cosmos.

The mineral cinnabar, or mercuric sulfide, is formed when mercury and sulfur combine. In alchemical tradition the world over, these two substances are considered indispensable, regarded as the ultimate expression of yin and yang, the masculine and feminine principles. Cinnabar represents the alchemical marriage, the *coniunctio*, the recombining of the masculine and feminine to create new life.

Mercury exemplifies the yin, with its watery, cold disposition. But mercury's silvery, quick and ever-shifting nature is also related to the yang male sexual fluids as well as to pure, unfettered consciousness. So mercury personifies the yin aspect of the yang that is central to sexuality and reproduction.

Sulfur, on the other hand, embodies the hot, dry, combustible qualities of yang. But sulfur's crimson, dense, opaque, inert quality is also related to the yin feminine menstrual blood and the heavy flesh of the body. Sulfur is related not only to the uterine blood and the ovum but also to pure matter. So sulfur personifies the yang within the yin that is central to sexuality and reproduction.

CINNABAR AS A MEDICINAL HERB

Cinnabar is paradoxical. Although it is poisonous, it can also heal, so cinnabar has been used for centuries in small quantities as a crucial medicinal. It is said that cinnabar sedates the heart, calms the spirit and reorders a scattered and fragmented psyche. Anxiety, insomnia, fright, obsessions and disturbing dreams are all symptoms that were said to indicate the need for cinnabar.

Due to its toxicity, cinnabar is no longer used in modern Chinese herbal preparations, but traditionally powdered cinnabar coated the classic formula for insomnia, the Emperor of Heaven's Special Pill to Tonify the Heart. It is also one of the chief ingredients in Cinnabar Pill to Calm the Spirit and Magnetite and Cinnabar Pill, both of which were used to help patients heal after sudden, terrifying experiences, shock, anxiety, phobias and uncontrolled emotion.

The Cinnabar Field

Cinnabar is found hidden deep beneath the earth. Its color is red, the color of the fire that burns in the darkness of the planet's core. In the metaphorical thinking of Taoist alchemy, the creative fire of sexuality and the transformative heat of the digestive processes are the bodily equivalent to the fire at the core of the Earth. In the metaphorical thought of the ancient Chinese, the human body is a microcosmic reflection of the planet. The part of the abdomen below the umbilicus, where this life fire burns, is the anatomical equivalent to the planet's core. It is the lowest of the three cauldrons or what Chinese healers call the "alchemical burning spaces" of the body. This lower part of the abdomen is referred to in Chinese medicine as the *tantian,* which literally means "cinnabar field."

The tantian is considered a furnace that empowers alchemical transformation, the power center of the body. It is the place from which Chinese martial artists move and the area where the awareness is focused in Taoist, Chan and Zen Buddhist meditation. The emptiness of the lower cauldron makes it useful because it is a space for the transformative fires of the spirits to burn.

Besides symbolizing the fire of the tantian, cinnabar symbolized the potent energy that is stored in matter. This "lower fire"—the power of the lower spirits—is the polar opposite and partner of the fire of the upper spirits that comes to us from heaven. While the fire of the upper spirits is initiatory and inspiring, the lower fire is the fire of potency. It is the power to do and to manifest as opposed to the initiatory spark or inspiring breath of the yang.

In alchemical terms, when we reach the farthest end of one polarization, there is a reversal. European alchemists referred to this as the *enantiodromia*. It is the compensatory function found in biological and psychic processes whereby some energetic event taken to its furthest extreme will spontaneously produce its opposite. Taoist alchemists recognized this compensatory function in every aspect of the cosmos. They made it the centerpiece of their philosophy, symbolized by the taiji, the graphic depiction of the swirling currents of yin and yang that, through the tension of their opposite polarities, create the vibrating field of life.

So, although the earth is associated with yin, with coldness, darkness and stillness, at its core we find the yang. The speck of fiery spirit in matter and the speck of dark matter in spirit are mysteries that fuel the engine of the eternal round, the dance of endless transformation. Without this speck of very special matter, the fire of spirit would have nothing to burn. And without its speck of special fire, the yin waters could not produce life.

Two Case Studies

In order to further clarify the differences between the restorative and transformational approach to acupuncture and to show how each is useful and appropriate in different situations, I offer two examples from my practice. Both cases involve the problem of adolescent menstrual irregularity yet needed to be approached quite differently. The first case required simply a realignment of qi in order for the patient to return to a basically stable wholeness. But in the

second case, the patient had no stable wholeness to return to. I needed to support her in assembling some kind of wholeness from the
shattered parts of her body awareness and the split-off chaos of her
repressed feeling for life. I do not believe that this second case would
have resolved without a deep working through of the chaotic emotions that were unleashed as the needles liberated the stuck qi in this
young woman's body.

Case I: Back on the Path

The first patient was a young woman whose period had begun when
she was thirteen. Her cycles had been increasingly irregular, and at
age seventeen the period stopped completely for five months. When
she came for treatment, her complexion was pale but her eyes were
lively and curious. She displayed an appealing adolescent shyness
combined with a dash of surliness and a healthy skepticism about
Chinese medicine. She asked quite a few questions about acupuncture and then agreed to tell me about her problem.

Among other things, she told me that she had become a vegetarian two years earlier because of her love for animals and a strong
commitment to animal rights. In addition to her menstrual irregularity, she complained of fatigue, lack of appetite and difficulty falling
asleep at night.

From a Five Element perspective, the element that was most
imbalanced was Earth. In addition, the Wood element was weak and
needed support. From a traditional Chinese medical perspective, her
menstrual irregularity was due to blood deficiency. I focused treatment on Spleen and Penetrating Vessel points and added direct moxa
treatment to Bladder 17 and Bladder 38 in order to build the blood.
We discussed her diet and she agreed to add a small amount of fish
to her vegetarian meals. I also suggested that she get in bed before
11:00 p.m. ("Wood" time). She was able to implement this earlier
bedtime program on weeknights and her sleep cycles improved. Her
period returned after three visits, and the menses settled into a rea-

sonably regular pattern after that. The patient came for a total of five sessions.

The last I heard from her, her periods were regular. She is currently majoring in physics at university, is an animal rights activist and works part time as a car mechanic. In the case of this young woman's treatment, there was no need to reintegrate the shattered parts of her being. Her problem was basically physical. Acupuncture, moxa,[15] dietary modifications, support and reassurance were enough to set things right, to restore the Tao and allow her to continue on with a unique and fulfilling young womanhood.

Case II: The Stone Gate

The second case was a nineteen-year-old woman, recently married, whose periods had stopped abruptly one year earlier. She was part of a very strict religious sect and was expected to become pregnant soon after marrying. Her mother made the initial appointment and came to see me first to discuss her daughter's problem. She told me that the whole family was desperate. They had yet to reveal the situation to the young woman's husband for fear that he would move to annul the marriage.

When the young woman arrived for treatment, her face was swollen, pale and puffy. She stared at the floor throughout the interview and answered my questions in monosyllables. On a physical level, this woman's symptoms included abdominal pain and extremely cold feet, hands and abdomen. Her belly was so tight she could hardly tolerate even light palpation. I diagnosed her as a Water causative factor and surmised that her amenorrhea was due to Cold in the Uterus. I felt that her problem was deeply rooted at the soul level and that she would not get better unless this level was addressed.

Our work proceeded very slowly. For the first few weeks, even the gentlest needling produced sensations of excruciating pain. Half the session was sometimes spent talking her through her terror and her resistance to the needles. She said that the taste of herbs I gave her was unbearable and she took them sporadically.

I found that moxa sticks on her abdomen relaxed her, as did rice grain moxa on Kidney 2 and 3 and Heart 7. After two months, there was no sign of change in her cycles but she had begun to be able to make eye contact with me. Gradually she started to talk about her feelings and to express her terror, rage and despair. For several weeks, she sobbed through the sessions and then became angry at me for making her feel these feelings when it "wouldn't do any good." After she saw that I was not upset by her strong feelings and anger, she began to trust me more.

In this woman's treatments, I combined work on a physical level with very deep soul level treatment. Her uterus was cold not only on a physical level but on an emotional and soul level as well. When I touched her abdomen, I got an image of something stuck there. I used moxa, gentle supportive touch and conversation to get things moving. Eventually she began to reveal some of her marital difficulties including her confusion and terror of physical intimacy. A pivotal moment came when I decided to use a point called Stone Gate. I applied moxa to this point and spoke to her about the image of the Stone. I suggested that she imagine softening the stone in her abdomen by breathing into it as I warmed the area with a moxa stick. For the first time, she agreed to "try breathing." This brought about a strong release of emotion. At the end of the session, her cheeks were rosy and she thanked me for my help. That week she was able to begin to talk to her husband about her problems.

I worked with this woman almost weekly for over seven months. At the end of that time, her periods had still not returned to normal. However, she looked different. Her cheeks had color and she was able to look at me when we talked. She was also communicating more freely with her husband and beginning to relax with him physically.

At this point, she decided to take a break from acupuncture. After conversation with her doctor and her husband, she decided to wait another month or two before inducing a bleed with hormones. Several weeks later, she called to tell me that she had gotten her period without medical intervention.

In some situations, it is not necessary to address a patient's problem from a transformational perspective. When a person's outlook on life, situation and behavior can "contain" them, energetic balancing with acupuncture and herbs may be sufficient to restore the Tao. When the container of a person's life is too small, does not fit, or is completely shattered, however, it is necessary to enter the terrain of alchemical healing. Although a rational, deductive approach to diagnosis and treatment planning is still important, this level of work also requires that the practitioner have the ability to organize treatment strategies according to mythical logic and to open to the nonlinear cognitive modes of intuition, instinct and emotional responsiveness.

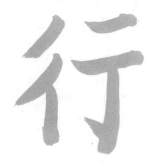

Chapter Three

The Axle and the Wheel:
The Five Elements and the Five Spirits

A t dawn, the sage stood at the edge of the road and watched the farmers as they headed toward the market. He watched as the carts passed, one after another, laden with fresh vegetables and rice. The farmers waved and offered him rides but the sage simply stood with his hands clasped behind his back and stared intently at the turning wheels.

When the sun had risen well over the horizon and the last cart had rumbled past, Lao Tzu turned and walked back up the mountain. When he got to his hut, he made himself green tea and poured it slowly into a cup. He pondered the tea in his cup, the motion of the carts, the spinning axle and the turning wheel. He pondered change and the turning seasons, and his own being. At last he picked up his ink brush and wrote:

> Thirty spokes converge upon a single hub,
> It is on the hole in the center that the use of the cart hinges.
> We make a vessel from a lump of clay.
> It is the empty space within the vessel that makes it useful.[1]

According to Taoist tradition, the cosmos began as chaos, an unbroken unity like the egg of Pan Gu. In the beginning was Tao, the unknowable wholeness beyond space and time, being and non-being, form and formlessness. Eventually the original unity polarized and the opposites of yin and yang came into being. After yin and yang appeared, heaven and earth separated and the world was born.

Just as the tension between positive and negative charges creates an electromagnetic field, the tension between the opposing polarities of yin and yang created a third phenomenon—the field of qi, the life force. As the field of qi was compressed and expanded by the tension of the opposites, it gathered potency and momentum and began to spin outward from its own center. The three became four and the compass points of the directions came into being.

As the centrifugal forces of the spinning qi increased, the heavier, coarser yin qi separated from the yang. The four directions further divided to form wuxing, the horizontal wheel of the Five Elements: water, wood, fire, earth and metal, the basic components of life on earth. The Five Elements went round and round, creating, destroying and transforming each other in endless cycles. The circulation of the Five Elements formed the Great Round, the Wheel of Life, which represents the cycles of the natural world, the seasons of life that spin in endlessly repeating rhythms of change.

In the middle of the Wheel, a vortex or empty center appeared. Here the lightest, most ephemeral yang qi gathered to create wushen, the vertical Axle of the Five Spirits. The Five Spirits animate the Wheel of Life and infuse the Five Elements with the light of the divine. At the center of the wheel is the empty space where the Axle of the Spirits spins its vitalizing and illuminating energies out into the material world.

The Five Spirits that gather at the empty center of the wheel make the Five Elements useful to human beings in a very particular

FIGURE 4: A TAOIST COSMOLOGY

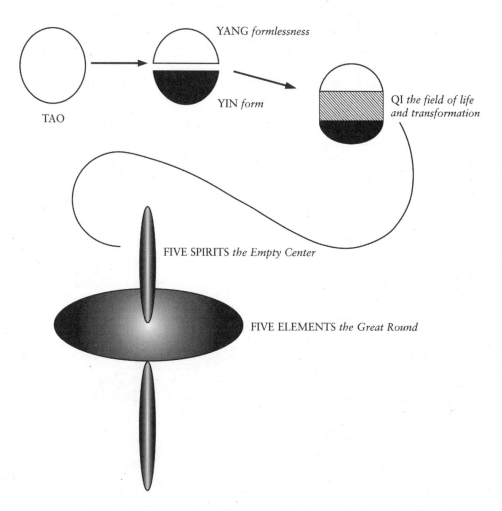

YANG *formlessness*

YIN *form*

QI *the field of life and transformation*

TAO

FIVE SPIRITS *the Empty Center*

FIVE ELEMENTS *the Great Round*

way. The spirits transform the material elements from dead weight into the vital matrix of the soul. As the spirits and the elements mingle, the earth becomes a sacred cauldron where the mystery of psychospiritual alchemy can occur. Through the influence of the spirits, lead becomes gold and an ordinary human being becomes a sage. By allowing the Great Round to travel through time, the Axle of the Spirits transforms the Great Round into a Spiral of Transformation that can break free from the endlessly repeating cycles of nature. Together, axle and wheel create the possibility for alchemical transformation: change that results in a permanent upgrade of the potency, complexity and quality of life energy.

FIGURE 5: THE AXLE AND THE WHEEL:
THE FIVE SPIRITS AND THE FIVE ELEMENTS

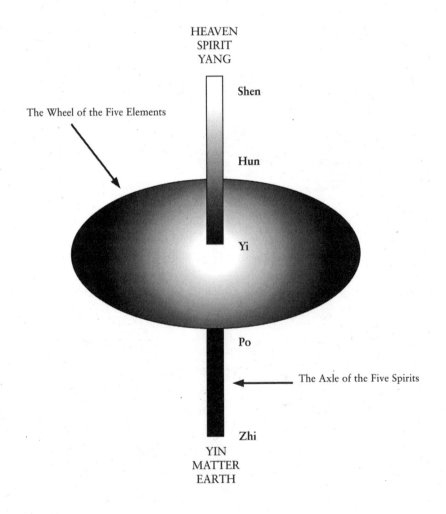

WUXING: THE CIRCULATION OF THE FIVE PHASES

The cosmic cycle of birth, growth, harvest, death and renewal has been an important aspect of human experience for millennia, forming the basis of rituals and myths for as long as human beings have told stories about the world and wondered about their relationship to the divine. This repeating circular pattern has determined the dance steps of shamans and the architectural designs of ancient temples.

The Chinese medical theory of the Law of the Five Elements is based on this same cosmic cycle. The Five Elements developed from a shamanic symbol into a philosophical idea around 300 BCE. The actual codification of the theory is attributed to the Chinese philosopher Tsou Yen. Today, Five Element Theory plays a significant role in the healing of symptoms that are rooted in emotional and psychosomatic distress.

The Law of the Five Elements describes the way organic processes occur on our planet. Each element characterizes a particular aspect of this energetic movement, relating to a particular vital organ, season, color, sound, odor and emotion. In this way each element crystallizes a multiplicity of associated correspondences into a single gestalt of meaning.

The term "Five Elements" is a translation of the Chinese term *wuxing*. The character *xing* is a picture of two footprints going forwards. It is also described as a crossroad where the path changes.

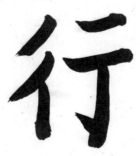

Xing, five elements

Although the Chinese word *xing* is usually translated as "element," many authorities acknowledge that other translations may be more accurate. Acupuncturist and classical scholar Kiko Matsumoto qualifies her use of the term "element" when she writes, "The Chinese character we translate as 'Elements' is sometimes rendered as 'phases' or 'movements.' In the ancient writings it meant 'crossroads.' This more literal meaning had the symbolic advantage of implying the energetic coordinates of a larger cosmological system."[2]

Whether we choose to translate *xing* as "element," "phase," or "movement," it is crucial to understand that the character implies a passage and a passing through. Xing is not thing but process, a noun that is at the same time a verb.

Wu means "five." The ancient character for this number was simply X. As previously noted, this character implies the idea of a center. Five is the number of the central position. X marks the spot. To the Chinese this is the place at the center is earth, the place where yin and yang meet to bring life into manifestation. X is a graphic representation of the idea that the Five Elements, the five evolutionary movements of life, emerge from the duality of yin and yang. At the crossing point of yin and yang, time and space, inhalation and exhalation (the two breaths of the qi), at the midpoint of the four directions, is the knot of life, the center point that is five.

The Correspondences

Each of the five phases corresponds to a particular natural element—water, wood, fire, earth, or metal—but the elements are only one of many associated correspondences connected to each of the five phases. Each phase contains a cluster of images and ideas that includes colors, seasons, times of day and flavors. Although these associations cannot always be rationally explained, for the most part they resonate with universally recognizable intuitive or somatic experiences.

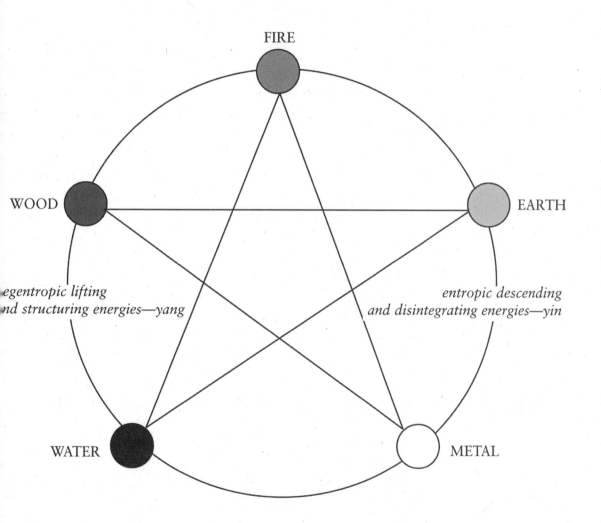

FIGURE 6: WUXING, THE WHEEL OF LIFE:
THE FIVE PHASES

FIRE

WOOD

EARTH

*egentropic lifting
nd structuring energies—yang*

*entropic descending
and disintegrating energies—yin*

WATER

METAL

ELEMENT	ORGAN	SOUND	CLIMATE	COLOR
water	kidney	groan	cold	blue/black
wood	liver	shout	windy	green
fire	heart	laugh	heat	red
earth	spleen	sing	dampness	yellow
metal	lung	weep	dryness	white

ELEMENT	PLANT PART	FUNCTION	SEASON	SPIRIT
water	seed	gestation	winter	zhi
wood	shoot	sprouting	spring	hun
fire	flower	blossoming	summer	shen
earth	fruit	harvest	late summer	yi
metal	compost	death	autumn	po

The *Sheng* and *K'o* Cycles

The Law of Five Elements describes the ongoing, repetitive cycles of gestation, birth, growth, transformation and death. The elements mutually create and destroy each other in the endless dance of life and death, entropy and negentropy. They create each other following the pattern of the *sheng* or life cycle: with qi moving clockwise, water nourishes wood, wood feeds fire, burned wood turns to ash and creates earth, and earth disintegrates into the minerals of metal. On the left side of the circle, from water to fire, the movement of qi is yang and negentropic as it lifts upward toward spirit, differentiated form, increased order, expansion and potency. But on the right side of the circle, from fire to metal, the forces of yin entropy take over. As the potency of the yang lifting energies run down, order, efficiency and complexity of form disintegrate back to chaos.

The phases control or destroy each other in the *k'o* or control cycle: with the qi moving in a clockwise direction along the lines of the inner pentacle, water controls fire, fire melts metal, metal cuts wood, wood contains earth, and earth limits and controls water. In the k'o cycle, the destructive aspect limits the powers of the creative aspect of matter.

The patterns of the sheng and k'o cycles can be applied not only to cosmic events like the seasons or to the emotions but to the progress of any creative project.

The sheng cycle is the outer circle of the pentacle diagram of the Five Phases. According to this cycle, anger gives birth to joy just as wood gives birth to fire. Sympathy is born of joy just as the ashes of burned wood give birth to the soil of the earth and so on around the wheel.

The k'o cycle or control cycle also unfolds in a cyclical pattern. It limits and qualifies the creations of the life cycle. The energy of this cycle moves across the crisscrossed inner lines of the star as water controls and qualifies fire, wood controls earth, fire controls metal, earth controls water and metal controls wood.

Without the limiting and qualifying effects of the k'o cycle, the sheng cycle would endlessly produce more forms and the cosmos would be choked in its own prolific productivity of form. Without the creative and quantifying effects of the sheng cycle, the k'o cycle would endlessly limit the production of form and the cosmos would dwindle away to nothingness.

Figure 7: Sheng and K'o Cycles

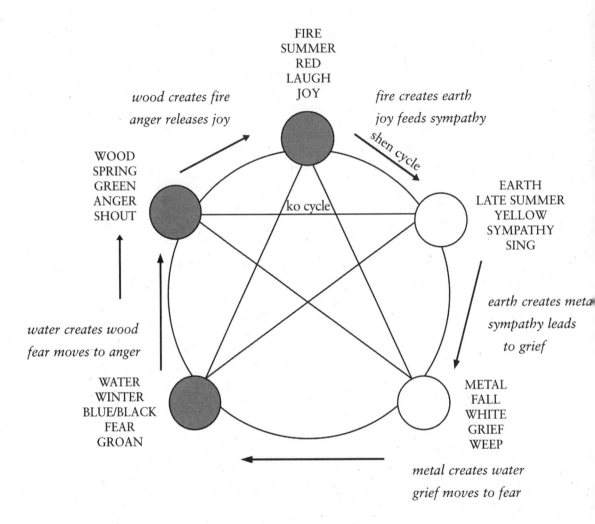

WUXING: THE FIVE PHASES

K'O CYCLE RELATIONSHIPS

wood breaks up earth	anger breaks up excess sympathy
earth absorbs water	sympathy absorbs fear
water extinguishes fire	fear extinguishes excess joy
fire melts metal	joy melts grief
metal cuts wood	grief cuts anger

Elements as Archetypes

When ancient Chinese physicians spoke of the elements, they meant the everyday natural elements: water, wood, fire, earth and metal. But they also meant Water, Wood, Fire, Earth and Metal—as first forms or universal essences. Each of the elements is a real but also a symbolic expression of how the life force moves and manifests on our planet and in our psyches. In Western psychological terms, the elements are what C. G. Jung describes as *archetypes*.

The term "archetype" comes from ancient Latin and refers to a divine form that exists outside of time and space. At the turn of the twentieth century, however, Jung began to use the term to refer to certain patterns and motifs that appeared in the dreams and fantasies of his patients as well as in the traditional artwork and legends of people from ancient and far-distant cultures. He noted that these recurrent motifs formed the basis of myths and religious symbols and appeared repeatedly in the individual as dream images and transcendent visions. Jung believed that these recurrent motifs and symbols were an inborn part of the human nervous system and emerged from a symbol-forming drive that was innate to the human psyche.

Although their expression reflects variations of time and culture, archetypes themselves exist beyond time and space. They are similar to biological instincts in that they are innate to the human organism and highly resistant to change. Just as sparrows build their nests in a particular way that does not vary through time or geographical location, so the dreams, myths and symbols of human beings form repeating patterns and motifs throughout space and time.

Archetypes constellate around astronomical, geological, meteorological and biological phenomena, yet their expression reflects the inner drama and development of the human soul. For example, when we see the symbol of the rising sun in a modern dream or carved on the side of an ancient bronze vase, we know we are in the realm of the solar hero, the one who overcomes the darkness of the night and re-ignites the forces of life. In Jung's words, "All the mythologized processes of nature, such as summer and winter, the phases of the moon, the rainy seasons and so forth, are in no sense allegories of these objective occurrences; rather they are the symbolic expressions of the inner, unconscious drama of the psyche which becomes accessible to man's consciousness by way of projection— that is, mirrored in the events of nature."[3]

Like acupuncture points on the body, the archetypes are points where the life force tends to gather in the soul. They are knots of concentrated psychic energy, accumulation points where very subtle levels of qi can be touched and moved. Archetypes attract, fascinate and even overpower us. They are a doorway between the everyday world of nature and the divine, invisible world beyond.

The Five Elements as well as other early theories of traditional Chinese medicine are rooted in archetypal consciousness. These theories contain universal truths that touch us at deep places in our being. Their imagery and poetry begin to heal us at unconscious levels long before we have any conscious understanding of the theories themselves. I have found that these archetypal images are another kind of needle that can be used to move qi on the level of the body and the soul.

Shui (water)

The element of water represents the water that pours down from the sky as rain and that we boil in a pot on the stove as well as the essence or original nature of water. The character is a picture of a river. It is a graphic expression of the flowing nature of water as it undulates between motion and stillness, this way and that. The element of water includes crashing waves, bubbling springs, steaming vapors, dew drops and ice crystals. It is the energy of winter, of the seed, of depth, darkness, dormancy and storage as well as the qualities of receptivity and gentle yet relentless power. Water gives an organism the ability to trust, to wait until the moment is right, and then to erupt like a geyser or a sprouting seed from the darkness of the earth into the light.

Mu (wood)

 The element of wood represents the wood we burn in the fireplace or use to build a table as well as the original nature of wood. The character is a picture of the trunk and roots of a tree. It is a graphic expression of the vertical thrust of the wood that shoots upward and moves with great determination toward the light, as well as the downward push of the roots sinking deep into the soil. The element wood includes the twigs and branches that quiver in the wind and the leaves that taste of the color green. It is the energy of spring, of new beginnings, progressive movement and reaching toward the future as well as the qualities of fiber and suppleness that give an organism the ability to maintain integrity through the storm winds of growth and transformation.

Huo (fire)

The element of fire represents the fire we use to warm ourselves or cook our food as well as the original nature of fire. The character is a picture of a dancing flame. It is a graphic expression of the expansive movement of fire as it flickers outward from its own center. The element fire includes the spark, the flame, the light and the heat as well as the dying embers. It is the energy of summer, of relationship and blossoming creativity as well as the qualities of spiritual warmth, initiating impulse and spontaneity that give an organism that ability to expand, to express its true nature and to reach out and connect with others.

Tu (earth)

The element of earth represents the earth beneath our feet, of fields and of gardens, as well as the original nature of earth. The character is a picture of the horizontal plane of the earth with a plant pushing upward from the soil. It is a graphic expression of the solid horizontality of earth as well as the capacity to support the upthrusting life of growing organisms. Earth includes the mountain, the meadow, the clod, the mud and the dry dust. It is the energy of late summer, of ripening fruit and ample productivity as well as the qualities of stability, fertility, nurturance and containment that give an organism the ability to sustain itself and others and to reap the harvest of its own life.

Jin (metal)

The element of metal represents the copper, iron and gold we use to make knives, pots and rings as well as the original nature of metal. The character is a picture of two nuggets of gold buried beneath the earth. It is a graphic expression of the inert, hidden nature of metal as well as its intrinsic value. The element metal includes the ores, crystals, minerals and stones found deep in the soil. It is the energy of autumn, of hardening seeds, falling leaves and sinking sap as well the quality of endurance and mysterious inspiration that gives an organism the capacity to crystallize its own structure and accumulate and maintain its quality and value.

THE ELEMENTS AND THE SOUL

Man's relationship to the elements has completely changed as we have moved more deeply into rational consciousness. Fire, water, wood, earth and metal are today viewed as unconscious matter, substances to be used by human beings for their own purposes, but for most of human history, the elements have been sacred. They often appeared in personified form in ancient myths and legend, and for millennia people paid homage to them as manifestations of the divine. If we shift our rational gaze and think of the elements from this more mythical perspective, their archetypal qualities rise naturally to the foreground of awareness. It is still possible for human beings to see the divine mystery of the elements, to become fascinated by their nature and movements and the forms that arise from them. At the moment when the elements come back to life in this way, we have reentered the sacred twilight domain of the alchemist and begin to see our soul reflected in the natural world.

Begin by observing the elements in nature. Notice the differences in temperature, movement, and color. Notice how you feel in the presence of these elements. Bring the elements into your living space: Put a shiny crystal on your desk. Keep a candle lit on your kitchen window. Watch how animals react to the elements. A cat holds completely still, staring in fascination as a drop of water drips from the kitchen faucet. She may become quite agitated by a lit candle. A breeze coming through an open window is full of messages and promise. In observing the elements, we discover forgotten parts of ourselves.

THE ALCHEMY OF EMOTION

Chinese medicine views the emotions as forms of qi, subtle energies that originate in the physical matrix of the organs of the body. Once they arise, emotions move through the body in waves of vibration that affect us on psychological and physiological levels. Like all other organic phenomena, emotions follow the predictable cyclical patterns of the Five Elements, simultaneously creating and destroying each other. The Five Elements give us a way to observe and work with the emotions as part of the dynamic, organic processes of life.

According to Chinese medicine, human emotions are animating impulses that move through the body in the same way that wind moves through the branches of the trees. Emotions are viewed as energies with specific qualities. They are related to colors, seasons, and elements and are conceptualized as interpenetrating agents of transformation that continuously engender and destroy each other.

THE ELEMENTS AND EMOTIONS

Fear is watery. It arises from the kidneys and bladder in the low back. Like cold and winter, it is constricting, limiting and deeply gestating.

Anger is woody. It arises from the liver and gallbladder in the diaphragm. Like wind and spring, it is energizing, propulsive and growth-promoting.

Joy is fiery. It arises from the heart in the upper chest. Like fire and summer, it is warming, circulating and blossoming.

Sympathy is earthy. It arises from the stomach and spleen in the center of the abdomen. Like humidity and late summer, it is gathering, nourishing and yielding.

Grief is metallic. It arises from the lungs. Like dryness and autumn, it is limiting, desiccating and completing.

Even in English the animating, moving nature of emotion is implicitly understood. The word "emotion" derives from the French *emouvoir*, which means "to stir up," and from the Latin *emotum*, "to move outward." Emotions move. They move out of us and through us. They cause us to move.

According to traditional Chinese medicine, emotions move in specific ways, in specific directions, at specific velocities. Anger rushes upward toward the head. Fear contracts and sinks down to a frozen grip at the base of the spine. Joy flickers like a flame in the chest. Compassion expands outward in ever-enlarging concentric circles. Grief floats like a mist until it is broken open by tears.

Despite their inherent conceptual differences, East and West share the universal understanding that emotions move. They move through the matter of our bodies and affect us. They engender impulses toward action and physiological responses such as tears, increased respiration, laughter, muscular tension and relaxation. In other words, emotions not only are qi, they also move qi. Like music, like poetry, like the atmosphere of the weather, emotions affect us and are the expressions of our soul. Like the elements of water (fear), wood (anger), fire (joy), earth (sympathy) and metal (grief), our emotions engender and subdue each other.

Each *zangfu* or organ has its own particular emotional resonance and psychic function. The liver relates to anger, the stomach to sympathy, the lungs to grief, and the kidneys to fear. But it is the heart that is most centrally concerned with the emotions and most susceptible to their effects. Although joy is its most specific emotion, the heart, as the center of psycho-emotional life, is immediately moved and affected by any shift in the emotional climate of the body. The lightning-quick shifts in heart rate and intensity that occur with loss, anger, joy or shock are the physical manifestation of the potent connection between the *zang* of the heart and emotional experience.

TRANSLATING PHILOSOPHICAL CONCEPTS INTO THERAPEUTIC STRATEGIES

Emotions are a form of qi, and like any form of qi they can become blocked from various psychological or physical factors. Just as a stream of water becomes blocked when choked with leaves, twigs and other woody debris, or when iced over in mid-winter, so can our water element become blocked when we are choked with anger and resentment or frozen with fear. Just as a fire grows dim when not fed with kindling, so our fiery joy becomes depleted when resentment smolders and rots our wood. Just as qi follows the path of the sheng or k'o cycle as it moves through the natural world, so qi moves through our body and mind. Stuck emotion, like any stuck qi, causes pain and disease. But once a blocked emotion begins to flow, we experience a renewed sense of well-being and clarity and are more capable of moving forward to the next chapter of our life.

Using Five Element Theory, an acupuncturist can discern which element is the source of a patient's distress. Points on the acupuncture meridian related to this element are used to move the stuck qi. The skillful practitioner also uses emotion, like a needle, as a tool to move qi. Meeting clients at the level of authentic emotional distress is a powerful tool in the healing process (see the case study that follows this section).

A blocked element is recognized by a particular hue or tone of a person's face, a particular sound of the voice, and an unusual preponderance or absence of a particular emotion. Bluish/black color around the eyes, a groaning voice, and an excess or absence of fear, for example, indicate a blocked water element. Some commonly seen associations are:

Blocked Water: Chilly hands and feet, urinary tract problems, low back pain, knee pain, anxiety, counterphobic behavior.

Blocked Wood: Tension in the diaphragm, bloating after meals, one-sided headaches, choleric temper, simmering resentments.

Blocked Fire: Overheated chest and head, palpitations, chest tightness, hysteria, manic moods, insomnia and dream-disturbed sleep.

Blocked Earth: Digestive disturbances, cold hands, excess hunger or lack of appetite, excess cogitation and worry, muddle-headedness and forgetfulness.

Blocked Metal: Chest tightness, irritable bowels, asthma, inability to reach out and make connections, depression and grief.

The very best way to begin to understand and recognize the elements in human beings is to follow the path of the ancient Taoists and watch the way the elements move and behave in nature. In this way the invisible Tao becomes visible to us through its reflection in the natural world.

CASE STUDY: USING THE K'O CYCLE TO SOFTEN RAGE

"I go around feeling pissed off," Jeff told me, "like I'm going to jump out of my skin. I used to like to be with people, to go out and have a good time. Now, as soon as someone gets close, I start feeling irritable and angry. I don't want to even try dating because I'm sure I'll just mess up other people's lives."

Jeff's chief complaint was pain and tightness in his back and shoulders, uncontrollable outbursts of anger and an inability to tolerate intimacy. Although he had a history of alcoholism and drug use, he had been sober for three years before I met him. But since he'd stopped drinking, his emotional life had deteriorated and he felt isolated and alone.

Through psychotherapy and talking to other alcoholics, Jeff had come to understand that rather than his psychological health deteriorating, he was in the process of healing and at last was seeing the emotional problems that drugs and alcohol had masked. Unfortunately, this intellectual understanding did not do much to alleviate his emotional suffering.

After his psychotherapist suggested acupuncture, Jeff decided to try a few sessions because he thought it might help his shoulder pain. When I explained that many of his emotional symptoms were classic signs for the Chinese diagnosis of wood or liver imbalance and that acupuncture might help him feel better emotionally as well as physically, he was not impressed. He made it clear he was anxious to get on the treatment table, close his eyes and, as he called it, "zone out." After a few treatments, his shoulders did begin to feel better and he claimed he was noticing an improvement in his sleep, but he felt as angry and irritable as ever.

About a month after his treatment began, Jeff came in looking worse than I had ever seen him. His jaw was tight, his eyes distant, and he sat hunched in his chair as he pounded a clenched fist against his thigh, but I had a peculiar feeling that there was something inauthentic about his anger, as if it was a caricature covering something more real. Under his shout, I heard weeping, and flitting under the greenish tone of his skin, I saw a pale white shadow.

"Stick a needle in my jaw, right here," he said, pointing to the corner of his chin. "I just can't take this anymore. I feel like I'm going to kill my boss. I want to bite off his head and chew him into little pieces. Just take your biggest needle and stick me. Make a big hole so this monster inside can get out of me. I just want to get rid of him."

I sat across from Jeff and listened to his words, but at the same time I remained focused on my breathing, my body, and the quality of the atmosphere in the room. I stayed with myself as I stayed in relationship to Jeff and to his "monster" inside. As I listened, I felt a deep sadness and heaviness in my heart as if I was going to start to cry. Beneath the angry voice of the monster, I dimly heard the voice of a young boy who had never been listened to. Slowly, from beneath Jeff's wood, I began to hear the voice of metal. I realized I had never really seen him. I had been misled by his angry exterior and missed the real energy necessary for his healing: the grief of his soul that was waiting to be recognized. Needles weren't what Jeff needed. At that moment, in order to resolve his rage, he needed to feel his sadness.

Through a combination of intuition, understanding, grace, and the profound psychological wisdom of Chinese medicine, I was able to see through Jeff's exterior symptoms to the underlying pattern below. As soon as I realized this, the energy in the room shifted. A part of Jeff felt the change in me before I said a word, and his face relaxed slightly and color came into his cheeks. From behind the blankness in his eyes, someone very young looked out at me, another Jeff peering out from the darkness. Using the feeling in my own body, staying close to the deep sadness I felt in my own heart, slowly and carefully I guided Jeff back to his own emotions.

"Have you ever felt really listened to?" I asked, saying the words to Jeff but speaking to the young boy hiding in his eyes.

For the first time since I had met him, Jeff took a really deep breath of air. His shoulders dropped and his jaw loosened. "Never," he answered. The intensity of his anger subsided as the healing energy of honest emotion, his loss and his grief, filled the space between us.

This single healing moment was not by any means a moment of cure, but it was the beginning of a shift, the softening of a painful, intractable emotional block. Without needles or herbs, simply through the alchemical power of emotion, Jeff's locked-up qi began to flow again. This moment was followed by months of work that included acupuncture, guided imagery, conversation and body psychotherapy, but from that moment on, our relationship was changed and we both knew that an important step had been made in Jeff's healing process.

My intuition and enlivened perception helped me reach the grief underneath Jeff's anger, but there was also a theoretical basis for the way this treatment unfolded. According to the Chinese law of the k'o cycle, grief is the emotion that limits or subdues anger, in the same way that metal shapes or cuts through wood. I was able to help Jeff through his chronic, debilitating anger by reaching the locked-up energy of his grief. I did this by bringing the energy of my own heartfelt sadness into the room. This enabled us to connect in a way that was healing for both of us.

In the case study above, the needles inserted into acupuncture points on Jeff's body helped him to relax and ease his physical discomfort, but Jeff's real healing began when I recognized the authentic arrested emotion hidden below his angry defenses. At that moment, both he and I had a shift in awareness. There was a pause, a not knowing, a silence, and then the spirits entered the treatment room. With his sudden insight, the shen arrived and movement and animation returned to Jeff's being. At that moment wushen penetrated wuxing, and the material world was illuminated by the lights of the divine world beyond.

The ancient Chinese recognized the crucial significance of relationship when working with the spirits. The *Neijing Suwen* emphasizes that it is the acupuncturist's open and attentive heart that allows the voice of the patient's spirit to be heard and seen. Ch'i Po, the ancient physician and teacher of the Yellow Emperor, states,

> Because of the fact that symptoms cannot be perceived upon the outside not everybody can see them. About those who are able to see with no need of symptoms and who are able to taste when there are no flavors—it is said that they make use of profound and mysterious knowledge and that they resemble those who are divinely inspired. . . . [I]f one pays close attention . . . *shen*, the spirit, becomes clear to man as though the wind has blown away the cloud.[4]

Chapter Four

Tao Lost and Rediscovered

The sage looked down from the mountain, out over the valley. In the distance he saw people rushing along the road and between the fields and houses. He leaned back against a stone and watched them.

A cloud moved across the horizon. The sun set slowly. The light grew dim. He wondered about the people rushing back and forth in the valley. How silly, he thought, when there is nowhere they need to go.

He dipped his brush in the ink but before he could begin his calligraphy he fell fast asleep. In the morning, he found these words on the scroll in front of him:

> Allow your life to unfold naturally
> Know that it too is a vessel of perfection[1]

TRANSFORMATIONAL HEALING

The first time I met Anne, her pulse rate was 115 beats a minute, and she had lost ten pounds in one month. My first impression of her was of Athena—a tall and thoughtful goddess with a distant gaze. So I was surprised to find her hands trembling when I took her pulses.

Ambitious and highly successful in her career, Anne spoke without emotion about her father, a lawyer, who although dead continued to look at her through his tortoiseshell glasses and ask what she intended to do with her life.

Shortly after her fortieth birthday, Anne's body temperature had skyrocketed. She broke into unpredictable sweats and her heart jumped erratically in her chest. Tests revealed that her thyroid was malfunctioning and her hormone levels were significantly out of normal range. After numerous conversations with her doctor and hours online researching her condition, Anne made an uncharacteristic decision to disregard the accepted medical route; something told her to try Chinese medicine before turning to standard Western medical interventions.

After the initial interview, our work began by using acupuncture to balance her qi, clear blocks in the meridians, disperse her excess Fire and tonify her deficient Water. The acupuncture lowered Anne's pulse rate and improved her sleep, but her thyroid was still unstable. I told Anne that I thought her problem was more than physical. If she was going to successfully stabilize her endocrine system using alternative methods, I thought she would have to include not only her body but also her imagination, emotions, dreams, desires and instincts in her healing process. The ancient Chinese referred to this kind of healing as "going to the level of spirit."

Despite her own uncertainty, Anne decided to take a leap of faith and trust her intuition, which told her it was safe to move ahead with the work we were doing together and refrain from standard medical intervention. Soon after that decision, Anne dreamed herself in a desert where she discovered a grove of trees beside a stream of cool blue water. I guided Anne through a process of active imagination[2] during which she was able to recognize the dream image as the voice of her own being—especially her overheated body—calling out for rest and the healing water of her unconscious. The dream image supported Anne's commitment to her alternative healing process and she came back to it many times during our work together.

I introduced Anne to Taoist breathing techniques and meditation practices, which helped her get out of her head and bring awareness to her body and the oasis of peace that lay deep in her own being. Dietary changes and Chinese herbs helped calm her spirit and gradually rebalance her endocrine system. I explained that small changes in behavior, made faithfully, day after day, would eventually result in changes in her physiology. I encouraged her to cultivate her yin—the embodied, receptive, lunar aspects of her being. She discovered gardening, tai ch'i, and the pleasure of consciously doing nothing.

One day, after about six months of treatment and slow but steady improvement, Anne came in pale and exhausted. Her pulse, which had been gradually returning to normal speed, had suddenly dropped to forty-eight beats per minute. A visit to her doctor revealed that her thyroid levels had plummeted. Her family became alarmed and urged her to begin medication immediately. Her doctor also felt that she should begin the medication, but he reluctantly gave her one more month to see if the acupuncture would work.

Anne, who at least on the surface was extremely self-contained, began crying on the treatment table. "I've had it. My life feels like it's falling apart," she said. "Everything that was right is wrong. I don't know who I am anymore."

I began to feel dread creeping up from the pit of my belly. I reached for her hand to check her pulse. Her hand was damp and clammy, and her pulse beat sluggishly. My dread increased and my thoughts began to race. By treating Anne with acupuncture, I was going against the grain of culturally accepted medical practice. What if something had gone wrong? What if, by her waiting to begin medication, some irrevocable damage had been done to Anne's body? I felt the entire medical establishment just beyond my office door, waiting to pounce on my first clinical screw-up.

Between Anne's emotional meltdown and the anxiety pulsing through my body, the atmosphere in the room turned thick with fear and confusion. The floor beneath my feet felt tilted. It was like being in a boat on a stormy sea, everything swaying, no place solid to stand.

"It's scary not knowing," I heard my voice say out loud. Anne looked at me and it was as if I was seeing her for the first time. A small, very frightened girl peered out from behind her woman's eyes. "You feel that way too?" the young part of Anne asked.

I nodded yes and then asked, "Do you want to turn back?"

Anne shook her head no. "It's OK. I can do this," she said.

I took a breath and felt the support of the earth coming back beneath my feet. "It's going to be all right," I said to Anne and to the terrified child who was hiding somewhere in the space between us. "You're in touch with your doctor. If you need to take medication, you'll take it, but meanwhile I think a part of you is coming back to life."

I decided to needle an acupuncture point called Spirit Storehouse, which has the effect of regulating the heart and relaxing the intercostal muscles of the chest. Spirit Storehouse is also a special kind of point called a spirit point, known to have psychological as well as physical effects. This particular point is used to help a person let go of the past and recover lost parts of the self, especially very old parts lost in childhood. When I needled the point, I knew I was treating both Anne and the frightened young girl who was also present in the room.

Afterwards, Anne looked different. She had more color in her cheeks and her eyes were softer. Something else changed as well, a subtle sense of emerging presence, as if Anne, who had always given the impression of cool aloofness, was actually making contact with me for the first time.

"After I got sick," she said, "I felt like such a failure, with my hot flashes, sweats, insomnia, and racing heartbeat. I couldn't work all night and keep the house in perfect order like I always had. I felt like I was disappointing my boss, my husband, my kids." The hint of a smile appeared. "For the first time in my life, I was completely out of control." Then, she laughed. "I have to admit, it's kind of a relief."

Soon after that treatment, Anne gave up her corporate job and took time off to rest. She continued to meditate and practice the deep relaxation and abdominal breathing techniques I had taught her. Like a gyroscope in search of its center pole, her thyroid gradually tilted its way back to a new center of balance. Anne also found a new center of gravity, one that was in her body and emotions instead of her thoughts and her will. During her convalescence, she had a vision of a new career, a consulting program that would teach others how to use intuition to solve problems as well as reduce stress. Now, several years later, Anne's thyroid is healthy and her consulting business is doing well. Her doctors were surprised that her thyroid levels returned to normal without surgery or pharmaceutical intervention, but ancient Taoist healers would not have been surprised at Anne's success.

In addition to the benefits she received from acupuncture, Chinese herbs, meditation and psychological insight, the alchemical wisdom of Chinese medicine helped me guide Anne through the chaos of a challenging transformational journey. In the process, Anne discovered the greatest medicine of all, the medicine Taoist alchemists called wisdom, the ability to align one's will with one's true nature. Although wisdom alone is not enough to cure every disease and solve every problem, its emergence from the chaos and suffering of illness marks a turning point in the healing process. Wisdom rises like light from darkness, a light that points the way to a new way of being. The emergence of wisdom is a crucial part of the journey Chinese alchemists called "the return to Tao," or "the return to Original Nature."

At one of our last meetings, Anne said, "If I find myself trying to impress people, getting wound up, pushing and rushing, I just think of water, how it goes its own way, flowing without effort towards the sea. If I go along like that, just staying in flow, everything I really need to do does get done. And what doesn't get done probably doesn't matter in the long run."

THE LOSS OF TAO

Although each patient in my practice is different, nearly all share one aspect of Anne's problem: a lack of relatedness between thinking and feeling, mind and body, action and imagination, will and receptivity. Rather than flowing easily between doing and being, following the natural biorhythms of their bodies and the planet, my patients' lives are characterized by abruptly changing rhythms and radical disharmonies, spurts of intense activity followed by passive exhaustion.

The lack of connection to natural biorhythms is not a new problem for human beings, but it is one that has gotten progressively more serious with the advance of modern technology. Today, Western holistic healers describe this problem as a split or rupture between the mind and the body. In the language of modern depth psychology, it could be explained as a disequilibrium between the conscious and unconscious forces of the psyche. In ancient Western traditions, this rupture was spoken of as a tear in the fabric of the soul or subtle body. However, by using the concepts of Taoist alchemy, we can have a deeper, more coherent understanding of what is going on. From a Taoist alchemical perspective, the mind/body split is the result of the yin and yang aspects of the qi separating. As the yin and yang or negative and positive poles of the energy body separate, the vital energetic system of the body no longer has a healthy, dynamic tension. A rupture forms between the yang, cerebral, psychic, spiritual pole of the qi and the yin, vital, sensational, material pole. In the language of the Five Spirits, the *hun* or yang aspect of the soul is no longer communicating with the *po* or yin aspect of the soul. The hun no longer inspires and enlivens the body with its healing visions and dreams, and the po no longer grounds and stabilizes the psyche with its reliable organic rhythms and infallible instincts.

Whatever terminology is used, this lack of tension in the qi or breath body results in a deterioration of the health and vitality of physical and psychological functioning. When the yang hun or spiritual soul no longer lifts and animates the yin po, the life force collapses toward the embodied or somatic aspect of the psyche. When the qi collapses towards the soma or po soul, we find chronic, unmoving physical blocks, rigidities and pain, regressive behavior and depleted psychic energy. This kind of collapse may lead to depression, obsessions, chronic muscular pain, exhaustion and hypochondria. Conversely, when the yin po or material soul does not tether the yang hun to the earth, the qi floats up and accumulates in the non-material or mental aspect of the psyche. In this case, as happened with Anne, the result is hyperactivity, insomnia, anxiety and heart palpitations. This overexcitation at the nonmaterial or spiritual pole is accompanied by an undercharged vital force that is unable to reestablish necessary natural rhythm to the functions of the body.

Most often, once the polarizing tension between the hun and the po diminishes, yin and yang continue to separate and the situation deteriorates. The hun rises toward spirit and the po drops down toward matter. The patient experiences erratic spurts of enervation and exhaustion. Unless communication between the hun and po is restored, psychological and physical illness develops, and ultimately the entire energy system loses its vitality.

The split in the soul or subtle body begins when human beings

FIGURE 8: YIN AND YANG POLES OF THE BREATH BODY

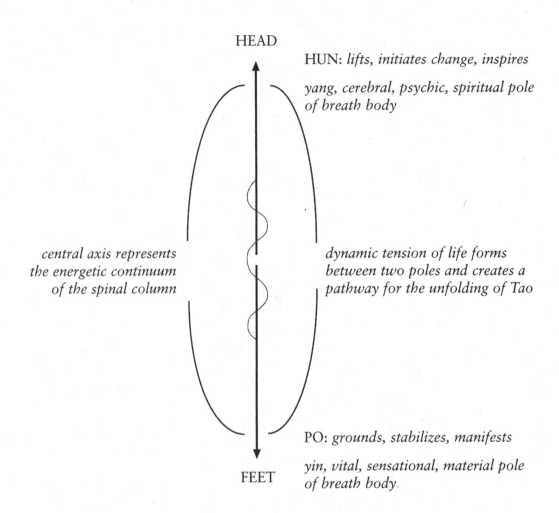

HEAD

HUN: *lifts, initiates change, inspires*

yang, cerebral, psychic, spiritual pole of breath body

central axis represents the energetic continuum of the spinal column

dynamic tension of life forms between two poles and creates a pathway for the unfolding of Tao

PO: *grounds, stabilizes, manifests*

FEET

yin, vital, sensational, material pole of breath body.

lose touch with the guiding light of spirit, the inspiration of dreams and the wisdom of the body. It begins when we lose touch with the natural rhythms of the earth and the ever-present ground of a harmonious cosmos. When I see this in my patients, I say they have lost their Tao. They are cut off from the inspirations of spirit, the enlivening movements of emotion, the organizing rhythms of organic processes and the vitalizing energies of the instincts. They have lost the capacity to connect with the flowing river of the life force and creative wisdom of the cosmos.

Much of the physical and emotional distress of modern Westerners is the result of a loss of integrity at the level of the subtle body. The language and mythical vision of Taoist alchemy give us a way to access this subtle level and to work with it in powerful ways. This ancient consciousness supports reorganization of the shattered parts of the self into a new, more efficient wholeness that can endure, and even flourish, in the face of the stresses and challenges of modern life.

The authentic rediscovery of Tao is more than simply giving up the thinking mind and surrendering to the whims of the instincts. Tao is not found through regression to an idealized child-like past or a progression forward to a future in paradise. The return to Tao transcends concepts such as young and old, body and mind, surrender and will, self and cosmos. The return to Tao is a spiraling backward return that brings us forward to a wholeness of greater complexity and quality than what was lost.

Anne, for example, lost her Tao and her sense of wholeness when her will-driven behavior overwhelmed the capacities of her vital body energies and she became ill. As her healing unfolded, she discovered a new and more efficient integrity as she came to a deeper understanding of her true desires and abilities and the authentic needs of her body. As the splits in her soul body healed, her life became infused with a new light, the glow of humor, acceptance and wisdom that she had acquired through the suffering and limitations of illness.

Tao is an old way of being and a completely new possibility, the unity that both precedes and is born from the tension of the irreconcilable contradictions of embodied life. Today the mystery of Tao has become the background illumination and supportive foundation of my practice, but before I could begin to work in this way I had to learn to lean into the Tao, not only as an idea but also as an embodied experience that takes me, as well as my patients, far beyond the limited range of three-dimensional reality and rational understanding.

THE REORIENTATION OF THE SELF

Alchemical Acupuncture supports healing that is not restorative but transformational. This kind of healing is not a return to familiar but no longer life-affirming patterns of behavior. It is a reorientation of the self to the inner and outer world. It results in unexpected new ways of being, new possibilities that resolve seemingly irreconcilable paradoxes. This kind of acupuncture goes beyond physical and even psychological healing to support the alchemical reorganization of the self.

Through this process, many of my patients have been able to give up the idea of getting back to their old selves again. As they open to the spaciousness of the unknown, they discover ways of organizing their lives that bring mind and body, being and doing, conscious and unconscious back into harmonious relationship. The result of this kind of healing is not always the alleviation of the original symptoms but it is always a fundamental shift in a person's relationship to his or her symptoms. Symptoms may gradually disappear, dwindle or simply become unimportant as wisdom, compassion, trust and acceptance replace resentment, suffering and power-driven will.

Alchemical Acupuncture is based on ideas and techniques drawn from Chinese medicine, Western depth psychology, and European and Taoist alchemy. The map I use to organize the process, however, is based on the Taoist description of the human psyche as expressed through wushen, the Five Spirits.

Generally, the process of Alchemical Acupuncture begins with a shift in awareness. Patients come to me because they have a problem they have not been able to solve. They have reached an impasse. Either the rational methods of Western medicine have failed to help them or they have been unable to figure out the problem on their own. They are stuck in a pattern of thinking and behavior that isn't working but they have been unable to find another way. So the first step is to discover a new point of view.

The tools of depth psychology open the door between the conscious and unconscious mind. In Taoist terms, this phase begins the descent process as we move from the shen, or realms of conscious awareness, to the hun, the realm of vision, images and dreams. Through active imagination,[2] the patient begins to relate to the life myths, images, dream symbols and creative impulses that constellate around his or her particular symptom. Drawing, painting and journal writing enhance this growing relationship, as does the healing partnership that gradually develops between patient and practitioner.

This work provides an entryway into the archetypal dimension of the psyche, the psychic unconscious where East and West meet in a world of ancient, universal symbols. Here patients begin to look at their symptoms and their lives in symbolic ways, to discover meaning in what before seemed like meaningless pain and suffering. Through this work they are able to identify their own life myth, the actions, behaviors and ways of being that have perhaps contributed to their illness or that may be interfering with their healing. In addition, this work provides a way for Western patients to bring the healing myths and symbols of Chinese medicine into their own lives and to recognize these ancient symbols through active imagination in their own dreams, body symptoms and fantasies.

At this point acupuncture takes up where depth psychology leaves off. Acupuncture opens the door between the mind and the body and enlivens an awareness of the body as a place of mystery and possibility. Patients begin to connect their state of mind, their feelings, visions and thoughts, to their physicality. They sense themselves differently and begin to see how their being exists in a flux of constant energetic change. Here the movement of descent is from the hun to the yi, the realm of thought, intention and embodied application of ideas and personal feeling.

The needle's ability to reconnect the mind with the body and the ever-changing field of qi is an important step in the transformational healing process. However, unless this new awareness is woven into a person's actual being through work with the body unconscious—the deepest, most unconscious level of the psyche—acupuncture may result in unstable physical shifts. For example, a stress headache that psychotherapy didn't cure may disappear after two or three acupuncture sessions. However, the patient's life has not fundamentally changed, and the cure remains incomplete if the patient does not address the unconscious neurological impulses, the tissue memory, emotions and compulsive behaviors that are tangled up in the physical symptoms. The person's body continues to be vulnerable to attack from what the ancient Chinese called the *gui*, the underworld demons that represent the energies of buried, unresolved psychological issues. This may result in short-lived successes or symptoms that disappear only to reappear later in new form. So the descent from the shen to the hun to the yi still may not complete the healing process if a patient's symptom is in fact rooted in chronic emotional or psychological distress.

In my clinical experience, I find that it is the hidden wisdom, the Taoist alchemical aspect of Chinese medicine, that makes truly transformational healing possible, healing that fundamentally changes—and most importantly, upgrades in value—a person's relationship to self, life and the outside world. In order for this kind of transformation to occur, old ways of being must be dissolved and new ways created, or at least seen as real possibilities. Self and noself must meet—an encounter with the mystery that resolves the paradox between them. This meeting occurs below the level of conscious awareness in the realm of the lower spirits, the po and the zhi. These lower spirits represent the underworld of the bodymind, the realm of the autonomic nervous system, the instincts, the animal impulses, the realm of karma and fate, and ultimately the alchemical cauldron in which the light of new life and wisdom emerges spontaneously from the void of Tao.

Transformation of this magnitude occurs in what the ancient Taoist alchemists called the *huntun*, or chaos state. In order to enter the huntun, we must leave behind rational thought and its distinctions of conscious and unconscious, body and mind. We descend to the realm of the bodymind or embodied psyche, a swirling universe of sensations, emotions, neurological impulses, dreams, memories, symptoms, visions, actions and desires. Here, the contradictions and dualities of self and no-self dissolve in a vast river of qi, which flows through body and mind, image and reality, time and space and beyond to the ocean of the life force itself.

True healing and transformation demand that we be willing to be changed by chaos rather than rushing in to impose a premature order. In Anne's story, the turning point in her healing came when we descended together into the huntun, where the earth shifted, real and imaginary merged, and the fearsome unknown became palpable in the treatment room. At that moment Anne surrendered to her despair. She stopped trying to hold it together and allowed the outmoded structure of her life to fall apart. It was only then that something new could emerge spontaneously from Tao. It is in this swirling universe, the embodied psyche or bodymind, that transformational healing occurs. This is the psychic space where individual identity comes closest to dissolution in primordial chaos. Here at the edge of the rational universe, when the needle slips between spirit and matter, there comes a shock and an inexplicable organizing principle enters the healing process. At that moment the self spontaneously realigns with the cosmos and a new possibility rises like a sprouting seed from the dark, fertile ground of a person's authentic nature.

This kind of healing cannot be forced or willed. It is a process that is surrendered to. This kind of healing can never be completely explained. It is and always will remain a mystery. This kind of healing is the embodiment of what the ancient Chinese called Tao.

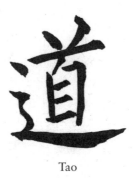

Tao

The character for *Tao* is comprised of two parts, one that signifies a head topped with two plumes and the other a foot. Plumes in ancient China were used to mark the rank of a military general. Thus "head" in this case also means "the leader" while "foot" means "to go," "to follow" or "to travel along a path." The character for Tao makes reference to the highest and lowest parts of our being, to the illuminating, initiating, spiritual or yang aspects of the mind and the grounding, manifesting, materializing or yin aspects of the body. What is between the head and foot is the universe, the "all that is" that is Tao naturally unfolding through our being and out into the world.

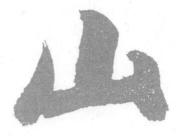

Chapter Five

The Mountain

> The Spirits. Oh! the Spirits! The ear cannot hear them, but the heart
> opens through the brilliance of the eye . . . only the bright flash can
> provoke the radiance; it is like a wind blowing away the clouds. This
> is called the Spirits.
>
> —Neijing Suwen[1]

THE LANDSCAPE BEYOND

From a traditional Chinese perspective, health arises from harmony—an attuned correspondence between the natural world and the life of human beings. Health is an inner and outer landscape where the Five Elements are in balance and the weather is in accord with the season. But there is still a further landscape beyond: the light-soaked radiance and misty vapors of the spirit world that shadows and illuminates the world we know as real.

Walking through life without the spirits, we cannot see the music of the moon or hear the bony branches of winter trees. Without the light of the spirits, we cannot see the Way, even as we walk on it. Without the darkness of the shades, there would be no wandering.

In our most profound experiences of health, the world we see and know as real is infused and sustained by the unseen world beyond. Every river, every mountain, every blade of grass has a divine breath: the heavenly light that calls it forth, the dark earth wisdom that gives it the boldness to be.

The Spirits

Hidden at the core of traditional Chinese medicine are wushen, the Five Spirits—the shen, hun, yi, po, and zhi, which are the resident deities of the Taoist psyche. They are our guides to the radiant landscape of the soul, the landscape that lies beyond the ordinary. During our lives, the spirits reside in the organs of the body. At death, they return to the divine realms of above and below.

The Five Spirits are the immaterial aspect of a human being, the finest, most ephemeral vibration of qi. They cannot be grasped, yet they are the foundation or root of all that can be grasped. They cannot be seen except as support for all that is seen, heard and felt by the senses. This level of subtle energy can be compared to the Western concept of the soul. However, the spirits, unlike the Western soul, are not abstract. They are the vital, energetic expression of psychic and neurological processes.

Each Spirit represents a particular psychological function and is related to a physical organ and one of the Five Elements—fire, wood, earth, metal and water. Disturbances of the elements can result in physical as well as emotional and psychological problems. Similarly, disturbances of the spirits result in physical, emotional and psychosomatic problems. Symptoms such as depression, anxiety, alcohol and drug addiction, allergies, chronic pain, eating disorders and phobias are typical spirit level problems.

The spirits affect many aspects of our lives on a subtle qualitative level. They affect the quality of our relationships, our creativity and our intellectual and emotional life. They affect our relationship to our bodies, our self-worth and our ability to make our impression

THE FIVE SPIRITS

Spirit	Psychological Function	Element	Organ	Polarization
shen	thought, consciousness	Fire	Heart	Yang Spirit
hun	vision, imagination	Wood	Liver	
yi	ideation, intention	Earth	Spleen	
po	emotion, instinct	Metal	Lung	Yin Matter
zhi	will, wisdom	Water	Kidney	

on the world around us. However, the distinguishing hallmark of a spirit disturbance is that individual symptoms are only one part of a global breakdown of a person's ability to continue on his or her life journey. When the spirits are disturbed, our lives lack inspiration, direction, intention, embodied knowing and instinctual potency. Our actions lack authenticity, spontaneity and authority. We are stuck and cannot move forward in the manifesting of our Tao.

An understanding of how to work with the Five Spirits gives a Chinese medical practitioner the ability to work with symptoms that might otherwise be impossible to heal. This understanding also supports us in helping ourselves and our friends, family and people in our community discover more graceful, efficient and satisfying ways of being and living. The spirits must be related to and cultivated. If we do not attend to them, their light dims and may even depart the body entirely. Then, although the physical body still walks about, talks and continues to breathe, we are no more than a dry husk, blown this way and that by the winds of fate, and are particularly susceptible to physical illness. Most often it is the person's life, the atmosphere and result of his or her actions that tell us about the condition of the spirits.

When the spirits are healthy and aligned, they transform the scattered winds of fate into destiny. Although they cannot be perceived with our ordinary senses, their effects can be known through our behavior and the qualities that emanate from our inner being. The spirits can be seen in the brightness of our eyes, the firmness of our identities, the clarity of our ideas, the strength of our compassion and the depth of our wisdom. Through the influence of the spirits, life takes on meaning, direction, purpose, integrity and spontaneous authenticity, and the landscape of the life reflects the luminous world of the divine.

The spirits are to human beings as a flame is to a lantern. When the flame is extinguished, the form of the lantern remains, but its essential beauty and meaning is gone. Similarly, when the spirits are ill or have fled the body, the physical structure may remain and even seem to function, but the luminous presence or soul of the person is lacking.

The Breath Body

In the Taoist imagination, the Five Spirits are bits of heavenly light that drop down into matter and take some of its weight and form. Through their contact with matter, the spirits become moistened by the essences of the earth and move through us as a kind of vapor or breath. As they accumulate color, moisture and form, they take on a subtle body that is neither pure spirit nor pure matter but a mixing of the two.

This subtle breath body forms a complex pneumatic system that both lifts and stabilizes the psychic and vital processes of the human organism. It is the emptiness at the center that animates the body, that turns flesh and blood from "mere dead weight"[2] into a vital, living being with a soul. The Five Spirits are a mythical expression of the undulating spinal column that extends from the earthbound tailbone to the heaven-bound crown of the head. They are the tiny deities, the animators of the fabulous Chinese dragon that lives in our soul with its turquoise fish tail swimming in the oceans of the instinctual animal body and its fiery crimson head facing upward toward the starlit regions of mind and spirit.

The breath body's movements do not follow the cyclical rounds of the Five Elements. Unlike the cycles of nature that go round and round, endlessly creating and destroying each other, the spirits follow a vertical trajectory as they move between the two poles of heaven and earth. Because of their breathy lightness and the pneumatic effect of their attraction to heaven, these psychic energies have a negentropic effect that lifts human beings up and beyond the downward pull of instinctual life. In this way, the spirits initiate the spiraling motion that permits the upgraded reorganization of alchemical or transformational healing.

The ancient Taoist alchemists referred to the spirits at the two poles of the pneumatic body as the hun and the po. The hun is the yang, cerebral, higher soul. The po is the yin, vital, lower soul. During a person's life, the hun and the po are in a dynamic dance as the qi, or breath of life, is polarized, first at one end and then at the other. As long as the qi continues to oscillate between the two poles of the subtle body, the natural forces of entropy are held in check and the human being continues to transform vital energy into psychic potency and vitality. But if the movement stops or the qi becomes bound at one end of the system or the other, the negentropic effect of the spirits drains away and psychological and physical disintegration follows.

The Five Spirits form a spinning axis of light that penetrates and illuminates our being. They are part of a complex alchemical system through which the divine is drawn down into our material lives and our material lives are lifted toward the divine. Beyond their function of animating and regulating the physical and psychic processes, the primary purpose of the spirits is to support the alchemical transformation of an ordinary human being into a spiritually enlightened sage.

Different wisdom traditions use different maps and symbols to describe the central axis of the breath body or vertical ridgepole of the self. In the Vedic tradition, this axis is represented by the sushumna, the ladder of the chakra system that runs from the bottom of the pelvis to the crown of the head. In the Hebrew mystical tradition, it is the Kabbalistic Tree of Life. In Chinese medicine, it is the conduits of the "Extraordinary" Acupuncture Meridians, the Governing and Conception Vessel, that run up and down the spine, and in the Taoist psychospiritual tradition the axis is Kunlun Mountain. Despite their differences, all these maps describe conduits and pathways that relate to the organs, glands and nervous system of the body and represent the tracings of vital psychic energies. These paths exist as qualitative experience between the real and the imaginable in the subtle body rather than as physical anatomical structures. They function to connect the material and spiritual aspects of our being through a web of psychic threads that cannot be apprehended with the ordinary five senses yet can be seen through the eyes of the imagination and known during heightened states of awareness. These psychic conduits support the animating breath of the life force—called qi in the Chinese tradition, prana in the Vedic, and quintessence in medieval alchemy—as it moves from spirit to matter and back again.

SPIRIT MOUNTAIN

In the dust-filled valleys and lowlands of our daily existence we have forgotten our connection with stars and suns; and so we need the presence of mountains—mighty milestones and signposts—to awaken us from the slumber of self-complacency. There are not many who hear the call or feel the urge under their thick blankets of petty self-interests, of money-getting, and of pleasure seeking. But the few who do form a perennial stream of pilgrims and keep alive throughout the ages the arcane knowledge of these terrestrial sources of divine inspiration.

—LAMA ANAGARIKA GOVINDA[3]

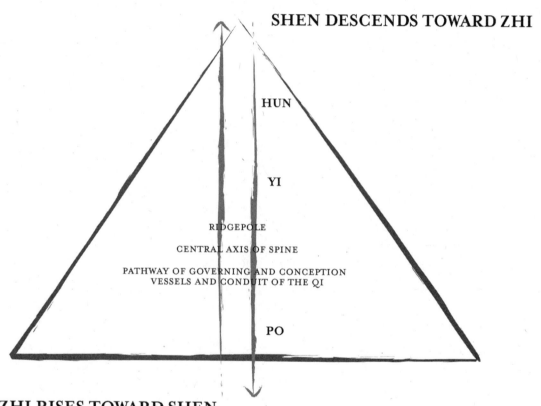

SHEN DESCENDS TOWARD ZHI

HUN

YI

RIDGEPOLE

CENTRAL AXIS OF SPINE

PATHWAY OF GOVERNING AND CONCEPTION
VESSELS AND CONDUIT OF THE QI

PO

ZHI RISES TOWARD SHEN

From a Taoist perspective, cosmology and psychology are fundamentally related. Taoists viewed the psyche as a reflection of the cosmos, as an inner world that mirrored the patterns and rhythms of the outer world. They imagined this inner world as a mountain inhabited by deities and spirits, the mountain a conduit of Tao, a numinous pivot that connected the human and celestial realms. The Five Spirits were the animating energies that transmitted the messages of the divine from heaven to earth and back again.

According to Stephen Little, Curator of Asian Art at the Art Institute of Chicago,

> The worship of sacred peaks can be traced as far back as the Shang dynasty (c. 1600–1050 BCE) . . . Mountains were venerated in China as numinous pivots connecting the human and celestial realms. Mountains were also seen as places in the terrestrial landscape where the primordial vital energy (qi) that created the world was particularly strong and refined . . . . Sacred mountains were also sites where one could find cavern-heavens (*dongtian*), grottoes deep in the earth that functioned as boundaries of the spirit world and gateways to paradise. . . . . It is especially significant that in religious Taoism, both the human body and the ritual altar are visualized as a mountain. Furthermore, the inner topography of the human body is perceived as populated by gods, who correspond to deities in the heavens. This imagery is fundamental to the Inner Alchemy (*neidan*) tradition.[4]

Taoist cosmology recognized five sacred mountains, one for each of the cardinal directions and for the center. Kunlun shan is the mountain in the middle, the empty center that is the spinning axis of the Taoist universe. In keeping with Taoist philosophy, this center was a point that was nowhere and everywhere at the same moment. For millennia, Kunlun Mountain traveled freely from one part of China to another, its geographic placement conveniently shifting as the centers of Chinese civilization moved from one province to another. But at the end of the nineteenth century, when Christian missionaries arrived in China, Kunlun Mountain finally settled down to a fixed location on a map—most likely because the missionaries succeeded in convincing the Chinese that mountains do not move and a center can only be at one place at one time.

Today, the name Kunlun is assigned to a range of desolate mountains on the western border between China and Tibet. The Kunlun Range is the original home of the Kunlun sect of Magical Taoism, a Taoist group of sorcerers, alchemists, and magicians who are heavily influenced by the Tibetan tantric tradition. The Kunlun sorcerers no longer live on Kunlun Mountain, but they continue to practice their rituals of healing and magic in Hong Kong, Taiwan, southern China, and southeast Asia. The mountain itself is abandoned and desolate.

But another Kunlun Mountain still remains. Shrouded in mists and dappled with shining groves of tea trees and gardenia flowers, this mountain continues to move from place to place and appears and disappears in dreams. This Kunlun Mountain is the mythical Taoist paradise. Deep below the surface of the earth, its caves and labyrinths burrow to the earth's core of fiery rivers. In the watery caves below the mountain, Xi Wang Mu, the Queen Mother of the West and the Goddess of Immortality, resides with her phoenix, the magical bird of death and resurrection. And Kunlun's snow-capped peak towers above the clouds, reaching to the stars and the realms of the gods. Here at the peak, in Kunlun City, are the palace and final resting place of Huang Di, the legendary Yellow Emperor. The lakes in the parks of the royal city are perpetually replenished by springs of yellow water laced with alchemical cinnabar, making immortal all who drink it.

To the ancient Chinese, high mountains were shrouded in mystery. They were unknown and unpredictable, their harsh and fickle weather conditions making them dangerous and inaccessible to all but the bravest adventurers. Mountains became symbolic of what lay beyond the veil of the visible world. Since the highest, most imposing were regarded as sacred, temples and shrines were built in their sheltered canyons, and stories and legends were told about the mystical occurrences that happened on their slopes.

Kunlun Mountain slipped easily back and forth between the world of matter and the world of dreams. The ancient Chinese regarded the mountain as the center of the world, the umbilicus of the universe, the connecting link between heaven and earth. Over centuries, Kunlun Mountain became a symbol for the unknowable wholeness of Tao, reflected in the unknowable mystery of the self. The paths along the mountain came to represent the paths we follow through life, the path of our destiny. The mountain is our being, the connecting link between our body, our spirit, our mind and our soul. The labyrinths below the mountain represent the primal, instinctual wisdom of our bodies while the North Star, which shines at the mountaintop, represents the speck of spirit whose light guides our journey from birth through life and back to our original nature.

Kunlun Mountain is a paradox. It exists both in and out of the world we know as real. The Mountain is and is not. It is ancient and it is not yet born. At the point of intersection of the four directions, the mountain is the unknowable empty center, the self that connects each of us to the whirling mystery of Tao.

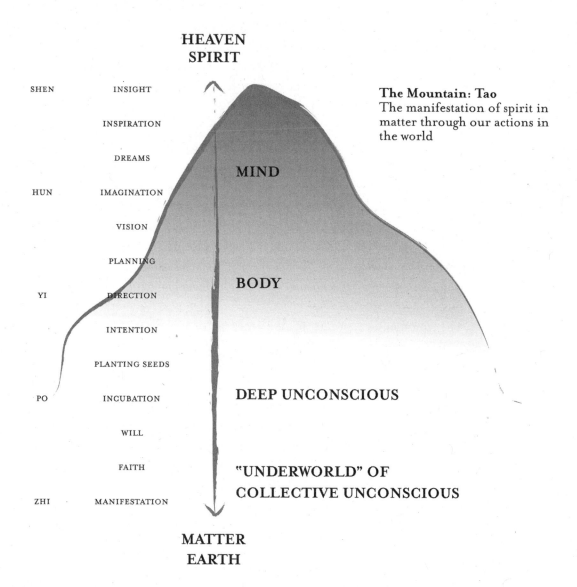

FIGURE 10: KUNLUN MOUNTAIN: SELF AS MOUNTAIN

HEAVEN
SPIRIT

SHEN   INSIGHT

INSPIRATION

DREAMS

MIND

HUN   IMAGINATION

VISION

PLANNING

YI   DIRECTION   BODY

INTENTION

PLANTING SEEDS

PO   INCUBATION   DEEP UNCONSCIOUS

WILL

FAITH   "UNDERWORLD" OF

ZHI   MANIFESTATION   COLLECTIVE UNCONSCIOUS

MATTER
EARTH

The Mountain: Tao
The manifestation of spirit in
matter through our actions in
the world

Keeping Still/Mountain

Hexagram #52 of the *I Ching* or *Book of Changes,* the much-revered ancient Chinese book of oracles, is called "*Ken / Keeping Still, Mountain*" and is described as an image of the centered person who has achieved a quiet heart and peaceful mind. In Taoist philosophy, this centered serenity is achieved through the practice of meditation or, in the words of the ancient text, by "keeping the back still." The commentary to this hexagram tells us that the mountain

> signifies the end and the beginning of all movement. The back is named because in the back are located all the nerve fibers that mediate movement. If the movement of these spinal nerves is brought to a standstill, the ego, with its restlessness, disappears as it were. When a man has thus become calm, he may turn to the outside world. He no longer sees in it the struggle and tumult of individual beings, and therefore he has that true peace of mind which is needed for understanding the great laws of the universe and for acting in harmony with them. Whoever acts from these deep levels makes no mistakes.[5]

The commentary points to the integral relationship between physical and mental processes that was clearly recognized by the ancient Chinese. By stilling the restless movements of the body, the agitation of the spinal nerves was quieted and the restlessness of the mind and heart was calmed. A person with a quiet heart could see beyond the endless desires of the personal ego. Such a person— referred to as a sage—could understand and act in harmony with Tao. Acting from this expanded viewpoint, the sage "makes no mistakes." Through every action, spirit manifests in matter and the way of heaven manifests on earth.

Kunlun Mountain

This legend of Kunlun Mountain provides a way to understand and make practical use of the Taoist alchemical ideas that are at the basis of traditional Chinese medicine. Kunlun Mountain was regarded as the mythical center of the Taoist cosmos, but like the vertical spinal column of the chakra system or the Sacred Tree of the Kabbalists, the mountain is actually an ancient representation of the self—a reflection in miniature of the divine wholeness of Tao.

According to the Taoist view, the self, like the mountain, extends in an uninterrupted continuum upward and downward between heaven and earth, spirit and matter. But over the past two thousand years through the influence of our Western, rational, analytic viewpoint, the mountain of the self has split into disconnected parts. While spirit and mind shine high above in the light of consciousness, matter and body have been shut away in the shadowy darkness of unconsciousness. Metaphorically, we could say that the mountain trails no longer lead from below to above. Alchemically, we could say that the interpenetration of heaven and earth, yang and yin, spirit and matter has been blocked and the cycles of life are drastically threatened. Yet the fundamental health of an organism depends on wholeness. The healthy ecology of the mountain requires communication between the dark caves and the bright summit, and our psychological health requires communication between our bodies and our minds, our unconscious and conscious processes.

The vision of the Five Spirits reminds me that "I" am the mountain. Like the mountain, I exist as a unity that reaches upward toward the bright, clear, fiery light of transpersonal consciousness and downward toward the fertile, swirling, watery darkness of the collective unconscious. Like the mountain, I exist at one pole as a single, bright peak, as conscious ego, as a unique point of recognizable individual identity. And at another pole, I exist as infinite, dark labyrinths, as unconscious instinctual impulses, as swirling, unrecognized collective drives. At one pole, I am yang fire; at the other, yin water. At both ends of the spectrum, I approach the divine. This vision of the unified psyche is beautifully expressed by C. G. Jung in his writing on the unconscious.

Water is the commonest symbol for the unconscious. . . .Water is the "valley spirit," the water dragon of Tao, whose nature resembles water—a yang embraced by a yin. Psychologically, therefore, water means spirit that has become unconscious. . . .The unconscious is the psyche that reaches down from the daylight of mentally and morally lucid consciousness into the nervous system that for ages has been known as the "sympathetic." This does not govern perception and muscular activity like the cerebrospinal system, and thus control the environment; but through functioning without sense-organs, it maintains the balance of life and, through the mysterious paths of sympathetic excitation, not only gives us knowledge of the innermost life of other beings but also has an inner effect upon them. In this sense it is an extremely collective system . . . whereas the cerebrospinal function reaches its high point in separating off the specific qualities of the ego."[6]

ALCHEMICAL TRANSFORMATION: DESCENDING THE MOUNTAIN

Unlike the wheel of the Five Elements, which begins in the yin darkness of the water, the journey of the Five Spirits begins in fire, in the infinite light of utmost yang, at the top of Kunlun Mountain, at the empty center of the universe, the spinning still point of the Pole Star. Their journey is initiated when the spirits are touched by the beauty of the yin essences of the earth and through this attraction the infinite activity of the yang comes under the influence of the limiting, downward-tending energies of entropy. At that moment, the descent of the Five Spirits begins.

Transformation occurs when the yang spirits enter the alchemical cauldron of the earth or of the human body, where they mix with the yin elements. Until the yang shen is called down to earth by the beauty of matter and the yin, it remains a perfect abstraction, with-

FIGURE 11: DESCENT OF THE FIVE SPIRITS

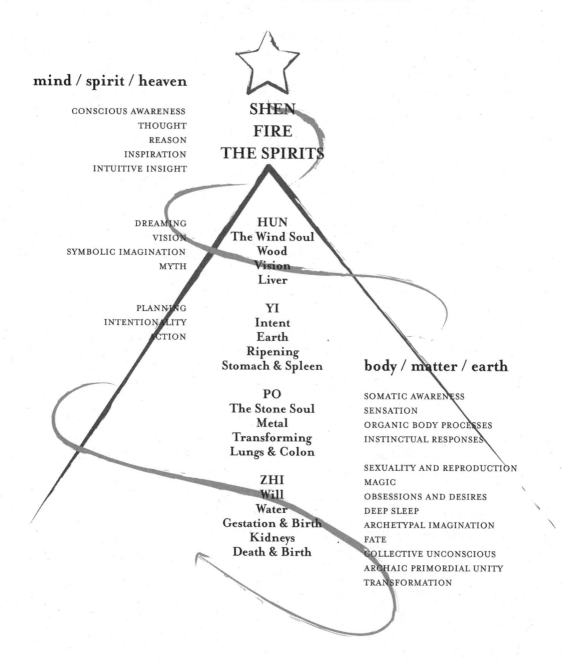

mind / spirit / heaven

CONSCIOUS AWARENESS
THOUGHT
REASON
INSPIRATION
INTUITIVE INSIGHT

SHEN
FIRE
THE SPIRITS

DREAMING
VISION
SYMBOLIC IMAGINATION
MYTH

HUN
The Wind Soul
Wood
Vision
Liver

PLANNING
INTENTIONALITY
ACTION

YI
Intent
Earth
Ripening
Stomach & Spleen

body / matter / earth

PO
The Stone Soul
Metal
Transforming
Lungs & Colon

SOMATIC AWARENESS
SENSATION
ORGANIC BODY PROCESSES
INSTINCTUAL RESPONSES

ZHI
Will
Water
Gestation & Birth
Kidneys
Death & Birth

SEXUALITY AND REPRODUCTION
MAGIC
OBSESSIONS AND DESIRES
DEEP SLEEP
ARCHETYPAL IMAGINATION
FATE
COLLECTIVE UNCONSCIOUS
ARCHAIC PRIMORDIAL UNITY
TRANSFORMATION

out heart or soul. The heart and soul of the divine come into being through the spirits' descent into the joys and suffering of time and space and life on earth. The ancient Taoists believed that the divine appeared when the sparkling, evanescent nothingness of the spirits mingled with the heavy, sweet, watery essences of the Mysterious Feminine, the yin elements of the earth. This alchemical marriage was for them the prerequisite for divinity: the crystallization of Tao living form, which the Taoists referred to as the "birth of the Golden Flower."

While this may seem beyond the scope of a human being's everyday life, we see the rising of the Golden Flower if we open our eyes to the true mystery of the healing process. When a bit of wisdom, insight or compassion sprouts up from the darkness of suffering, the spirits have been transformed by life on earth and something new and divine is born in human life. This birth comes only from "down below," from a willingness to descend to the realm of the underworld, to endure the suffering and not knowing of embodied healing.

This understanding led the ancient Chinese to a reverence for the yin—matter, the earth, nature and the body. They called the natural world the Mysterious Feminine and referred to it as the "visible face of Tao." Taoist alchemists believed that all transformation as well as all healing depended on the healer's ability to understand and work with the divine energies that stream through matter, which they recognized as the cauldron in which all alchemical processes occur. Only through our willingness to immerse ourselves in the cauldron of matter, to surrender to the powerful instinctual energies of the Mysterious Feminine, can we experience healing that is transformational, that results in ways of being more effectively, more authentically, and more gracefully who we truly are.

To experience this immersion, we begin our journey through the realm of the Five Spirits at the top of Kunlun Mountain. We begin with the North Star, the fiery home of the shen. As we move downward through the terrain of the spirits, we descend to deeper strata of the body, the psyche and the nervous system until we reach the deepest place of all, the abode of Xi Wang Mu, the Queen of the Underworld, the Goddess of Life, Death and Transformation, and the Mystical Sister of Taoist alchemy.

Descent is counter-intuitive or, in alchemical language, *contra natura*. It is a conscious decision to go against the natural flow, to turn away from expansion, freedom and the windy, sunlit heights of the upper spirits. When we descend, we turn away from the insights of the mind and from conscious control of our lives and environment. We go down backwards into the watery unknown of unconscious processes, back to our beginnings in the womb-like darkness of the body, the breath, the viscera and the sympathetic nervous system.

Following this downward path, we eventually encounter another aspect of the divine, the yin spirits. These lower spirits are responsible for the involuntary movements of the autonomic nervous system and the endless flux of the emotions and hold the key to psychospiritual transformation. Through them we experience the suffering, joys, losses and lessons of life on Earth. And through them we gain the compassion, embodied insight and wisdom that will bring us back to ourselves, transformed.

MOUNTAIN MEDITATION

In many Taoist alchemical practices, one's inner being is visualized as a lush mountain landscape populated by deities. The image of Kunlun Mountain is often used to channel energy through the spinal column down into the lower body, where it is made potent by the fires of the pelvis, and then back upward to the heart, where it is transformed into the light of wisdom and compassion.

For this meditation, you may sit in a chair or on a cushion on the floor. What matters is simply that the back is straight, forming a vertical axis between the top of the head and the bottom of the tailbone.

Begin the meditation by visualizing your body as the mythical Kunlun Mountain, your peak reaching up to heaven and your base planted deep in the earth. Feel the mountain's beauty and power, feel the mists swirling around you and the clear streams of water and light rushing through you. Now bring your awareness to the top of the head, the highest point of the mountain peak, the realm of King Mu, the King of the Eastern Sky and Emperor of the Rising Sun. Visualize a single star shining just a few inches above your head. Feel the light of this star pouring down on you in a radiant shower of liquid gold. This is the light of the shen spirit, the yang light of heaven and conscious awareness.

Feel the golden light of the shen drift down through your body, coming to rest in the space at the center of your heart. As you breathe into the heart space, visualize the shen spirit taking on form and color, drifting and changing like the mists and clouds on the mountainside. As the yang light of awareness grows moister and more yin, we enter the realm of the hun, the spirit of vision and imagination.

Follow the light as it drifts downward, coming to rest in the solar plexus. As you breathe into the solar plexus, feel the light gathering potency and weight as it descends toward earth. Feel the light take root in your belly like a seed taking root in the fertile valley at the mountain's edge. This is the realm of the yi, the spirit of embodied action and intention.

As your awareness drops deeper, it dips below the horizon line, down into the dark caves below the mountain, into the labyrinth of the viscera of the pelvic basin. Bring your awareness to a point about three inches below the umbilicus and take a moment to feel the powerful energies that reside there. This is the realm of the po, the yin spirit of the animal body, the breath and the autonomic nervous system.

Now go deeper as your awareness follows the labyrinths of the viscera deep below the mountain, down to the darkest cave, to a point at the base of the spine. Feel the energies that pulsate here, ebbing and flowing, as the tides of the cerebral spinal fluids expand and contract. Feel the darkness envelop you as the yang light of consciousness is swallowed in the dark ocean of the yin fluids of life. This is the realm of the zhi, the spirit of the collective unconscious, the Spirit of archetypes, cell memories, genetic codes, primal symbols and the luminous threads of fate that are the yin reflection of the Tao.

In the darkest cavern below the mountain, at the base of the spine, we come to the cinnabar throne of Xi Wang Mu. Here we come to the center of the alchemical mystery, the dark womb of the Mysterious Feminine. Now, breathe and wait and do nothing. Surrender to her power. As you breathe into the deepest, most hidden point of the body, you will gradually feel a tingling begin at the base of the spinal column. This tingling is the fire of the yin, the light that rises from down below, the fiery spring of the life force, the river of liquid light that gushes up from the heart of darkness.

Breathe this underworld fire upwards, up through the pelvis and the solar plexus. When it reaches the heart, feel the luminous yin fire of the zhi spirit mingle with the radiant yang light of the shen. As you breathe into the heart, feel the light pour in from above and below. As upper and lower lights mingle, you will feel subtle streams of pleasure radiate from the heart and fill your entire body. Compassion and love pour through you as you continue to breathe the two lights into your heart. You are now experiencing the sacred union, the alchemical marriage of yin and yang. Let the dance of this union continue as you open your eyes and let the light of the Five Spirits shine from your heart outward to the world.

Part II:

Descending the Mountain

師曰此經乃九天八會

道元始天尊昔經歷千

備生死五運遷變萬變

唐景雲之上上清之境

詳生火慈不舍吾

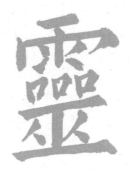

Introduction to Part II

[The adept wishes to] dwell forever on the summits of the Great Void, in the Chamber of the Precious Palace; in the morning to take his pleasure with the Jade Emperor and in the evening to rest with the Mysterious Mother, when thirsty, to drink his fill among the jade plants of the Immense Spring of Lang Well on the cosmic Mount Kunlun.

—SHANQING TEXT[1]

To the ancient Taoists, Kunlun Mountain was the still point or center pole of the spinning world as Tao was the still point of the spinning cosmos. In the inner world, the mountain was regarded as the center pole of the self. It was related to the brain and nervous system and recognized as a miniature expression of Tao within. This inner mountain was a metaphoric expression of the vertical axis of the spinal column, the conduit through which human nervous and spiritual energies flowed between heaven and earth. The mountain within was the terrain of inner alchemy and psychospiritual transformation. Aligning the spine meant aligning the mountain. Aligning the mountain meant aligning earth with heaven and human life with Tao.

Taoists regarded Kunlun Mountain as the home of the deities and a place of retreat and revelation. Similarly, the mountain within was regarded as the home of wushen, the Five Spirits.

The system of the Five Spirits is a symbolic representation of human consciousness. Each spirit presides over a particular aspect of the nervous system, a specific form of awareness and a precisely defined level of the psyche. Each spirit not only has its own function and terrain but also functions as an expression of the divine in human life.

In Part II, we follow in the footsteps of the Taoist alchemists as they journey up and down Kunlun Mountain. The book will take you on a journey, a vision quest that will help you, like the sage, to discover the sacred mountain that is a symbolic expression of your inner self. In the process, you will gradually discover ways to bridge the gaps between your spirit, your mind and your body. Through traversing this mountain, you will rediscover the innate wholeness of who you are. You will come to understand the connection of your being to the earth beneath your feet and the heavens above your head. In addition, you will learn how:

- to use an understanding of your own inner landscape to gently guide the unfolding of your destiny
- to become an alchemist, a transformer of your own life
- to consciously interpret the wisdom of your body
- to heal psychological and psychosomatic symptoms and resolve emotional conflicts in new, holistic ways
- to enhance the effectiveness of your actions
- to commit to your own visions
- to get more of what you want from your life and your relationships
- to know when to do nothing but wait and make room for the mystery

Each of the five chapters in Part II focuses on one individual spirit as well as how the system of the Five Spirits works to integrate the body and the mind. Each chapter includes:

- A description of the spirit and its relationship to the natural environment
- An introduction to the spirit and its territory on the inner mountain of the self
- A look at the related Chinese character
- A list of associations and correlations, including the element, organ, emotion, psychological function and psychospiritual issue related to the spirit
- A description of the physical, emotional and psychospiritual problems and symptoms related to the spirit
- Suggestions about how to work with the spirit
- An in-depth case study that demonstrates the problems that can come up when a spirit is disturbed and the process through which the spirit can be healed and psychospiritual vitality restored to a person's life

In the alchemical traditions, it was believed that transformational processes occur when the yang spirits of heaven descend into the alchemical cauldron of matter where they mix with the yin essences of earth. For this reason, the chapters of Part II follow a downward trajectory and are arranged according to a pattern of descent from heaven to earth, spirit to matter.

Our journey begins at the top of Kunlun Mountain, at the North Star, the fiery home of the shen. In Chapter Six, we will explore the Spirit of Fire, the psychological counterpart of the sun and the stars that shower the mountain with golden light. The shen represent the function of conscious awareness, insight and illumination. They inform and direct the cosmos of the human psyche and maintain the integrity of individual identity.

Following our downward path, in Chapter Seven, we encounter another aspect of the divine, the hun, the winged messengers of the shen. The hun are the spirit of wood, the psychological counterpart of the breezes and winds of the mountain cliffs. Through their wind-like nature, the airy hun blow the light of the shen into our lives in the form of visions, foresight, dreams and imagination.

Midway down the mountain, in Chapter Eight, we come to yi, the spirit of the earth. The yi are the psychological counterpart of the fertile fields and rich soil of the mountain meadows. The yi endow us with intention and purpose and give us the ability to plant our ideas into our actions so that they can manifest as the harvest of our lives.

In Chapter Nine, we drop below the horizon line and enter the domain of po. At this level, the psychic functions of the upper realms—our inspiration, vision and intention—are buried below the ground, in the underworld of the body, the unconscious and the involuntary responses of the autonomic nervous system. In this darkness "beneath" the earth, the golden light of spirit descends into the underworld, where it crystallizes and hardens and waits in silence. Here, outside of time, the light endures in a death sleep and burial that is the prerequisite for its transformation and rebirth.

As we descend to the labyrinths at the lowest depths of moun-tain caves, we enter the realm of the zhi, the spirit of water. The zhi are the psychological counterpart of the thermal geysers, the fiery springs that spurt up from the darkness at the center of the under-world. They represent the potent energies of the instincts, the forces of sexuality and survival. The zhi open the door to the palace of the dark goddess, the place of transformation and return, where yin becomes yang and inert matter comes back to life. Thus, in the place of deepest darkness, our return journey to the light begins.

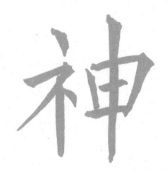

Chapter Six

Shen: The Spirit of Fire—Inspiration, Insight, Awareness and Compassion

> We know that the *shen* are the messengers of Heaven. . . . Heaven is
> not in myself without some kind of intermediary and the intermedi-
> ary between Heaven and myself is *shen*.
>
> —CLAUDE LARRE[1]

POLARIS

I am alone in the darkness, with only the garbled songs of
frogs in the woods and the hollow whoosh of waves in the
cove. When I look up, I am less than a speck beneath a black
sky whirling with stars. On a summer night in Maine, when I step
outside the back door of my house, I am swept up in a chaos of con-
stellations and galaxies interspersed with meteors and vapor clouds.

In the midst of this circus of lights, always shining in exactly the
same place, just at the tip of the Arnie McGraw's chimney, is Polaris,
the North Star. It's not very glamorous at first sight. It's not one of
the brightest stars in the sky. But, unless the clouds or mists have

come in from the sea, this little star is always where I left it, pointing reliably to the north.

When I need to find my bearings in the night, I look for the bowl of the Big Dipper and follow the line of the pointer stars to Polaris. This is the pole star, the pivot point, the still center around which the night sky turns. Once I have found it, I know where I am and which direction to go next.

But when I need to orient myself in the swirling confusion of my life, the tumult of desires, possibilities, expectations, hopes and dreams, I look to the star within me, the guiding light of my own heart. The ancient Chinese regarded this inner guiding light as the light of the shen, the heart spirit, the most yang, heavenly aspect of the Five Spirits. According to myth, this light is a spark of heavenly fire that comes to us at birth directly from the stars.

Just as we look to Polaris to discover true north, so we look within to the light of the heart to discover our direction in life. The shen, the shining light of spirit, will always guide us reliably if we take the time to listen. And as the Pole Star directs us to true north, the shen will always direct us toward Tao, the path of our true nature.

According to modern astronomy, the entire universe began with starlight. The first star that exploded from pre-cosmic nothingness provided the ingredients that eventually became the basic elements of all that is. So we are star people and the world we inhabit is made of stars. The shen are the star spirits that connect human beings with the cosmos.

THE SHEN

If we look at the map of Kunlun Mountain, we find the shen at the highest point. They are the starlight and sunlight that stream down from the sky and illuminate the mountaintop. They inhabit the realm of the divine fire of the sun and the initiatory energies of dawn, the home of King Mu, the king of the eastern sky.

In Taoist tradition, it is said that when the yang and yin essences of the parents unite at the moment of conception, the star seeds of the shen are scooped up in the ladle of the Big Dipper and poured down into the heart of the developing embryo. In the alchemical vessel of the heart, this pure light mixes with the essences of earth and eventually becomes the stuff of awareness, intelligence and consciousness as well as the basis of our own unique sense of self.

The light seed of the shen first sprouts when a child is about three months old, when the smile reflex signals the infant's first delighted recognition of the parent as an "other," a discreet and separate being. At the same time as the other is identified, the first, embryonic inkling of "I" comes into being. This moment is marked by the appearance of a new luminosity in the child's eyes, the bright light of recognition and conscious awareness.

This sprouting of the shen is the first break in the wholeness of Tao. It is the beginning of the journey of individual life—the journey away from original nature that eventually leads back to Tao and a new, more complex wholeness. If all goes well, this sprouting of the shen seed is imbued with feelings of joy, delight, love and wonder, all of which will mark the eventual return to wholeness when the tiny seed of the shen eventually grows into the great tree of the self.

During our life, the shen resides in the empty center of the heart, where it continues to grow as it guides us along our path through life. Although it is invisible, its presence is reflected in the light that shines from the eyes of a healthy human being. In the presence of healthy shen, there is a luster and brightness to the disposition, a feeling of connection and awareness. Most of all, the presence of healthy shen results in a life that is uniquely suited to the individual and a person whose actions make sense within the context of the surrounding environment.

The shen in their purest form are divine light. They are the first intimation of possibility, the first "wink of an eye," intuition, insight, the light bulb that goes on in the brain, the "got it!" that "gets" a whole project in a flash. They are the bright idea, the illuminated understanding that sets the course for the long journey to come. Shen is the electric current of the lightning bolt that initiated the first spark of life in the primordial waters. As pure yang, pure light, the shen are energy without mass. Faster than sound, faster than anything we can know, shen is spirit, the closest we can come to knowing what is essentially unknowable.

WHAT IS SHEN?

The Five Spirits are the finest, most ephemeral expressions of qi. Each spirit represents an aspect of awareness and consciousness, and as aspects of consciousness, all are expressions of the element of fire and all come under the jurisdiction of the heart, the center point of human awareness. So in a way, all the spirits are shen!

But when we speak of the individual spirit shen, we are speaking of the most yang, most fiery aspect of the Five Spirits. During our life, the shen are said to reside in the heart. At death, they rise up through the crown of the head and return to the distant starry realms they came from.

The Chinese character *shen* has several meanings. While they are interrelated, each meaning has its own particular use. Shen can mean

- **spirit as infinite cosmic light** outside and beyond the scope of human experience

- **the yang energy that enlivens the psyche.** Therefore, as a generic term, *shen* is used to refer to all of the Five Spirits.

- **the activity of thinking, consciousness, insight and memory,** all of which are related to xin, the heartmind

- **an intangible yet recognizable quality of luminous vitality that is seen in a healthy human being**. The shen manifests in the radiance that shines from the eyes and a vibrant, flourishing quality of the complexion.

- **spirit, god, deity or divinity.** It is the spirit of enlightened awareness, inspiration, insight and love that comes to us from the divine.

- **the name given to one specific expression of the Five Spirits,** the finest, most active, most yang of the five, and the one closest to the realm of heaven. In this case, it refers to the fiery, yang spark of conscious awareness that is said to reside in the human heart.

(Because of the nature of the Chinese language, the same character can be used as a singular or plural noun. In the case of the shen, the same character is used to mean all the infinite bits of golden light that shower down on earth from heaven as well as the single infinitesimal speck of divine light that illuminates the human heart. For this reason, in the text, we will at times use shen as a plural and sometimes as a singular noun. This same rule will apply to all of the Five Spirits.)

A Look at the Chinese Character

The character for *shen* is formed of two parts. *Shih,* the radical on the left, means "altar," "to divine" or "influences from above." *Shen*, the radical on the right, means "to extend or expand."

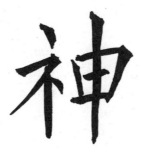

Shen

The radical on the left, *shih*, was once pictured as seen here on the left, and progressed to the character on the right:

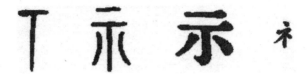

The two parallel horizontal lines at the top of a character mean "high" or "superior." In this radical, they specifically mean "heaven." The three vertical lines hanging down from the heavens represent the heavenly lights, the sun, the moon and the stars, which reveal the distinctions of life to human beings and illuminate our way, the path that will lead us back to wholeness and Tao.

Shih symbolizes the "celestial influxes from heaven," "the signs by which the will of heaven is known to mankind." An altar is the horizontal plane on which the influxes of heaven extend down towards the earth. The "diviner" is the sage through whom the influxes of heaven are voiced or made visible on earth. This character is sometimes translated simply as "to divine."

The second element of the character *shen* was originally a picture of two hands extending a rope, thus the idea of something reaching or extending. For example, lightning or a thunderbolt is a storm cloud extending itself toward earth.

Combining the two elements of the character—shih and shen— gives us shen, the heavenly light that extends itself downward through spirit. The shen "gives the orders" that precipitate each human life. But the shen also gives us our "heavenly mandate": It is the "heavenly star" that is the guiding light of our individual destiny. In this way the shen is both our origin and our destination. It has to

do with the shedding of light, the gift of perception and conscious-·
ness. The coming and going of the shen mark the beginning and end
of a person's life.

Shen is the seed mantra "I am," which is the initiatory spark of
human self-awareness. It is pure potentiality, the breath or active
impulse that initiates, instills and maintains the appearance of a particular human form. But if we look again at the character, we see
that shen is also the way that the light of heaven extends itself into
us and then through us to manifest through our actions on earth.
Shen is the extension of the light of the cosmos through us. The shen
or active spirits in heaven give us signs that help us to "see" or
"divine" which way to go to keep to our path of Tao.

ASSOCIATIONS AND CORRELATIONS

Shen is related to:

Element: fire
Organ: heart
Emotion: joy
Psychological function: awareness, inspiration, insight
Psychospiritual issue: knowing true self
Cosmological associations: starlight, lightning
Chakra: seventh—Thousand Petal Lotus: Enlightened Mind
Alchemical virtues: compassion and love

Organ Correspondence

During our lives, the shen are said to reside in emptiness at the center of the heart. From a Chinese medical perspective, the heart is not

only a physical organ but also the emperor/empress, the "supreme sovereign" of the body and the mind. The heart, as sovereign, is responsible for the circulation of the blood and the overall state of the emotions as well as the well-being of the shen.

In ancient China, things with similar functions were looked upon as aspects of a single unity. The heart—as organizer of all aspects and activities of the bodymind—performed the same function as the emperor of a kingdom. The emperor of a kingdom performed the same function as the sun, the still point, like Polaris, around which the solar system turns and an entire whirling universe spins. Polaris, sun, emperor and heart are united by their centering, organizing function. Each holographically contains the other, and at the center of them all is a golden light, the light of the shen, the scintillant spark of spirit.

Heart, emperor, sun and North Star control, harmonize and unify an infinite number of separate individual energies. This task of joining the many into a single unity while allowing each to retain its own particularity is accomplished by each of them in the same way: wuwei, the way of emptiness. It is the way of wisdom, the way of the sage. Zen meditators, tai ch'i artists and calligraphers, Native American shamans and the very greatest African dancers know this way of being, this way of the heart, this way of paradox where the most powerful doing is accomplished by doing nothing at all. It is the way that heaven extends itself effortlessly into the environment through the illumination of the shen.

Through wuwei, the heart is able to pump blood effortlessly through the body for the span of a human lifetime. Through wuwei, the heart coordinates and organizes every aspect of the bodymind. Thus the greatest emperors' rule their kingdoms without effort, simply by maintaining their position of perfect equilibrium between earth and heaven. Sunlight informs the vibrancy and movement of every aspect of life, yet the sun itself does nothing but hold steady while the light of its fire showers the solar system with energy and the pull of its gravitational weight locks each planet in perfect orbit. Similarly, the North Star shines motionless at the hub or pivot point of the night sky as the stars spin in the great echoing silence of eternity. Such a "form of government," writes Lao Tzu, "is what people hardly even realize is there."

According to Hindu science, the element of the heart chakra is air. In her book about the chakra system, Anodea Judith describes the heart's relationship to air. She says that air implies space and a certain kind of emptiness. It represents freedom, as shown by the birds that fly.[2] In the airy space of the heart, there is room to breathe, room for the self and the reflection of another. The airy space of the heart is the space of wuwei, the space of emptiness, the space of unknowing and of awe. It is into this empty silence that the shen come like birds alighting on a branch at dawn. Without this spaciousness the spirits will flee and the light of the divine will no longer illuminate our consciousness and actions. In such a state, a desperate effort to control the environment replaces the effortless nondoing of wuwei wisdom. In this state, the empress cannot fulfill her crucial organizing functions on the physical, psychological and environmental levels.

EMOTIONAL AGITATION AND THE HEART

The shen are yang. They are polarized toward heaven and their natural tendency is anti-gravitational and negentropic. In their book *The Heart,* Claude Larre and Elisabeth Rochat de la Vallée describe the shen as a precious, wild bird. Like birds, "the shen are free to come and go, to come into myself or to quit this place and to fly away. . . . The shen go up, they want to go back to heaven."[3] Unless they are entranced and nurtured by the yin essences of the earth, the shen rise up and fly off, back to the heavenly realms. In a healthy human being, the yin lower spirits magnetize the yang shen downward, allowing them to rest in the inviting hollow of the heart space. In order to maintain a suitable resting place for the shen, the heart must remain in a state that is close to its original nature, serene, accepting and open. The light of the shen radiates from such a tranquil heart to illuminate the lives of all those it touches.

If the precious wild birds of the spirit burst prematurely from the heart, the light of the shen will no longer be present to guide and inform the movements of qi. All bearings lost, the breaths of qi become chaotic, the fire of the heart grows dim and we wander in a daze from one meaningless project to the next, wondering how we found ourselves in this or that predicament. No matter how we try, nothing can fill the emptiness that is left once the spirits have departed. Life on earth is filled with events that elicit powerful emotions, but according to the Taoist tradition, the sage or wise one does not become overly attached to these passing storms. Rather, the sage's one and only concern is maintaining the tranquility of the heart so that the luminous wild birds of the shen will have a suitable resting place. As long as the shen remain in the heart space, the direction of our lives will be clear and our paths will be illuminated. Through wuwei we will naturally and effortlessly create order and harmony in our environment.

When strong emotions come, the way of the sage is not to try to stop them but to observe their rushing passage. We watch them from the top of a high hill, as we might view the magnificent passing of towering thunderclouds on a rainy summer evening. In this way, we can allow emotions to move through us while still maintaining our serenity.

Chuang Tzu, one of the great early Taoist sages, describes the heart as a reflecting pool. When this pool is calm and still, it is "the mirror of heaven and earth, the glass of the ten thousand things."[4] In this state, the heart reflects the truth, beauty and intrinsic order of the cosmos as an undisturbed pool of water reflects the forest glade. The movements of our lives will be based on this accurate observation of the world around us. But when the heart is disturbed by violent emotion, it is like the wind-tossed sea. All images are fragmented and unclear, and the truth of heaven and earth cannot be perceived. Actions taken at such a time of fragmentation will only further the confusion and unrest. However, if we hold ourselves back from action and do not get attached to the emotions as they pass, then the heart will grow calm again like water after a storm and can once again reflect the truth and wisdom of the Tao.

SIGNS AND SYMPTOMS OF SHEN DISTURBANCE

Common Symptoms

insomnia

dream-disturbed sleep

anxiety

palpitations

inability to concentrate

timidity, being easily startled

being overly talkative

forms of schizophrenic mania

incoherence

hyperactivity

restlessness

Spirit Level Signs

- lack of coherence to life; the person's personality does not fit the life he or she is living

- lack of inspiration and insight; "deadness"; no "heart and soul" to life

- no sense of unique person with a unique path; "ambivalence"

- much activity but no center so activity turns to anxiety, restlessness and, eventually, fatigue

- no ability to discern what is truly "right for me"

- no self-reflection

- inability to distinguish true from false, real from unreal

Possible Causes

- constitutional or "karmic" issues that are part of person's "work" in this lifetime

- "narcissistic injuries": parents who couldn't see the child and consistently inhibited the expression of true nature

Anything that upsets the heart upsets the shen! Emotional trauma, shock and abuse can cause a shen disturbance, as can recreational drugs such as cocaine, nicotine, and amphetamines.

HEALING THE SHEN

In Chinese medicine, when we say that the shen is disturbed, we are saying that a person's consciousness is disrupted; the mind is not at ease. This is one of the most commonly used descriptions of psychological and emotional disturbances. No matter what the causes and no matter what the specific symptoms, a person whose shen is disturbed exhibits an odd energy and generally elicits uneasiness in those around him. It is exactly the opposite atmosphere to that produced when the shen are in harmony and the light of divine is reflected in the material world.

When a person's shen is disturbed, the light in the eyes (a reflection of the light of the shen of the heart) may be dim, as if the person is not really present, or it may be strangely bright with a hard-edged glitter. Making real contact is difficult. Another characteristic is frequent, inappropriate laughter or other signs of a split between the content of a person's conversation and their emotion/affect. Nightmares and sleep disorders are also common. People whose shen is disturbed are like a candle in the wind, at one moment flaming with a wild brightness, sputtering down to near extinction the next. There is no steadiness, no reliability, no sense of a stable identity. Nonetheless, people with a propensity to these disturbances are often fiery, bright, charismatic, fun and full of creative ideas. They live intensely, very close to the edge of their skin.

The shen flickers like starlight. Like the fire element it is related to, the shen responds quickly to stimulus. In my experience, the shen moves more quickly than any of the other energies of the bodymind. When using needles, it is extremely important not to over-treat. The fragile flame can all too easily be extinguished by too much stimulation. By understanding the nature of this quick-moving, fiery energy of consciousness, however, it is possible to help someone feel better within moments. Trained acupuncturists can use needles, non-professionals can safely use certain teas in highly diluted potencies, but even without needles or herbs, it is possible to settle the shen simply by helping a person bring the fiery energy of awareness down from the yang domain of the mind (the head) to the more yin matrix of the body. If the shen is disturbed by acute shock or intense emotion, it will often respond very quickly to gentle, conscious touch or a well-placed word of comfort.

The shen spirit has a special relationship to the element of fire. In the *I Ching*, we read that *li*, fire, relates to the sun. It dwells in the eyes and is the divine substance that protects us against evil forces. Fire is related to intuition, to magical wands and to spiritual transformation. Like fire the shen respond quickly to subtle stimulus. Like fire, the light of the shen flares up quickly, disappears, and then flickers up again. Sometimes a thought, even unspoken, is enough to set them moving. They respond to insight and to laughter but most of all they respond to being recognized, to being seen, to being illuminated by the light of another being's eyes.

WAYS TO HEAL AND CULTIVATE THE SHEN SPIRIT

The first and most important step in working with the shen is the realization that we are working with a living, vibrant substantiated light that responds to being seen and related to.

When there has been a shock to the shen, an upsetting experience or emotional trauma that has frightened the birds of the spirit away from their nest in the heart space, we as healers must embody the energy of the ling. We are the sorceresses beckoning the cooling rains down from the clouds, calling the scattered spirits back to the realm of matter. Meditating on a candle cradled in a ruby red votive glass is a good way to begin this process since red, the alchemical *rubedo*, is the color symbolic of the marriage of spirit and soul in the palace of the Heart.

You might begin by placing the hands gently and with consciousness on the body. This invites the shen to settle back into the matrix of the material world. A gentle foot massage with olive or almond oil or careful, intentional touch or energy work around the heart chakra may also help, but sometimes the most effective method is to call the awareness back into the body by asking the person to simply notice what is going on in the legs, the tantian (the cinnabar field of the lower abdomen), and the edges of the skin where their body meets the surrounding environment. Since consciousness follows the direction of awareness, relocating the focus will often be enough to shift physiology, to soften the breathing, normalize the heart rate and thus settle the disturbed shen.

In addition, Bach Flower Rescue Remedy is very effective for shock and disturbances of the shen. A few drops administered under the tongue every few hours until the person feels calm can help enormously. Rescue Remedy is available in most health food stores and even some pharmacies that sell homeopathic remedies.

Once the shen has settled back into the heart, it is important to give it some space. Encourage the person to rest for a few moments without talking (talking tends to stir the shen and may not be helpful immediately after this kind of treatment). Quiet music, peaceful sounds coming through an open window, and non-intrusive relatedness are all good ways to close the treatment and make a transition back into the world. This shift in awareness can be done anywhere, any time. It is a gift we can offer to ourselves and to others.

OUR COLLECTIVE CRISIS OF THE HEART

According to the psychology of the ancient Chinese, the heart is the mediator between above and below, within and without. Because of its position at the boundary and shuttle point between realms, it is the shock absorber that bears the brunt of our emotional agitations. Although it is scrupulously protected by the pericardium or heart protector and other ministers of protection and defense, the level of shock that is prevalent in our modern world has increased far too rapidly for the bodymind to evolve adequate psychological protection. The result is that many people actually exist from day to day in a state of numbed-out, unconscious shock and disassociation from the self, in Zen Master Robert Aitken's words, "rationalizing themselves into insensitivity."[5]

We live in a world where assaults to the heart come at us from every direction. Violence is all around us, if not in our immediate environment, then constantly tapping at the windows of our lives in the form of images in movies, on TV and in the newspapers. The endless, impersonal strain of modern culture creates an atmosphere that is the antithesis of the atmosphere required for the heart's tranquility. The delicate fire of the shen has been nearly extinguished by the garish, artificial lights and harsh noises of our technological world. This state of desensitization and objectification of our selves and our world is accompanied by tight breathing, contracted chests and closed hearts. In such a state, the illumination of the shen is at best a dim and distant memory. That most of us are cut off from the light of our hearts and the ability to see with clear, true sight hampers attempts to solve our problems on a personal or global level.

We see symptoms that result from the ongoing attacks upon the shen and the shutting down of the energies of the heart in every aspect of daily life. Psychologically, we are plagued by a lack of closeness and intimacy in our relationships and a lack of meaning in our lives. Physically, heart disease is the deadliest of all killers in our country, taking the lives of more than seven hundred thousand people every year. And beyond the realm of personal suffering, our inability to see the world around us with the eyes of our hearts results in the abuse and destruction of our living environment.

The sacred wild birds, the lights of the shen, have fled, not only from the hearts of individual human beings but from the heart of Western culture. In our perpetual shock, we are blind to the true light of the living world. The more we rush about, vainly searching for solutions to our innumerable problems, the further we get from the answers that might well be waiting for us in the tranquil, empty silence of our hearts. But if we take a moment to sit quietly and turn the light of awareness inward to the heart, the shen will return to guide us forward on our path.

CASE HISTORY: LITTLE RUSHING IN— THE SLEEPLESS POET

The following case history is as an example of how an acupuncturist can use needles to work with the shen. It is one of those peculiar but true acupuncture "miracles" that makes no sense from the perspective of Western science, conventional medicine or psychology and yet makes perfect sense from the perspective of the synthetic, right-brain logic of Chinese medicine.

Phil arrived at my office looking harried and disheveled. His hair was standing up from his head in thin wind-blown silver spikes, his cheeks were flushed, and his bright blue eyes sparkled a bit crazily from behind his glasses. I think he could best be described as the typical absentminded professor, and I have to say I fell in love with him the moment he walked through my office door. Within minutes we were discussing the poetry of Shakespeare, Milton, Pound and Mary Oliver. Following his short but brilliant course in the history of modern poetry, Phil treated me to an improvised dissertation on dogs that was akin to the ravings of a *New Yorker* essayist on a late-night bender.

I quickly realized this man could talk a mean streak and keep me laughing, but if I was going to help him I needed to make a radical intervention! Underneath his zany, captivating intellect, there was a feeling of confusion and enervation.

I finally managed to get Phil focused on why he had come to see me. Intractable insomnia was the first symptom he mentioned, insomnia so bad that he had given up on sleeping at all and just watched television until three or four o'clock in the morning while semi-reclining in his armchair. Phil told me that he was in the middle of writing a book, which always "made things worse." The "things" that got worse turned out to be red, painful sores on his tongue and a habit, which had plagued him since adolescence, of chewing the skin at the sides of his mouth until it was raw and bleeding.

I felt that herbs and acupuncture would probably help with his sleep problems as well as the sores on his tongue, but getting to the root of his compulsive habit was a long shot. However, it didn't take me long to make a diagnosis. Phil was a classic case of "rising fire of the heart" and disturbed shen. The heat was showing up in the red, painful canker sores; the shen disturbance manifested in his entertaining but compulsive conversation, his insomnia and the energetic impulses behind his self-inflicted injuries to his mouth.

On a psychological level, Phil was suffering from a painful malaise. His busy mind and cleverness were a fragile cover for a lack of meaning, coherence and intimacy in his life. His spirit (consciousness) was over-fired to the point of burnout. It was like a flame sputtering wildly on its last bit of oil. There was no place of quiet wisdom, no orderly space of ritual, no cooling waters where his shen could settle and rest, so this energy rose and fueled the tension and heat in Phil's mouth. He turned the fiery agitation and frustration of his heart inward in the way that young, poorly nurtured children sometimes do, mutilating himself as a form of perverse self-soothing. I felt strongly that what he needed was an opening, a doorway between his heart and the world, in part to let the steam out and release the excess rising fire from his body but also to create a conduit through which the energies of the shen could return to his heart.

I asked Phil to lie down on the table and explained to him about the diagnosis I had made. As a poet, he appreciated the metaphoric nature of Chinese medical language and was struck by how the phrase "rising fire of the heart" so accurately described how he felt.

I told Phil that I was going to insert a needle into a point at the corner of the nail of his little finger. I explained that the translated name of the point was "Little Rushing In" and that the rushing referred to the qi that rushed through the meridians at the fingertips. This point would clear the excess heat that had accumulated in the heart meridian, which was causing the sores in his mouth, but at the same time it would settle his shen and calm the agitation of his mind.

Phil lay back but he didn't relax. He watched carefully as I located and applied alcohol to the points. As I inserted the first tiny needle into the point on his left hand, he continued watching. No sooner did the needle make contact with the qi than a smile came to his face. His body relaxed and his breathing pattern shifted. I walked around the table and needled the same point on the other hand then turned away for a moment while I disposed of the used needle. I knew that the points at the tips of the fingers could have powerful, almost instantaneous effects but I didn't expect to see what I saw when I turned back to check on Phil—he was sound asleep!

Phil slept for the remainder of the session. When he woke up, he looked different. The patches of red on his cheekbones were dispersed and his eyes were focused. "I can't believe this!" he said. "I haven't felt this relaxed in years. Hey! Can I just move in here?"

A week later, Phil came back. He still looked like a professor but not nearly as absentminded. He told me that he had slept three or four hours every night since the treatment. His mouth sores were getting better. Most amazingly, he said, he had almost completely stopped biting the sides of his mouth. "I can't understand it," he said, "but somehow it just stopped. My body doesn't want to do it any more."

Over time, the sores in his mouth improved. For several months he took a low dose of herbs to continue clearing the rising fire from his gums and tongue. He still worked until late at night, but he usually slept at least five to six hours after he was done. He no longer stayed up all night watching TV and began instead to take a half-hour walk after he finished writing. He said he had forgotten how beautiful the sky was at night and enjoyed looking at the stars. He started a series of poems about his late-night rambles through the sleeping suburban streets that were published a few years after I met him.

Phil made a habit of coming to see me every few months, even after his problems were more or less "cured." He claimed he came in for a "tune up," not only because he "needed the rest" but because he got new ideas for poems from the names of the acupuncture points! And he added that since he had started acupuncture he saw, for the first time in his life, a reason for having a body.

In this case study, healing resulted from releasing the agitated emotions and energies from the heart space so that the shen could settle in the "nest" or crucible of matter and illuminate Phil's life. In this way, communication was reestablished between body and mind and the light of heaven could extend downward to manifest through identity in action in the world.

BEING WITH YOUR HEART LIGHT:
CHECKING IN WITH THE SHEN

"Checking in with your shen" is simple and yet easily forgotten, especially in the midst of emotional upset or the excitement of a new project. However, it is a good idea, any time you are beginning something important, entering a new relationship or just starting out the day, to take a moment to notice how the shen feel about what you are up to.

This is actually not as mysterious as it may seem. Even without learning to meditate or to do inner visualizations, you can make it a practice to note how you feel when you think about a particular person or project. Are you relaxed, infused with a steady, gentle warmth? Or are you jumpy and agitated? Is your excitement like the quick flash of a match (that will soon burn itself out), or is it a flame that glows steadily and grows as you continue to move along this path?

You know your shen are disturbed if you experience anxiety or palpitations when you think of a particular person, project or idea. If your sleep becomes disturbed by upsetting dreams or if you can't sleep, your shen are probably trying to tell you something. If you feel muddled and confused when you think about this issue . . . oops, you know the birds of clear awareness have flown the coop! Take some time out. Don't move forward until you have clarity. Walk. Breathe. Get calm and wait until the shen have settled down before making any important decisions.

Pay attention to the voices in your head. After a while, you may recognize one that is like a clear bell, not loud but somehow brighter than the others. This is the voice of the shen, the voice that organizes the others into a pattern that makes sense. This voice may come as a flash of intuitive knowing ("I don't know how I knew to stop at the post office at just that moment!") or of sudden insight ("I get it! That's what I need to do to pull this party together"), or as a gradually gathering clarification of an unclear situation.

Avoid repeatedly returning to situations or relationships that you know disturb your emotions or your mental clarity.

If you have had life experiences or used substances that have damaged or upset the shen, seek the help of a licensed, well-trained acupuncturist to help you clear the heart so your spirit birds can return to the nest.

If you are taking prescription medication that makes you feel muddled, unclear or lacking joy or a zest for life, you know that this medicine is affecting your heart spirit. Seek the assistance of a skilled acupuncturist or Chinese herbalist. With help, the shen can return to their original luminosity. If your practitioner suggests it, speak with your medical doctor to see if another medication is available or if it might be possible to lower the dosage of one you are on.

Find a contemplative practice such as meditation, prayer, drawing, journal writing or mindful walking in nature that will clear a space for the shen. In this tranquil quiet, you will be able to hear their voices. Take time to look in your own heart and your true identity will be illuminated by the light of your awareness. This is the practice of cultivating shen.

WHAT TO EXPECT AS YOU HEAL
AND CULTIVATE THE SHEN

As you become familiar with your shen, learn to recognize their voices and understand their messages, you will notice changes in your life, such as

- Better sleep and a sense of ease as you live in alignment with your true nature and cultivate your own authenticity

- More integrity and honesty in your relationships as you know and express who you really are and what you really want

- Less time doing things that really don't matter to you or being with people who really aren't part of your Tao

- Increased sense of your Tao or path so you are less easily distracted by extraneous events or tempted by dead-end streets and convoluted alleyways

- A light or glow infusing your life with the magic of the heart

- An increase in illumination, intuition and insight in your everyday life, guiding your decisions

- A greater ease in loving as you can more clearly discern "I" from "thou" and appreciate the differences

Shen in its pure form is invisible light. It has no quantity or quality and cannot be felt or touched or seen. It is infinite momentum, nowhere and everywhere at the same time. It is absolute yang, absolute negentropy—completely free from the effects of time, space and gravity.

As soon as the tiny fiery spark of shen settles in the heart at the time of conception, it encounters the limitations of life on earth, the limitations of the yin. The effects of the flesh and the blood take hold and the movement of the shen is slowed. Yin mixes with yang and the alchemy of the spirits in this particular life has begun.

In a very young child, the shen shines out from the heart as the light of curiosity, joy and delight. Later, in the adolescent, it ignites the sparks of intellectual curiosity, idealism, passionate friendship and romance. And with maturity, the shen becomes the illuminating light of insight and the flame of intuitive knowing. Gradually, the yin effects of embodied life temper the wild fire of the yang. Then the light of the shen softens and transforms into the illumination of self-awareness and introspection. The shen, as pure yang consciousness, depends on the structuring capacities of the other spirits to give it form.

It is only after the shen has been bathed over time in the yin waters of life on earth, after it has endured the losses, disappointments and suffering of its "descent" into the realm of time, space and gravity that the true alchemical transformation of the shen occurs. This is what the Taoists referred to as the "birth of the golden flower"—when the heavenly light of spirit, after long immersion in the transformational darkness of the earth, rises up from matter as a flower: the enlightened soul of the sage. This is when the true virtue of the shen comes into being; when after all the challenges, disappointments and pain of a lifetime, the fiery flower of compassion and unconditional love blossoms from the depths of the heart space.

The Taoists regarded compassion and love as substantiated light, illuminated matter that is no longer subject to the effects of time and gravity. They recognized this light in the effortless benevolence of the Taoist sage and in the infinite healing capacities of Quan Yin, the Taoist goddess of healing and compassion. Only rarely do we encounter this light in its fully substantiated form, but sometimes a drop of it will fall into our lives and everything is changed. As a touch, a tear or a ripple of laughter, the healing presence of love, the light of the shen takes form and we know, without knowing, that the spirits are passing by.

LING: THE RAIN DANCERS

Shen alone is like fire without eyes to see its brightness or a body to know its warmth. Shen, the yang aspect of spirit, can only be perceived in complement with ling, the yin aspect of spirit, the embodied reflection of heavenly light in the world of matter and form.

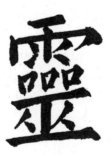

Ling

The character for *ling* is the rain radical above three raindrops, above two sorceresses doing a rain dance. Ling is related to spirit, but its yin nature is indicated by its relationship to water and rain. The raindrop is the shorthand sign that indicates ling's feminine, reflective nature. As rain brings down the virtue of heaven in the form of water, ling carries down the virtue of shen so that its invisible brightness can than be perceived. Ling is the shimmering reflections that dance in the raindrops, the colored lights that swim in clear pools of water. As shen is the spirit, ling is the soul.

The swirling rain dance of the water sorceresses does more than simply mirror the beauty of the shen. Ling has a beauty of its own, a lunar light that catches the attention of the shen and entices it down into the net of reflections, which is the material world. The fire of starlight dives into the depths of watery darkness in search of itself, its opposite reflection. This diving down of the shen into matter initiates the spiral dance of the individual soul along the path of Tao. It is the beginning of the alchemical journey of life.

In some traditions, all five of the spirits are considered ling, since all five are denser and more yin than the original spirit, more earthbound than the pure golden light of the stars. It is more useful, I think, to regard the ling as the hun and the po, the dual expression of the soul in its yin and yang aspect. (We'll look closer at the hun in the next chapter and the po in Chapter Nine.) The character *ling* can then be understood as a picture of the dance of the two souls, the po and the hun, as they carry the messages of the spirits into the world: the dance of the clouds carries down the rain, the dance of the water springs upward from the stones.

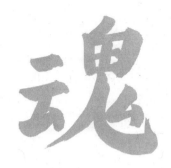

Chapter Seven

Hun: The Spirit of Wood—Vision, Imagination, Direction and Benevolence

> Penetration produces gradual and inconspicuous effects. . . . If one would produce such effects, one must have a clearly defined goal, for only when the penetrating influence works always in the same direction can the object be attained.
>
> —THE I CHING, HEXAGRAM #57, "THE GENTLE (THE PENETRATING, WIND)"[1]

CLOUDS

I watch the clouds gather as I paddle out across the cove to Darling Island. Behind me, a torn sheet of gray approaches from the west and shadows the sun. Slightly to my left, coming in over the southern tip of Mt. Desert Island, a mountain of round, towering heaps tumbles forward in a slow-motion avalanche of late-afternoon cumulus clouds. I sit and watch as the wind churns these endlessly changing forms up from the thin air. Ephemeral, they are no more than the reflection of light in water vapor. Yet in their patterns I see images come and go like dreams: a castle rising above my head evaporates into a mare's tail that moments later becomes a wave rolling away into the upside-down ocean of the sky.

Clouds brush the hem of the stars, then swoop down to linger inches above the surface of the sea. They capture our imagination and determine our moods. In the form of fog, they disorient us. Bringing rain, they nurture the arising of life, and in fair weather they temper the intensity of the sun. No way to pin them down, they go with the breezes up to the highest breath of the sky, then down to the boggy corners of the marsh. Whirling demons, transparent melusines, white-winged angels, genies appearing and disappearing out of invisible bottles . . . like the spirits, clouds go and come with the wind.

THE HUN

As we continue on our journey down Kunlun Mountain, we leave the starlit region of the shen and enter the realm of the cloud forests where the winds wreath the trees with scarves of mist. This is the upper soul realm, the transitional realm that exists between heaven and the horizon line where qi solidifies into matter and form. This is the realm of the hun.

In the microcosm of the psyche, the hun is the ethereal soul: the yang, breathy, spiritual aspect of the soul. It has three aspects: a vegetative aspect common to plants, animals and humans; an animal aspect, common to animals and humans; and a human aspect that is particular to the human psyche. In humans, the hun inhabits the vaporous, ever-changing region of our visions, dreams and imagination and is the animating agent of all mental processes. The hun are said to enter the body shortly after birth and follow the shen back to the heavenly realms after death. Unlike the po soul that decomposes after death, the hun are believed to carry an appearance of physical form back to the stars.

The hun is a slightly more materialized psychospiritual substance than the shen. Although they live quite close to heaven in the upper spirit levels of the mountain, a bit of yin sediment infiltrates the hun's yang. This infiltration of matter and vapor into the pure white light of the shen creates the hun. The bit of matter makes the hun more susceptible to the pull of gravity and the emotional life. Pure spirit becomes cloudy as we drift down through the upper soul realm towards the earth, and the pure, clear insight flash of the shen becomes shaded and colored by refraction and reflection.

Claude Larre and Elisabeth Rochat de la Vallée write:

> The shen are free to come and go, to come into myself or to quit this place and to fly away. The hun are more like a shadow depending on an object moving under light. They are some sort of escort. The shen go up, they want to go back to heaven, then in myself, a part of my animation which is called hun is on the verge of leaving my body. My family will try to call back my hun so that I will not be a dead person. For myself, if I want to save my life then I am recalling myself my hun. And if you are lacking energy because you are too weak, or you have been ill for too long then you have no more strength, no voice strong enough to call back your hun. Then you die.[2]

The hun are related to the liver and the element of wood as the shen are related to the zang of the heart and the element of fire. Wood is yin in respect to the fire. Its quality is less active, more dense, and thus more influenced by the constraints of time and space. In the same way, the hun—while still yang, expansive and active—are a bit slower and denser than the shen.

With the hun, we see form beginning to emerge from formlessness, manifestation beginning to emerge from pure possibility. Although the hun are free-flowing shape shifters that come and go with the winds of heaven, they whisper at the edges of matter. Unlike the absolute light of the shen, which is infinite and limitless, the illuminated vapors of the hun are susceptible to the influences and limitations of the earth.

In the macrocosm of the mountain, we see the hun in the clouds that hover around the peak. They are the mists and vapors that flit in and out of the trees and tint the atmosphere with colors as the sun rises and sets. They are the intermediaries between above and below as they lift moisture from the air and release it again in the form of rain and as they soften the blinding white light of the sun and refract it into an ever-changing play of rainbow colors. The hun are also the spirit of the wood, the potent directionality of the tree branches reaching toward the light, the strength of the tree trunks swaying with the wind yet steadily holding their own ground.

In human beings, the hun represent the psychological faculty of vision, imagination, clear direction and the capacity for justice. They endow us with the ability to discern our path, stay clear on our direction, imagine possibilities, move forward toward our goals and take a stand for what we believe is right. While the activity of the imagination—especially day or nighttime dreams—is energized by the coming and going of the shen, it is also influenced by the airy hun who follow the shen as they fly between the earth and heaven.

FUNCTIONS OF THE HUN

- **Sleeping and dreaming.** The hun are responsible for maintaining sound, peaceful sleep with dreams that are beneficial to the soul.

- **Emotional balance.** The hun maintain the balance of the emotional life. If the emotions are repressed, over time, the qi of the liver will back up and stagnate. Physical symptoms such as indigestion, abdominal bloating and headaches may result from emotional repression. Depression is another possible complication. On the other hand, excess emotion disturbs the shen and exhausts the qi.

Thus the hun's ability to appropriately maintain emotional balance is crucial to our overall health.

- **Decision making and planning.** The hun support the psychological function of decision making and planning. They carry the insights and intuitions of the shen into the realm of matter and manifestation by creating a course of action and deciding on priorities. They give us a sense of direction and a vision for our life.

- **Vision and imagination.** The hun are responsible for our ability to see the colors of the world through our eyes. They are also responsible for the inner vision and imagination, which bring creativity and growth into our lives.

A Look at the Chinese Character

The character for *hun* is made up of a combination of the radical for *yun* (clouds) and the radical for *gui* (discussed below). It reminds us that the hun are related to the breaths and to the spirits, and that the hun, like the shen, are free to come and go.

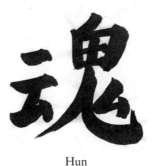

Hun

The top of the character represents the head of a person while the bottom is the body of the disembodied spirit, a ghost. *Gui* is often translated as "ghost" or "devil," but at a lecture given in London in 1985, Claude Larre had this to say about the gui:

Opposite to the *shen* Spirits, there is a world of creatures of a lesser quality . . . and I have to care for them too. And they are not called *shen*, they are called *gui*. These are just strolling on the air, these are walking more or less on the ground, and they have something contradictory, they go this way and that. [They have] a big head and something on the top. . . . For convenience sake, when we say Spirits we always refer to the *shen* and when we have to deal with the *gui*, we just say *gui* because it's not safe, not good, to call them bad names. You never know exactly how they would accept it. If you say devils, it's not proper. If you say genii, genii is vague. If you say *gui*, it's exactly that.[3]

The character for *po*, the spirit we will look at in Chapter Nine, also contains the character for *gui*. If you look carefully, you will see a small angular twisting figure at the bottom right corner of it. Some authorities say this twist indicates the shadowy comings and goings of ghosts.[4] Others believe it represents a tiny whirlwind, the swirling emptiness at the center of matter, the chaos of the Tao that the gui emerge from and where they return.

Like the clouds, the hun cannot be pinned down. Yet, also like the clouds, they are influenced by the vicissitudes of life on the material plane. They do have some relationship to time and space. Unlike the pure infinite light of the shen, however, which comes from heaven, the light of the hun is partially dependent on the nourishment of the earth. It must be fed by matter in order for it to shine. Like clouds, the hun must be fed by a constant swelling of earthly influences, the watery vapors and essences of the earth.

ASSOCIATIONS AND CORRELATIONS

Hun is related to

Element: wood
Organ: liver
Emotion: anger
Psychological functions: vision, imagination, direction, decision making
Psychospiritual issue: finding true path
Cosmological associations: clouds, mists, tree branches
Chakra: sixth—Third Eye: Perception
Alchemical virtues: benevolence and justice

Organ Correspondence

Traditional Chinese medicine relates the wood element hun to the liver and to the wind. By day, the classics state that the hun reside in the eyes, where they help us to see and think clearly, to make wise decisions and to direct our actions in the way that is best for our soul's purpose. By night, the windy hun descend downward, sinking to the fleshy organ of the liver where they are weighted down by the yin essences of the blood. At night, while we sleep, the hun actively organize our dreams and imagine our plans for the future.

The hun inform the shape and direction of our lives as the winds determine the shape and direction of the growth of the pine trees, the rippling patterns in the sand or the shape of billowing clouds. As the wind blows heaven's breath into every nook and cranny of the earth, the hun are the agents of penetration who bring the spiritual resonances of the shen down to the earth so that they can enter into form, space and time.

According to the *Neijing*, the liver "has the function of a military leader who excels in his strategic planning."[5] The hun carry out the liver's function on a psychological level by endowing us with the capacity to organize the chaos of random possibility into meaningful patterns, which give organization and direction to our lives. As the wind disperses clouds and leaves the sky clear and serene, the liver cleans our blood and the hun clear away the clouds of muddled thinking and help us see the big picture of our lives. We are then able to see into our future and, like a great military leader, create the strategies that will help us the most. Like the wuwei action of the heart, when the hun is in a state of equilibrium, its activities may never be noticed because they are achieved easily and are perfectly synchronized with the righteous unfolding of our destiny.

Symptoms of Hun Disturbance

When there is a disturbance or weakness in the liver or the body-mind is overwhelmed by longstanding emotional distress, the hun cannot fulfill their task as messengers. When the liver is weak, the hun follow their predominantly yang impulses and fly out of the body to their home in the cloud lands. The signs of chaos and confusion that result from this disturbance are unmistakable. When the hun are disturbed, they cannot carry the illumination of spirit into our lives. They no longer sweep away the clouds so that the light of the shen can guide our path. Our capacity for clear thought and vivid yet grounded imagining is "gone with the wind." Without the hun, we cannot know our true selves. We cannot organize and plan our lives and put things in motion, implement bright ideas or carry through on promises we've made to ourselves and others.

Without the hun, our lives become chaotic and confused. We have lost our vision. We cannot see the forest or the trees, and we cannot find the inner light that will guide us toward the orderly and graceful unfolding of our destiny, our journey through life back to the stars. Instead, no matter which way we turn we run into a brick wall, which may result in feelings of guilt and self-recrimination—a feeling that we are at fault, that nothing works out right. Or it may result in feelings of irritability, repressed anger and blame. A person whose hun is disturbed may constantly be in a state of righteous indignation, ranting and raving about the unfairness of the world, unable to take responsibility for his or her own life.

When the hun are in harmony and health, our lives are grounded in a deep trust in the intrinsic wisdom of the cosmos. Our decisions are not controlled or forced but unfold organically and spontaneously from the peculiar inner logic of our personal stories. This is the "free and easy wandering" for which the healthy liver is known. This kind of decision-making is not the logic of reason or analysis but the logic of divine chaos.

What does this kind of divine chaos look like? To answer this question, look up to the sky. The answer is there in the clouds.

SIGNS AND SYMPTOMS OF HUN DISTURBANCES

There are two basic categories of hun disturbances: the excess pattern and the deficiency pattern. Sometimes a person will have a mixture of both. This mixed pattern most often shows up in women and often correlates with the menstrual cycle. In the excess pattern, people often feel angry and experience life as one injustice after another. Whichever way they turn, there seems to be a brick wall, and they often inappropriately express extreme emotion. In the deficiency pattern, people feel timid, depressed and confused. They lack emotional expression and are usually too weak to even try to start a project. If they do make an attempt, they often cannot get past the decision-making stage.

Common Symptoms

- depression
- insomnia / excess dreaming / absence of dreams
- erratic emotions
- disorientation/disorganization
- repressed emotion
- excess sleeping
- vague anxieties, especially at night
- digestive disturbances related to emotional upset
- lack of clear vision on physical or psychological level
- outbursts of anger

Spirit Level Signs

- timidity, inability to take a stand
- "lack of color" to life
- wandering aimlessly with no direction
- starting projects but moving on before they are done
- always "running into brick walls"; can't seem to "get anywhere"
- obsession with injustice, which interferes with moving ahead with life

Possible Causes

- constitutional or "karmic" issues that are part of person's "work" in this lifetime
- exposure to violence, drug abuse or alcoholism in family during childhood
- lack of guidance and direction from family
- recreational drug use, especially alcohol and marijuana
- malnutrition, eating disorders, anemia
- repressed emotions, especially anger
- exposure to environmental toxins or toxins at the work place—i.e. paint and paint thinner, industrial cleaning products, artist's materials, urban pollution

In Chinese medicine, disturbances of the hun, like all psychological distress, may be caused by inner organic weaknesses or external stresses that overwhelm the bodymind's defenses. Thus we see disturbances of the hun in cases of drug and alcohol abuse and other physical illnesses affecting the liver, such as chronic hepatitis and cirrhosis. This typically results in a person's inability to organize his or her own life.

MARIJUANA AND THE HUN

Although marijuana has not been proven to be as disruptive as alcohol to the physical structures of the liver, it has an equally if not more disabling effect on the hun. Steven, a charming, warm-hearted man in his late thirties, was a patient who exhibited many of the problems of a disoriented hun spirit. Steven could be characterized as a master of disorganization! He worked as many as fourteen hours a day as a self-employed builder and contractor but still was unable to pay his bills. On a typical workday, if he didn't forget his appointment book, he couldn't read what he had written in it. His truck, which was his mobile office and supply station, was a total disaster and the mess spilled over into his desk at home. His wife had had it and was threatening to find another place to live.

I liked Steven immensely, but working with him was next to impossible because he would call to change appointments two or three times before he finally showed up. When he did show up, he was inevitably late. What finally helped was explaining to him the soul function of his liver and helping him see the correlation between his recreational use of marijuana, his inability to organize his life, and the effect this was having on the unfolding of his destiny.

Malnutrition and eating disorders such as anorexia and bulimia will also deprive the hun of the rich blood necessary for their renewal and dreams. Here the symptoms are more often extreme timidity and a lack of self-confidence, "muscle" or drive to bring dreams to manifestation.

The hun will also be unable to function properly if a child's growth is stunted by a lack of psychological support. The hun require the nurturance of love, mythology and beauty in the same way that the physical liver requires food and rest. When a child has been emotionally deprived or constantly criticized or there is violence or alcoholism in the home, the hun will flee or not develop properly. The child will be unable to concentrate on schoolwork, will procrastinate and complain of boredom. Such a child will be particularly susceptible to the temptations of drugs and alcohol.

Overwhelming emotional experiences will also unsettle the hun, especially if the liver is already vulnerable. This vulnerability is often seen in women after childbirth when there has been loss of blood and insufficient time for recovery, in teenagers, and in anyone with a sensitive constitution. The activities of these people may become chaotic, and it may seem as if no one is home inside their being. Their behavior is unpredictable, and their lives lack direction and point.

Those whose hun are disturbed and have flown off, most need support to see themselves clearly. When the hun are out of balance, we are unable to see either our true weaknesses or our true strengths. In my experience, in our culture, women with disturbances of the hun are especially susceptible to the problem of not seeing their own strengths. Because of their monthly loss of blood, chaotic diets and repressed anger and aggression (emotions of the liver), women easily lose touch with the power of the hun. They lose touch with the "military leader" inside their psyches, the ability to strategically plan their lives and the power to thrust themselves forward into their destinies. Instead, they stagnate in indecisiveness, passive-aggressive self-pity and muddled thinking, which are the psychological equivalents of "deficient liver," or are plagued by hyper-emotionality, psychosomatic complaints, irritability and PMS depression, which are symptomatic of "constrained liver qi." It is crucial for women in this state to express their authentic feelings as clearly as possible and to find ways to release emotions on a regular basis. Authentic movement (see Appendix ii for more information on this technique), natural voice work, martial arts and journal work are all practices that can help restore the health of the hun.

In addition to acupuncture, herbs, breath work, and nutritional support, one of the most important steps in healing the hun is to dare to see yourself realistically, especially to see the gifts and talents no one has ever taken the time to recognize. Look at yourself clearly. Be firm with the negative voices in your head that criticize and demean. Keep your eye on the light of your true nature, the light of the shen. Then the hun will again be guided along by the spirits and can resume their free and easy wandering along the path of the Tao.

WAYS TO CULTIVATE THE HUN SPIRIT

When the liver is disturbed, the hun fly away and the soul is confused and disorganized. Acupuncture and acupressure are effective ways to heal and strengthen liver function. If you have a history of drug use or alcoholism, or if you have or have had hepatitis, a well-trained acupuncturist can help you cleanse and tonify your liver so your hun will have a peaceful home and resting place in your body.

It is crucial to clear the bodymind of toxic substances and to recognize alcohol and mind-altering drugs as the potent soul-disturbing influences they are. If you have an ongoing problem with drugs or alcohol, AA, NA and other Twelve Step Programs will help you let go of these self-destructive behaviors as well as regain a connection to the light of your own spirit.

Cleansing and tonifying herbs are also extremely potent ways to heal. Dandelion, peppermint, chelidonium and milk thistle are effective and safe herbs that can be taken over long periods of time. Look for organic, wild-crafted herbs, available at most health food stores (or refer to Resource Guide in Appendix ii).

- Dandelion is an overall liver cleanser and tonic. It is particularly effective for PMS mood swings accompanied by bloating and breast tenderness.

- Peppermint is a mood-elevating, invigorating herb that will also help with digestive disturbances, bloating and poor appetite. Take as a tea and drink freely throughout the day.

- Chelidonium is one of the best overall liver tonics. It should be taken as a tincture—a few drops in a tablespoon of water—three times a day before meals and will quickly clear digestive and appetite disturbances, enhance clarity of vision and ease emotional strain.

- Milk thistle is the premier herb for anyone who has been exposed to toxic chemicals and should be taken for at least two months after exposure. In addition, for people who work with chemicals or are routinely exposed to pollution, milk thistle can be taken on a regular basis with a one-week break every six weeks.

A person with problems of the hun will greatly benefit from good nutrition. Foods that nourish the blood and liver, such as dark leafy greens, grains and fish, are especially important. Smaller balanced meals at regular intervals will keep the liver content and well supplied with nutrients.

Adequate sleep and time enough for dreaming will help to make the liver a good home for the hun and encourage them to roost again at night.

Meditation and adequate, moderate exercise are also important, as these help reestablish the rhythms the hun require in order to do their job.

Natural beauty also helps to heal the hun, which need to be in the contact with the life force of the wood, feel the breezes of the air and feast their eyes on the colors and movements of the trees. Birdsong is their favorite music, and a day spent watching the shapes of clouds move across the blue sky will sometimes do more for them than any medication.

Visionary healer Rudolf Steiner points to the healing influence of light and color in working on the "astral" or soul realms. The hun, as the agents of clear sight and unclouded vision, are especially receptive to work with active imagination. Taking the time to paint pictures of your dreams and fantasies and meditate on these inner images often helps entice the hun back to the bodymind.

WHAT TO EXPECT AS YOU HEAL
AND CULTIVATE YOUR HUN

As you become familiar with your hun and learn to recognize their voices and understand their messages, you will notice changes in your life. Some changes you may experience are:

- Clarity about your direction and purpose in life

- Increased ability to achieve your goals. Fewer problems with procrastination and getting side-tracked. An ability to move forward with power.

- Richer imagination. An ability to envision possibilities and weave dreams.

- Emotional stability. An ability to identify what you are feeling, to state your feelings clearly and to stand by your feelings and beliefs.

- Less wobbling and indecisiveness

- Less guilt, timidity, irritability and depression

- Increased passion, excitement, joie de vivre. Life regains its zest and color.

- Greater capacity to "go with the flow" while staying focused on ultimate goals

- Less need to blame others and less focus on the injustices of the world

- Increased self-responsibility combined with increased ability to know one's own values and to take a stand for one's beliefs

The following case tells of the healing of a young woman whose hun had been damaged by early childhood exposure to parental violence and alcoholism. This early trauma was compounded, as is often the case, by a complete lack of supportive direction during adolescence. Although her initial complaint was headaches and abdominal bloating, the deeper issue was that she had no conception of her real talents, brightness, intelligence and charm. She had no idea who she was or where she was going. It took the re-illumination of her inner vision to turn the corner in her healing.

Camilla's initial complaint was one-sided headaches that began with dizziness and visual disturbances and proceeded to debilitating pain over her left eye. Sleep was the only thing that helped. She also complained of bloating and indigestion after eating. Otherwise, she said her life was "OK." She had a boyfriend she liked and a job in a health spa selling natural cosmetics.

Camilla was twenty-eight years old. Since she had graduated high school, she had worked as a model in a department store, a dentist's receptionist, a veterinarian's assistant and a water filtration systems salesperson, to name only a few of her jobs. She had never gone to college because she "couldn't figure out what she wanted to do." When I asked her if she had any visions or dreams, she replied, "I'd like to do something in health. Or maybe Tim and I will have a baby."

It took me a few months to realize what a bright, talented and creative woman she really was, but this was only after I put together the pieces of her childhood. At first, she said she couldn't remember much, but as we talked, memories of waking up at night to the "sound of shouting and banging downstairs" began to surface. Dreams came of being chased by "gangsters with knives" and finding children under the sink or in the liquor cabinet. After her parent's divorce, Camilla spent her adolescence shuttling between her grandmother's apartment and her father's house while her mother struggled to create a new life for herself. Later Camilla and her mother became quite close, but this was after Camilla had spent her teenage years in a haze of drinking and vague dreams of becoming a songwriter.

Camilla had the quality of a lost soul and exhibited the timidity, absence of vision and lack of an organizing sense of self typical of a hun disturbance. Her soft voice and lack of irritability belied a well of repressed anger that was pushing against her wall of defenses in the form of headaches and abdominal bloating (both signs of the liver qi constraint that often accompanies a hun disturbance).

The first thing I did was tell Camilla that I thought her problems were multi-leveled and not just physical. I wanted her to come regularly—every week at the same time on the same day. (Although I did not share this information with her until later, this regularity was important in order to set up a rhythm for her hun. It was a pattern that was dependable and could become an organizing influence on her life.)

Camilla had stopped drinking and smoking three years earlier, so I immediately got her on a program to detoxify and tonify her liver. This included a glass of lemon in spring water every morning upon arising, an herbal tincture of dandelion and milk thistle, and abstinence from food preservatives and caffeine. With acupuncture we focused on freeing up her liver qi and gently tonifying her liver and gallbladder.

Over several months, I noticed she was beginning to express her opinions more strongly. She told me she was becoming annoyed with the women at the spa whose "only concern was their appearance." Color was coming back to her cheeks and brightness to her eyes, and she looked more animated, like there was somebody really there inside her—someone who could express her own thoughts and opinions, someone substantial that it was possible to "push up against." According to Chinese medicine, this is the quality of a healthy liver, nourished blood and strong wood. In Western alchemical terms, one might say she was regaining her soul.

Through relaxation techniques and guided visualization, Camilla began to be able to listen to her body, which resulted in her recognizing the tightness in her stomach as a sign that she was upset or angry rather than that she had simply "eaten something too fast."

I encouraged Camilla to keep a journal, suggesting she write, draw and paint her dreams and thoughts with complete abandon—but I insisted that she keep to a regular schedule, to make her journal writing a ritual that, like her acupuncture sessions, would help her organize her time into a rhythmic pattern. Keeping to a schedule was difficult, but Camilla managed it and the accomplishment gave her a tremendous sense of satisfaction.

I knew our work was coming to a close when she came in one day and told me that she was thinking about going to college. She said she had been reading back over her journal and it had occurred to her that she had opinions and thoughts of her own.

"I was so excited," she said. "I never realized that I had something to say. I figure if I can do this, I probably could manage to write papers for school."

I asked Camilla how her headaches had been. "Oh, I got one last week," she said, "but it wasn't so bad. I just took a nap and when I woke up, it was better. Maybe I was just tired."

Although it was crucial that I know the story of Camilla's early life, very little of our work together actually focused on her history. By using the theories and tools of Chinese medicine, we were able to accomplish a great deal simply by "staying in the present" and working with her immediate issues. This is one of the interesting and complementary differences between the Western and Chinese approach to the psychological healing. Western psychology emphasizes the history and development of the personality while Chinese medicine tends to focus on harmonizing the energies of the soul as they manifest in the here and now.

The goal of my work with Camilla went beyond her physical problems. Ultimately she needed help to develop her capacity to organize her life, to envision goals for her future and to begin to manifest her dreams. In short, she needed to heal her hun. Eventually, it will be important for her to dig her creativity out of the tangled roots of her anger and to understand certain aspects of her complex history. But at her age and stage of life, I felt it was most important that she "get on with it" and begin to develop her own rich potential. For this, she needed not so much to understand her past as to clear away the clouds so that she could see her own future.

ALCHEMY: THE RAIN OF BENEVOLENCE

As psychic messengers, the hun carry the illuminations of the shen down toward the earth so that we can manifest the divine through the path we follow in the world. They also carry the moisture and essences of the earth up to the sky so that matter can be refined into activity and light. They endow us with the power to transform the insights of spirit into new possibilities and to envision ways to implement them.

Like the blood, sinews and tendons of our body, which are the physical manifestation of the wood element, the hun are the blood, sinews and tendons of the psyche, the psychospiritual manifestation of the wood element. Through the hun, we are able to imagine, envision and recognize our life path. They give us the ability to choose the path through which we will realize our potential, to set out on a project with certainty and determination, and to manifest heaven through our right action in the world. They are the soul forms through which the light of spirit, the shen, can shine.

Like the shen, the hun represent an aspect of consciousness. However, the hun are closer than the shen to the yin manifest embodiment. The shen arrive in a flash of bright light, a dazzling *Aha!*, a joyous revelation of selfhood, an infusion of gold in the heart. The hun drift and dance, turn and return, hide behind shadows and trees. Hovering close to the emotional life and the daydream mind, the hun are related to sleep, imagination, mythmaking, poetry and fantastical visions, where all inspired tactical plans, acts of genuine creativity, and clear decisions are born.

According to Taoist mythology, at the end of our days the hun follow the shen, rising back to heaven through the acupuncture point One Hundred Meetings, which is located at the top of the head. From there, they ascend with the shen back to the stars of the Big Dipper. But when the hun leave the body, they do not leave empty-handed. If the alchemy of the soul has been successful, the hun carry with them something eternal, some lesson learned from their sojourn on the earth.

The hun are not only the messengers of the heavens to earth but of the earth to the heavens. Through them, we here on earth gain consciousness and self-awareness and the ability to make decisions, which help us turn the fickle winds of fate into the currents of our destiny. But through the stories of our lives that the hun carry back to heaven, the spirits gain other lessons, lessons that can only be learned in a physical body through the experiencing of emotion and the passage of time in the temporal realm of the earth.

Through the alchemy of the spirits, the propulsive, yang, forward directionality of the hun is tempered by the yin through the challenges and resistances of embodied life. The original nature of the wood, which shoots forth in spring and pushes forward against all obstacles to achieve its own purpose, is alchemically transformed into the movement of clouds. The quality of benevolence is the rain that showers down from the cloudy hun as we gain the ability to move in ways that not only benefit the self but also benefit others. The emergence of benevolence marks the transformation of the hun from yang windy potency to illuminated soul. The golden gift of the hun is the quality of justice, the ability to weigh the righteousness as well as the effectiveness of our decisions and our actions in the world.

A person of the Way fundamentally does not dwell anywhere. The white clouds are fascinated with the green mountain's foundation. The bright moon cherishes being carried along with the flowing water. The clouds part and the mountain appears. . . . [T]he six sense doors are not veiled, the highways in all directions have no footprints. Always arriving everywhere without being confused, gentle without hesitation, the perfected person knows where to go.

—from Hung-Chih's Practice Instructions:
The Clouds' Fascination and the Moon's Cherishing[6]

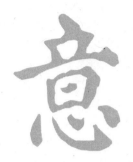

Chapter Eight

Yi: The Spirit of Earth—Integrity, Intention, Clear Thought and Devotion

> What is well planted cannot be uprooted.
> What is well embraced cannot slip away.
> —Lao Tzu, Tao Teh Ching, Chapter 54[1]

GROUND

On Darling Island, cormorants stand on the black rocks, drying their ragged wings. The rocks are piled up, fragmented abstractions against the pale sky. At the other side of the cove, stunted birches, bayberry bushes and the skeletons of dead spruce make a boundary between the beach and the impassible thicket that forms the core of the island's vegetation. Here the sea breathes in and out, covering and then uncovering the barnacles and kelp at the tide line. Between the salt spray and the incessant ocean wind, only the hardiest plants survive.

So I am surprised each time I look down and notice the sea lavender . . . the way it stands so precisely between the jagged rocks, its head covered in a veil of purple flowers and flanked by golden honeybees. Rooted in the coarse sand and clay, turning its leathery leaves upward to the light, it is undeterred by weather or waves and devoted wholeheartedly to its purpose. Persevering with single-minded determination, year after year, it continues to bring forth its unique form into the wild windswept light.

This faithful, steadfast, purposeful application of the creative force toward a single goal, the bringing forth of the spirit in the infinite and glorious diversity of form, is yi—the spirit of intention.

THE YI

When the heart applies itself, we speak of intent.
— NEIJING SUWEN[2]

In our descent, when we reach the yi spirits, we have arrived on solid ground. On Kunlun Mountain, we find the yi at the horizon line, at the boundary point between spirit and matter, above and below. When we arrive at yi in our soul's journey from the high peaks down to the labyrinths below Kunlun Mountain, we leave behind the fiery golden regions of the shen and the cloud realms of the hun where mists swirl through the trees and tangle with the sky. With the yi, we begin to feel earth beneath our feet. It is no longer enough for us to know, to intuit, to envision and to dream. Now we must put the solid weight of our being, the power of our intention, behind the knowing that is in our heart. When the yi is fulfilling its function, we fully commit ourselves to manifesting our destiny and to bringing the light of our spirits into the world around us. The yi is the soul aspect that lets the world know that we mean to stand by our dreams.

Yi is the middle, the earth, the celestial pivot. Above is heaven, light, formlessness, infinite possibility and the yang spirits of the shen and the hun. Below is matter, darkness, density and finite form, manifestation and the yin spirits of the po and the zhi.

In the macrocosm of the planet, the yi are related to the fertile fields and meadows of the middle regions. These spirits of earth are enlivened by the sunlight and breezes of the heavens and fed by the minerals, waters and essences of the underworld. The yi are the spirits of the receptive, creative energies of the earth. Their function is to receive the messages of the shen through the imprint of the hun and then manifest the way of heaven in concretized form.

In the microcosm of the human bodymind, the yi represent the powers of the earth in us. They are the spirits that give us the capacity for sustained intention, purpose, clarity of thought, altruism and integrity. They are related to the emotions of sympathy and the organ of the spleen. They support our capacity for thought, intention, reflection and the act of applying ourselves to our heart's purpose. They give us the ability to concentrate, study and memorize data for our work, and they endow us with the capacity for clear thought. In other words, they allow us to apply our spirit to the world of forms.

The yi endow us with the power to stand behind our words through committed, persevering action. Through them, we stay with our task and stay on our path. And through them we gain the capacity to digest experiences and impressions and turn them into usable ideas that empower our action in the world. The yi endow us with the intent, purpose, integrity and devotion necessary to plant and tend the garden of our lives. Once we are familiar with their territory and nature, we discover a powerful ally who can help us bring our dreams to fruition.

Yi is the psychic counterpart of the earth, the rich soil of our purpose that nourishes the gestation of our ideas so that they can ultimately manifest in our lives. The yi allows us to bring our ideas and visions down from the windy skies of the hun so that they can be digested and nurtured in the yin matrix of the earth. The yi keeps us hoeing, watering, feeding and weeding the soil of our dreams so that one day we can present them to the world in substantial form, as a project, a creation, a fully worked through idea. The yi is the spirit that moves us as we say, "Here, this is the unique gift that I bring forth."

A Look at the Character

The character for *yi* shows us the picture of the open bowl of the heart. Above it is the radical indicating an uttered sound, poetry or a musical note.

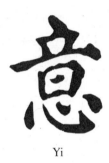

Yi

Sound is vibration. Like the wind, sound creates movement through the air, a breeze. Like the wind, it is a messenger between realms. Sound, in the form of prayers, chanting and poetry, carries our hopes and desires into the world and up to the heavens. The vibrating sounds of our hearts and our spirit are also carried "down," extending spirit into matter through the words we speak and the actions we commit to. This is yi. As indicated by the musical note above the heart in the character, yi is the connecting link between the heart and the spleen, between inspiration and intention, bringing the limitless, infinite energies of the heart into time and space. In our own Biblical creation myths, this manifesting sound is called "the Word."

The yi spirits are the gardeners of the soul who plant the light seeds of the shen in the soil or matrix of the earth. Singing and humming as they work, the yi nourish the spirit seeds with their own vibrations. They work steadily, with untiring dedication, until the light seeds sprout into manifestation. The excessive sympathy and caretaking that can become such a problem for people with an "earthy" constitution is an imbalanced expression of this sympathetic resonance between the yi and the shen. In a healthy state it vibrates between the light fields of heaven and the material fields of earth in a continuum of light to music to form. The "sound" that manifests from this is your word, your declaration: This is where you stand. This is what you stand for. There is what you will stand behind.

Yi gives us the power not only to sing the music of our spirits but to persist in singing, to apply ourselves to singing, until the vibrations of our heart songs have crystallized into material form. Yi is the original "I am" of the shen as it moves down through vision and imagination and finally manifests through enduring intention. Yi gives us the power to say our own name not just once, but many times over. Yi enables us to impress our unique signature into the world, as we manifest heaven through our actions on the earth.

> In the center of the heart, there is another heart.
> Intent [yi] precedes declaration.
> After intent comes form.
>
> —CLAUDE LARRE AND
> ELISABETH ROCHAT DE LA VALLÉE[3]

Organ Correspondence

In Chinese medicine, the earth element yi is related to the stomach and spleen, these organs that digest our food and distribute the nutrients through our bodies. They create the nutrients we need to do what we do in the world. On a psychological level, this process enables us to digest our experiences and impressions and to turn them into usable ideas and concepts. In a healthy state, we readily absorb the impressions that we need for psychological growth and development, and let go of those that are not useful so we do not take on concepts that do not "belong" to us. We have a clear sense of what and how much we need to grow.

Yi resides in the zang of the spleen just as the hun resides in the liver. The spleen and the yi are related to the element earth as the liver and the hun are related to wood. Earth is yin in respect to wood. Its quality is less active, more dense, more material, more influenced by the constraints of time and space. Unlike the wood, the earth cannot reach toward the sky to actively gather up the qi that pours down from heaven in the form of sunlight. The earth's nature is rather to keep still, to receive, absorb and contain the qi, and to nourish life from its resources.

The Yi as the Pivot Point of the Soul

Earlier, we learned that the heart, as the resident of the spirit, is at the center of the spiritual, atemporal realm, the "upper heaven." Similarly, the earth is at the center of the material, temporal realm, the "middle ground." According to the alchemical text *The Golden Flower,* the yi is the heavenly heart of the middle house. So, as the shen is the heavenly heart or spirit of the upper house, the chest or upper alchemical cauldron, the yi is the heavenly heart or spirit of the middle house, the abdomen or middle alchemical cauldron. With the zhi, the heavenly heart or spirit of the lower house, the pelvic bowl or lower cauldron, these spirits form the axis, a celestial pivot, a conduit for Tao.

The yi is also at the pivot point between the two aspects of the soul—the yang hun and the yin po. Between the shen and the yi, the hun drifts up and down between heaven and earth. And between the yi and the zhi, the po soul rises and falls like the breath between the earth and the underworld.

How does this work? The hun are the psychological manifestation of the heavenly qi—qi in its vaporous form—and in the form of wind and clouds, vision and imagination, are the messenger between above and below, carrying the fiery light of spirit down from the upper skies to the intermediary cloud zone between spirit and matter. Here in the cloud realms, the heavenly qi mixes with the essences and fluids of the earth. It becomes denser and heavier, more susceptible to the pull of gravity and time. In the process it is able to bring the messages of spirit down to the yi. In the impressions left by the wind on the material world and in all the structures and forms of life, we see the light of spirit concretized. The wind, as the gentle penetrating messenger of the shen, leaves the spirit's imprint all around us: in the ripples of the sand dunes, the waves of the seas, the billowing forms of clouds.

On a psychological level, the hun carry the light of the shen into our lives as vision, clear sight and imagination, inspiring us with the breath of spirit. The yi are the psychological force that impresses these visions and patterns onto the material substrate of our lives, which manifest as the patterns and actions we commit to over time that ultimately determine how our destiny unfolds.

According to the Taoist viewpoint, our true destiny is the materialization of our original nature, our celestial sound, in time and space, which reflects the intrinsic beauty and order of the Tao. It is a mantra, a word, a sound seed in us that is waiting to be unfolded. The yi, as earth, is the intention and purpose in us that creates the possibility for this seed to sprout.

WORRY

Worry—persistent, anxious thinking about unpleasant things that have happened or may happen in the future—is a mental state that has a direct and very negative effect on the yi. This mental attitude may arise from a constitutional weakness of the spleen or it may be a patterned, habitual response to excess stress and insufficient life supports. Whatever its cause, worry is part of a self-perpetuating, vicious cycle. The more qi we expend in this useless mental activity, the less we have available to nourish our yi and to take steps to create the life we really want to live. As the yi is weakened, we have less and less capacity to move forward on our life path and manifest our Tao, the heavenly mandate of our destiny.

A central principle in Chinese medical psychology is that for every thought we have in our minds, there should be a corresponding action in our bodies. This unimpeded movement from the mind into the body, from shen to hun to yi and down into the nerves, muscles, tendons and instinctual impulses of our body allows our Tao to flow effortlessly through us and out into the world through our words and our actions.

Worry interferes with this natural flow. It ties the psychic qi into knots and causes it to stagnate. Eventually the knotted psychic qi transforms into denser qi and manifests as physical symptoms such as chronic muscle spasms, digestive and appetite disturbances, epigastric discomfort, abdominal pain and distention, and fatigue. Over time it can affect the heart and lungs, disturbing the shen and the po and eventually causing such stress-related symptoms as insomnia, palpitations, breathing difficulties and chest tightness. When we worry, rather than allowing the initiating energies of the shen and the visions and plans of the hun to animate the yi, we block these energies, perseverating and worrying rather than taking action. The qi backs up and the yi becomes paralyzed or stuck in repetitive, obsessive thought patterns.

Brooding, mulling over past events or people in our lives, nostalgic longing and obsessive analyzing have similarly destructive effects on the yi. In fact, any way of being that keeps a person stuck in excessive thinking, rather than in spontaneous living, will affect the yi. As the yi grow weak, they have less ability to move thoughts into actions.

It is crucial to interrupt this cycle. Various strategies are effective, and usually it is necessary to employ more than one at a time. In addition to the suggestions given at the end of this chapter, meditation and movement are indispensable. Through meditation, we discover a way to quiet the mind's random chatter and to channel psychic energies more effectively. Whether we engage in moving meditation practices such as tai ch'i, qi gong, or yoga, or our movement takes the form of jogging, walking, aerobic dance, or simply getting up and getting something done, motion magically quiets the mind as psychic qi is drafted by the moving body and pulled back into the vital cycles of life.

SIGNS AND SYMPTOMS OF YI DISTURBANCE

According to Chinese medicine, yi disturbances, like all psychological problems, can have internal or external causes that exacerbate a constitutional vulnerability. A person who has an earthy constitution will be more prone to these problems than others. The following common behavior patterns of earth types are also common symptoms that appear when the yi is afflicted.

Psychoemotional Signs

- obsessive thoughts and repetitive thought patterns
- worry, obsessions and a continual focus and brooding on one's own problems
- excess thought and cogitation and insufficient movement or action
- eating disorders such as anorexia, bulimia and binges
- muddled thinking; an inability to make logical connections between ideas or to order thoughts in logical patterns
- over-nurturing of others to avoid one's own responsibilities and growth

Spirit Level Signs

- stagnation in the zone of manifestion, inability to transform ideas and thoughts into commitments and actions
- continually generating new ideas but not taking action on any of them

Problems with the yi are actually problems of "psychospiritual digestion," a disturbance in our soul force's ability to digest experiences and impressions and transform them into values, ideas and actions. A block has formed where spirit is attempting to enter into manifestation in our material lives.

Possible Causes

- constitutional issues that begin in utero or stem from genetic makeup and karmic issues that become central psychological problems needing work over a lifetime

- excess worry, excessively thinking about the needs of others at expense of one's own

- improper eating habits

- anemia and vitamin deficiencies

- excess sugar. Sugar does give an energy rush but weakens endurance over time so the vibration of the self does not get firmly planted into matter.

- codependency. Early childhood exposure to alcoholism and family dysfunction can result in a coping strategy of attention focused on others. People who are forced to be overly involved in other people's stories will not be able to hear the sound of their own heart's voice.

- exhaustion and long-term strain. The yi is also impaired by any weakness in the shen or in the hun, so if the heart or liver is under strain, the yi will have difficulty standing by the spirit's vision.

CULTIVATING THE YI

Symptoms of disharmonized yi revolve around the disturbed digestion and assimilation of psychospiritual experience and impressions. These disharmonies result in our inability to transform life experience into ideas and intentions that are the vital expressions of our souls. Problems with the yi are actually problems of psychospiritual digestion, creating a blockage or disturbance at the point where our soul and spirit forces are attempting to enter into manifestation in our material lives. The primary symptom of a yi disturbance is a thought pattern that goes around and around. Worrying, obsessing and focusing continually on one's own problems are examples of this unproductive mental state. There is thought but no movement or action.

According to Chinese medicine, yi disturbances, like all psychological problems, can have internal or external causes that exacerbate a constitutional vulnerability. A person who has an earthy constitution will be more prone to these problems than others. People with a weak center and unclear sense of self will not be able to set a clear intention. Those who choose or are forced to be overly involved in other people's stories will not be able to hear the sound of their own heart's voice. Exhaustion, eating disorders and long-term strain will affect the yi, as will any weakness in the shen or in the hun. So if the heart or liver is under strain, the yi will have difficulty standing by the spirit's vision.

Healing involves strengthening a person's center. It means being able to listen inside to one's own voice. And it also means having the power to move from the realm of abstract ideas into concrete action. Thus we nourish the seeds of our dreams.

Because our relationship to food has a significant effect on our yi spirit, any abuse of food can muddle the heartmind and interfere with our ability to set a clear intention. Food abuse includes over-focusing on what we eat, dieting and fasting, which can be ways to distract ourselves, to go in unproductive circles around our stomachs instead of moving out with our ideas and actions in the world. So the very first step in cultivating the yi is to honor our relationship to nourishment, which is the way we are fueled to manifest spirit in our lives. If food and eating habits are a problem in your life, you already know that the yi are disturbed. If these devoted spirits do not have the strength to help you "stand by" what your heart knows you need and want to eat, how will they have the power to help you stand by your word in other areas?[4]

The first step in cultivating the yi is to make food sacred! Make it a practice to say a brief prayer of gratitude before eating or just take a moment to center yourself and appreciate the beauty of the food that is bringing the forces of life into your body. Once you have a delightful, gracious and joyful relationship to the foods that you nourish yourself with, you are well on the way to cultivating the yi.

The following are additional ways to support and nourish these spirits:

- Avoid clutter. When you work, clear a space so that there is room to think. Don't work in a cluttered, messy atmosphere.
- If you are expending a lot of energy taking care of others, make time to take care of yourself! Take time to rest, to walk, to just be quiet.
- Take your own words seriously! If you say you are going to do something, hold yourself accountable. Remember that with the yi, we come down to earth. We mean business. Dreaming and random conversation are not yi. Yi means saying it and staying with it, so be mindful not to over-commit so that you fail to carry through. Each time we do not keep our word, we create a chink in our own integrity and weaken the yi. If this is a problem for you—as it is for so many people in our busy, overextended society—try to following practices:
  - Say "NO!" as a full sentence. The next time someone asks you to do something you can't or don't want to do, say No without any explanation. Notice how hard that is to just stop right there!
  - Take small bites. Give yourself a very small task to accomplish within a set amount of time. Write your commitment down. Sign the paper and hang it up where you can see it. Hold yourself accountable. For example, "I will clean out the glove compartment of the car by 5:00 this afternoon." Once the job is done, appreciate yourself for the accomplishment. Small practices are push ups for the yi spirit. As you go along, you can take on bigger projects with more complex schedules and feel the satisfaction of knowing you can carry through.

ONE-BOWL EATING MEDITATION FOR THE YI

An ancient Zen practice is called the one bowl eating meditation. In this practice, you find a single bowl that becomes your eating vessel. For each meal, fill this bowl with any foods you want to eat and eat them mindfully. Then you stop until it's time for the next meal. This practice is harder than you might expect, and even if followed just one day a month it will change your attitude toward food and the way you eat.

What to Expect as You Heal
As you develop a relationship with your yi and work to heal and strengthen them, you will notice changes in your life. You may, for example,

- take on less but stay with the projects you start
- be able to say what you think and express yourself more clearly
- take the time to listen to your own inner voice and take its messages seriously

- feel more centered in your own self and be less thrown off balance by other people's problems, needs, demands or opinions.

- begin to feel a sense of solidity. When you meet an obstacle, you stay clear on your intention and work to find a way to solve the problem and move ahead with your project.

- hold your ground

- begin to feel as if your actions in the world result in a bountiful harvest. The world becomes a fertile ground for your ideas and actions.

SPIRIT POINT: THE CELESTIAL PIVOT—
EARTH EXPRESSES HEAVEN

Stomach 25, *tian shu* or Celestial Pivot, is located at the center of the body, on the abdomen about two inches lateral to the umbilicus. The point is commonly used to treat physical symptoms such as constipation, diarrhea, nausea, poor appetite and other intestinal and digestive problems. The point is also indicated for the Chinese diagnosis of "running piglet qi"—a symptom commonly but not exclusively experienced by women where there is sensation of agitation and tightness in the central part of the torso as if tiny squealing piglets were racing madly between the umbilicus, chest and throat. "Running piglet qi" is known to be a symptom that is exacerbated by stress, sexual repression and unexpressed emotion. Thus, it is generally accepted that Stomach 25 can be used in the treatment of psychological and psychosomatic problems especially when they appear in the form of abdominal distress. However, this rationale only begins to touch on the point's preciousness at the spirit level.

We find a doorway to the secret power of this point by taking a closer look at the symptom of "running piglet qi." The symptom arises from an imbalance between the energies of the the lower abdomen—the tantian or cinnabar field—the chamber of the uterus and sexual organs and the energies of the chest or upper palace, the chamber of the heart. The symptom often appears when the blood of the uterus dwindles, either due to excessive menstrual flow or due to the natural tidal shifts of menopause when the blood moves upward to nourish the growing wisdom of a mature woman's mind and heart. With the dwindling of the blood in the tantian, the nest or bodily home of the spirits is lost. The yang energies of the shen uncouple from the yin essences. There is a lack of harmony between above and below and a breach of communication between the upper and lower spirits When this situation goes untreated, not only is there an uncomfortable physical sensation in the torso, there is a spiritual crisis. When above and below are not in harmony, Tao is lost. Our feet and our hearts take us in opposite directions. We cannot access our authentic desires or get in touch with our true purpose. Our lives feel chaotic and meaningless and there is no comfortable place to rest, no place to sit quietly with the self.

Restoring harmony between above and below and communication between the upper and lower spirits is the sacred task of the yi spirit. The yi holds the center. It is the connecting link between the hun and po souls. It maintains the viability of earth, the middle ground between heaven and the underworld, between the wisdom of the heart and the potency of our instinctual nature.

We can call on the restorative capacities of the yi by gently needling, touching or warming Stomach 25, the point at the center of the body. This point not only calms and harmonizes physical digestion it also supports us in digesting the experiences of our lives. It allows us to transform experience into wisdom and to let go of ideas and feelings that no longer nourish us. It brings us back to our own intention, to our own song, to the garden of our own life.

In stimulating this point, we reconnect above and below and bring the energies of the bodymind back to the center. In this way, we restore the power of the Celestial Pivot, the power of Tao. . . .

CASE STUDY: VISITING THE HUT OF THE YI

Emily sat on the couch in front of me rummaging through an enormous pocketbook. "I know I have that list here somewhere," she said in a thin, plaintive voice as she pulled out a handful of notepaper. "I wrote everything down so I wouldn't forget what I wanted to tell you. But now I can't find the paper."

She shuffled the pile of notes and then put them down on the couch next to her. I suggested she try to tell me in her own words about her symptoms but she seemed too distracted to think. "This is how it is," she said. "I try to get organized but then there are a hundred other things I have to do. Getting the kids to their activities, food shopping, paying the bills, taking care of the dog. And Marty's been working all the time, trying to get money together for Alex's college next year. I'm afraid it's going to be too much for him. It's just one thing on top of another and I don't get to any of it. . . . I wish I could find that list." She sighed and turned the pocketbook upside down. The entire contents tumbled out onto the floor in front of her: keys, lipsticks, half a dozen pens, receipts, rolls of Life Savers, cell phone, notepad, business cards, change purse, wallet and several crumpled balls of tissues. "This is my life," she said. "What a mess!"

Emily was forty-seven, the mother of four children between the ages of six and fifteen. The youngest two were identical twins. As a young woman, she had traveled widely and been an avid photographer. She had a master's degree in art history from an Ivy League college but had given up her career to raise her children. She strongly believed that a mother's first responsibility was to her family. She loved her husband and children but said that lately she had felt no sense of connection to them. Several months before she came to see me, her periods had become irregular with missed cycles interspersed with excess bleeding. She had begun to feel overwhelmed with fatigue and struggled to get out of bed in the morning. She lost her appetite and was unable to take care of her home or children or fulfill her multiple community commitments. "I'm too tired to move," she said. "I keep pushing but it's harder every day."

I knew that Emily's fatigue was due to deficient spleen qi, probably exacerbated by her late pregnancy with twins. She needed to be supported with acupuncture and herbal formulas that would build her blood and restore her spleen qi. But I suspected Emily's problems were not just physical. I felt that there were spirit level issues that we would need to address before her fatigue lifted and her sense of well-being returned. In order for her to hang in for the duration, to complete the task of bringing her four children up and out into the world, Emily would need to discover some new place of strength and commitment. She would have to reconnect to her own center, her own intention, her own yi. Otherwise, I was afraid she was going to fall into a bottomless pit of chronic fatigue and depression.

Emily responded to the initial sessions of acupuncture and herbs. She regained energy and felt less overwhelmed, but she still felt no connection to her family and was unable to find a way to prioritize her many tasks. She still described her life as "one big mess."

Emily appeared to have no center. She was "all over the place," nowhere and everywhere, trying to do too much while actually accomplishing very little. Her words and her actions were out of sync. Her life didn't hold together. While she claimed to believe that a mother's first commitment was to her children, in fact she could not even get their breakfast made in the morning. An accomplished scholar and art historian, she could not keep track of her shopping list or the notes she made for her appointments.

After a few sessions, I felt that I had established a solid rapport with Emily and decided to take a risk and mention my observations. When I questioned her about the discrepancy between her words and her actions, she grew thoughtful.

"You're right," she said. "It's just that nothing comes from me. Nothing comes from my heart. It's all about *should* and *have to* and everyone else's needs. I think one thing and do something else because my heart isn't in any of it. And then that makes me feel worse, because if there's anything I care about, it's my family, my kids."

I suggested that she take a minute, right where she was, to check in with her body, just bring her awareness down from the swirling

thoughts of her mind to the waves of her breath, the rhythmic pulsing of her heartbeat. I suggested she try bringing her awareness to
her feet and notice the way it felt just to have them planted on the
floor in front of her.

She took a deep breath. "I never do this," she said. "I never take
time for me. I've just been trying to do too much, to take care of
everyone without taking any care of me."

I began to talk to Emily about the yi, about ways she could nurture her own spirit. I suggested that in addition to the Chinese herbs
and acupuncture she was already trying, she might reevaluate her
diet, eliminate sugar as much as possible and add a lot more iron-
rich foods. I suggested that she simplify her life, beginning by taking
a few minutes a day where she did nothing but notice the rhythms
of her body and her breath.

Then I had Emily lie down on the treatment table. The point I
decided to needle was on her back, a Spirit Point: Bladder 49, *yi she*,
Hut of the Yi. I think of this point as a humble abode, a small her-
mitage where the yi spirit sits in quiet contemplation. It is a quiet,
down-to-earth place that suits the unassuming nature of the yi.
Needling this point does not usually result in big, immediate shifts,
shattering insights, or dramatic emotional releases. Rather, it seems
to support a quiet presence, an ability to be with the self and to get
in touch with one's own life purpose.

After removing the needles, I added tiny bits of direct moxa to
spark the spirit. The muscles of Emily's back relaxed and her breathing slowed. She stopped talking. I let her rest a few minutes and then
asked her to turn over. She moved slowly onto her back and then
stretched her body carefully. "After you needled that point, I felt like
my breath got deeper," she said. "I could feel the air go all the way
down."

I let her rest a few minutes and then came back to the side of the
table. "The thing is, I really love them. I want to be a good mother,

a good wife, but I have to find another way to do it. The way I've been trying just isn't working."

Over the next months, Emily worked to find a balance between her commitment to her family and her commitment to herself. She realized that it would still be many years before she would have real time for her career or her own interests but she also came to understand that pushing beyond her own limits without taking time to rejuvenate herself was not going to work anymore.

She continued to come for acupuncture treatments once a month, as I explained to her that the yi thrive on consistency. I also explained that since her problem was deep and chronic, it would take some time to shift it completely. Her treatments included the ongoing use of spleen tonics[5] and acupuncture to build qi and blood, but our primary focus was on the yi—helping her learn how to bring her heart's desires, her words and her actions into harmony. We used many spirit points, including Spleen 1, Hidden White, Spleen 45, Stomach 36 and Leg Three Miles, a point that is known to have a regulating effect on the mind, subduing excess thinking and gently moving the blood and qi. We never needed to return to the Hut of the Yi. It seemed that once the yi spirit had been reinstalled, she was happy to stay in quiet contemplation in the "middle house."

ALCHEMY: DEVOTION

In the Taoist alchemical text *The Secret of the Golden Flower,* we discover the spirit of the yi at the center of the inner alchemical opus. The yi is what allows the yang energies of the mind to mix with the yin energies of the body. It is the agent of integration that folds the initiatory impulses of our insights, inspirations and visions seamlessly into our consistent and ongoing actions in the world.

In the first half of life, the yi is our intention and we call on it to support our projects, to remain loyal to our goals and to plant and nourish the seeds of our lives. As "intention," the yi gives us the capacity to stretch our will outward into the world. It allows us to direct the energies of our mind toward a goal, to direct the course of our journey. But at a certain point, sooner or later in life, the entropy of matter takes a toll on the yi. Its potency is weakened by the effort of pushing up against the resistance of the environment. If we fight the yi's dwindling potency and continue to try to use the yi as a way to bring our personal will to bear on the outer environment, eventually our spleen qi is depleted and the yi grows weak.

If, however, we turn our thoughts, away from our outer worries, plans and goals, and reflect inwardly on the true desires of our hearts, a new kind of energy infuses the yi. This is the yin power of devotion. Devotion means that we surrender our personal intention to the greater wisdom of Tao. With devotion, we totally give ourselves up to a greater power. Our devotion is a vow, a profession, a prayer that opens us to another way of being. Devotion is the way of the middle, the wuwei of the fields and the gardens that receive the seeds and rain and sunlight and rest in the peace of perfect receptivity. In the words of the *Golden Flower*,

> When one sets out to carry out one's decision, care must be taken to see that everything can proceed in a comfortable, easy manner. Too much must not be demanded of the heart. One must be careful that heart and power correspond to one another. Only then can a state of quietness be attained. . . . I do not mean that no trouble is to be taken, but the right behavior lies in the middle way between being and non-being. And if one can attain purposelessness through purpose, then the thing has been grasped.[6]

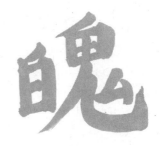

Chapter Nine

Po: The Spirit of Metal—Animal Wit, Embodiment, Sensation and Appreciation

A stone is frozen music.

—ANONYMOUS

STONES

The stones face us across a vast gulf of silence. Their wisdom can only reach us through our dreams and the murmurings of our bodies. All across the face of the planet, stones bear witness to the mystery of time. The idea of the "magic stone" is found in the myths and stories of aboriginal people the world over. Megalithic standing stones at Stonehenge, Avesbury and dozens of other sites across the British Isles stare blankly at the modern world, watching and waiting for the day when human beings will once again understand their language. Soul stones charged with *mana* have been found stored in secret caves at ancient sites in Europe, Australia and Polynesia. The world over, when ancient people looked at stones, they saw magic. In the stones they saw the entranceway to the underworld, the caverns where the mysteries of life, death and transformation occur.

The Po

On our journey down Kunlun Mountain, we have passed the sunlit regions of the shen, the windy cloud forests of the hun, the fields and gardens of the yi. Now, in order to meet the po spirits, we must descend below the horizon line.

The po is the yin, materialized aspect of the soul. In the macrocosm of the mountain, the po spirits are discovered beyond the dark gate that leads to the caves and labyrinths of the underworld. Deep in the darkness of the caves, amidst the minerals, stones and decaying compost of matter, the po spirits exist in a state of half-slumbering silence. The po are the animating agents of vital life processes that take place beyond our conscious awareness and control. They are closely related to the autonomic nervous system, the sensory receptors—especially the primitive touch responses of the skin—and the interior sense receptors of the visceral organs. Just as the shen and the hun can be correlated with the frontal lobe of the brain and the conscious mind and imagination, the po and the zhi can be correlated with more primitive aspects of the brain such as the limbic system and cerebellum.

The po are the buried light of spirit. They are the complexes, psychosomatic symptoms, emotional blocks and intuitive knowing that lock in psychic energy that can be later unraveled and used for our psychological development. The treasures of our embodied soul hide in these crystallized structures, the tangled psychic knots of consciousness.

In one of the earliest translations of Taoist alchemical terminology, Richard Wilhelm's translation of *The Secret of the Golden Flower,*[1] the word po is translated as *anima*, the Greek word for the feminine aspect of the soul. C. G. Jung, in his later Commentary on the text, develops this association to support his own ideas about the psyche. "The anima," says Jung, "is the energy of the heavy and turbid: it clings to the bodily, fleshly heart."[2] This association evokes images of the heavy, earth-bound nature of the po, the mood shifts, murkiness, depth and vast fertility of its nature.

The po are our embodied knowing, our animal wit, our street smarts, the part of us that can sniff out what's right or wrong, good or bad, safe or unsafe. Deep below the level of our conscious ability to articulate in words what we think about a person, place or situation, the po spirits already know—and, whether or not we realize it, our body has begun to respond by contracting or expanding, hardening or softening.

The silent murmurings of stones echo the murmurings of the po as they follow their path through the dark recesses of our somatic unconscious. Part animal, part human, part spirit, part stone, part flesh, part bone . . . these mysterious animators of the deep psyche represent the aspect of our unconscious that speaks to us through our desires, obsessions, psychosomatic symptoms and the wordless stories of our bodies.

The Po and the Essences

The po spirit is closely related to the jing, the essences, the yin, ungraspable, quintessential life substance of earth that supports the vitality of all living organisms. The po are created from the essences of the parents at conception, and from conception to birth the po direct the creation of the physical structures of the body, which are constructed from the essences of the mother. After birth, the po helps animate the body and enlivens the post-natal essences as they are incorporated into a person's physical being. "Without the Corporeal Soul the Essence would be an inert, albeit precious vital substance,"[3] for although the po is yin, it is yang in relation to the essences.

The po spirits represent the wisdom of the earth and the body. Just as the hun are the messengers of the upper spirits of the shen, the po are the messengers and handmaidens of the lower spirits. As the hun and the shen are guided by the golden radiance of the stars, the spiritual light of heaven, the po and the zhi are guided by the silver luminosity of the essences, the spiritual light of the earth.

The Po and the Emotions

In Chinese tradition, it is said that there are seven po. There are seven sense orifices through which a person relates to the outer world (the two eyes, the two ears, the two nostrils and the mouth). And there are seven emotions: fear, fright, anger, joy, worry, sadness and grief. The expression of emotion is related to the po since emotions are intrinsically related to the sympathetic and parasympathetic nervous system. Emotions elicit involuntary instinctual responses at the level of the breath, the hormones, fascia and muscles, and these involuntary responses are all related to the movement of the po soul.

Emotions are our organic response to the impressions of the world that we perceive through our seven sensory orifices. Chuang Tzu, an early Taoist sage, spoke of the emotions as winds. He described the human being as a tree with its roots sunk in the earth, its branches reaching toward the sky. When winds pass by, they rustle the branches of the tree and blow through all the little cavities and hollows of its trunk. He spoke of this wind blowing through the hollows and openings of the tree as earthly music and likened this music to the emotions that are stirred as the qi streams through the cavities and hollows of our bodies.[4]

As we have already seen, in Chinese medicine each emotion arises from a particular organ and has its own particular energetic character. Anger shoots upward from the liver like the wood in spring. Joy emanates outward like fire from the heart. Sympathy clings to the spleen like the humidity of late summer. Grief lingers like the autumn vapors in the lungs. And fear sinks like water and freezes in the lower back and kidneys. Oppression and overthinking are two other psychic functions that the Chinese considered emotions, and both have the effect of causing movement to stagnate. All emotions are viewed as psychic winds that arise from the organs of our bodies in response to our interactions with the outer world. Emotions, like breezes rustling the leaves of the trees, move us as they move through us.

The character for "seven" is drawn with a horizontal line representing the earth and a vertical line springing up from beneath the ground, moving toward the sky. Similarly, the emotions arise from the fleshy underworld darkness of the organs and move through us, eliciting actions that connect us to the outer world. They are an aspect of qi, the life force. As they rise up from the living sap of the body, they are connected to the *qing*, the blue-green life-giving essences of the vegetative world.

The emotions are the aspect of psychic life that connects us "horizontally" to the world around us. They are the result of our visceral responses to the people and events we come in contact with and they are the way we move out from our centers toward the world. They are the result of the interaction between the winds of life and the physical structures of our being. The organ structures, like the structure of the tree itself, the trunk and branches and hollows through which the winds blow, are the material, corporeal aspects of the soul. The organs are an aspect of the po soul, the embodied aspect of the spirit.

The Dual Expression of the Soul

Like the hun, the po is spoken of as a soul rather than a spirit. The hallmark of the two souls is their breathy, oscillating, up-and-down, coming-and-going quality. While both are also considered spirits and are yang, entropic and breathy relative to the essences and physical structures of the body, the hun are yang relative to the po. The hun regulate the coming and going of the mind,[5] while the po regulate the coming and going of the *jing qi* or essences.

The hun oscillate between the eyes and the liver. Residing in the former by day and the latter by night, they envision and plan in the light and dream in the darkness. The po journey from the lungs to the intestines, lifting upward with the first breath of life and dropping downward with the last. In life, the po resides in the lungs and is responsible for vital involuntary physical functions such as breathing, peristalsis, and evacuation as well as sensation, balance, and muscular coordination. At death, the po descends with the decaying bones of the body to the underworld where it is reincorporated into the inert structures of the earth, the stones, crystals, and minerals of the soil "whose richness they renew in the process of slowly decomposing and disappearing."[6] Life and death, movement and inertia, lungs and colon—these are the polarities of the po.

The two souls function together as pneumatic regulators of the breath body. The hun's activities are negentropic and lifting while, relative to the hun, the po's activities are entropic and grounding. Any abstract thought, idea, fantasy or vision we have produces a physical response in the body. Any movement of the hun—any inspiring or initiating thought or image that comes and goes through the mind—has a complementary response at the level of the po, some neurological, muscular or biochemical shift. In other words, when the hun moves, the po responds, even if we are not consciously aware of it. In a state of health, the complementary responses of the souls have the graceful movements of a dance. Led by the light of the shen and supported by the potency of essences, the dance of the hun and the po carries us forward along the path of Tao.

Ordinarily the hun leads and the po follows, but when there is dysfunction, the easy reciprocal play between the two souls is disrupted and the po is unable to manifest the hun's plans and visions. The hun, disconnected from the grounding, entropic influences of the po, fly up out of the body, into a whirl of useless ideas and grandiose fantasies. No longer supported by the buoyant, negentropic influences of the hun, the po succumb to their natural tendency to fall. "They tend to bury themselves in the depths,"[7] slow down, get stuck and revert to a state of inertia and congelation in the unlit regions of the somatic unconscious. The light of the po, the shimmering light of crystal and precious metals, cannot be seen when it is hidden beneath the earth. In order to be seen, the lower light of the po must be illuminated by the upper light of the hun and the shen, the golden light of the sun and conscious awareness.

Psychological issues at this level are very difficult to see because they are hidden in the darkness of matter. These issues may manifest as psychosomatic pain, eczema, asthma, incontinence, obesity, depression, lumps, tumors and bowel disturbances. In order to heal and reenter the cycle of life, the po spirit requires a restoration of animation and illumination of the shen and the hun.

In alchemical transformation and healing work, we recouple the two souls by allowing the yin wisdom of the body to lead and the yang mind to follow. In meditation, for example, we begin by consciously stilling the movements of the body, by keeping the back still and calming the central nervous system through the breath. As the po calms, the hun also becomes quiet, and in this space of silence the voice of the body becomes audible to the mind. This is why Lao Tzu says that enlightened action and leadership depends on our ability to "hold fast to the power of the One," to "maintain perfect harmony between the hun (Ethereal Soul) and the po (Vital or Corporeal Soul)," to "merge the body with the spirit."[8]

A Look at the Chinese Character

Like the Chinese character *hun*, *po* contains the radical *gui*. As we saw in Chapter Seven, this character means "earthbound spirit" and is sometimes translated as "ghost." The top part represents the head of a person while the bottom is the vaporous body of a spirit. The gui is the sign that reminds us of the po and the hun soul's breathy, come-and-go quality.

Claude Larre speaks of the gui as "just strolling on the air, walking more or less on the ground, and they have something contradictory, they go this way and then they stop."[9] Through his poetic description, we begin to get a picture of the gui as ephemeral mists that float lightly about the surfaces of things. Like ghosts, the gui are vaporous spirit beings, yet like ghosts they are still uncomfortably tethered to the world of matter. They are mysterious yet real, delicate and sensitive yet very powerful and especially worthy of great respect. Larre pays special attention to the curlicue, the spiraling tail at the lower right side of the radical *gui*[10] on the right side of the character for *po*. He refers to this curling line as the whirlwind, the chaotic energies that we feel as the souls pass by, the tiny dust storms and mists that swirl and spiral as one form changes into another, as the souls oscillate between vapor and form, carrying the messages of the spirits between above and below.

Po combines the radical *gui* with the radical *bai,* meaning "white." White is the color of the metal element. In the Chinese tradition, it is also the color of death, the color of the bones buried beneath the earth. Paradoxically, however, the character for "white" is a pictograph of the rising sun. The line at the top of the character *ba* represents a ray of light. Ba, the color white, is associated with brightness and is related to the color of the eastern sky at dawn.

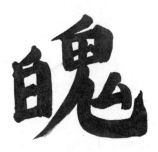

Po

The character *po* contains a paradox that gives us a clue to the mystery of the stone soul, the soul of matter. Clustered around the character *po* are the images of bones buried beneath the earth, ephemeral spirits floating this way and that, breaths, death, the underworld and the rising sun. So what we see in this character is an image of death and resurrection. This cluster of contradictory images has implications in terms of our collective attitudes toward the yin, the feminine, the body and the earth.

ASSOCIATIONS AND CORRELATIONS

The po are related to

Element: metal
Organ: lungs (and large intestine)
Emotion: grief
Psychological Functions: animal wit, embodied knowing, sensation
Psychospiritual Issue: discovering the preciousness of the moment
Cosmological Associations: stones, gems, minerals, caves, labyrinths
Chakra: first/second—Matter
Virtue: appreciation of preciousness

THE PO AND THE ELEMENT OF METAL

While we are alive, the po resides in the zang of the lungs as the shen resides in the heart, the hun in the liver and the yi in the spleen. The po are related to the element metal, as the shen is to fire, the hun to wood and the yi to earth. Metal is yin in respect to the earth. Its quality is even heavier than earth, less active and less susceptible to the influences of the outer environment.

In the metal is a stillness and slowness found nowhere else in nature. Here we enter the shadow land where the yin—the downward pull of entropy, matter, gravity and decomposition—has overpowered the upward, forward movement of the yang spirits. Metal is associated with the color white, the emotion grief, the season of autumn. It is associated with death, the endings of cycles, the coming and going of life, the rhythms of the breath and the excretory functions.

Like metal, the po are related to the coming and going of life; the *Lingshu* links them to the "exiting and entering of Essence." Unlike the hun, who fly off to the heavens with the shen when the physical body dies, the po are indissolubly connected to the body and accompany it as it disintegrates and descends back to the underworld at death. And at birth, they gather again as the earth essences restructure to form the body of a new embryo in the uterus.

Like metal, the intrinsic nature of the po is yin. Thus, like crystals, precious metals, minerals and mists, the po is fond of the secrecy and shadows of the cave world. In the microcosm of the body, the po's natural habitat is in the depths of our being, the anus and intestines—the deepest parts of our bodies—and in the mysterious labyrinths of the unconscious.

SIGNS AND SYMPTOMS OF PO DISTURBANCE

Common symptoms are:

obsessions, depression, anxiety

chronic tension and pain

eating disorders

undiagnosible lumps and benign tumors

impaired balance, movement, coordination

stress-related skin problems

asthma

bowel disturbances

restlessness during the day

clouded mind

Spirit Level Signs:

- a vague feeling that "something isn't right" but no clear sense of why

- physical pain that takes over entire life yet seems to have no identifiable cause

- extreme sensitivity to outer influences on a psychic level; for example, other people's negativity "gets in" without awareness and creates somatic disturbances such as digestive upsets, headache, etc.

- unexpressed somatized emotional issue and "stuck destiny"; the person doesn't ever seem to move on in life

IDENTIFYING PO SPIRIT-RELATED PAIN

When is chronic pain a calling out of the somatic soul? When is an aching or gnawing discomfort in the body a "crystallized emotion" waiting to be discovered? When does a patient need support, not only to feel better physically, but to dare to shine the light of awareness into the dark death sleep of a denied truth?

There are four signs that indicate a psychosomatic disturbance at the level of the po. The first three require careful history taking and patience on the part of the practitioner. The last requires what the *Neijing Suwen* describes as "profound and mysterious knowledge," "divine inspiration," or what we in the modern world call attention, experience and intuition. If you or someone you know has chronic pain that fits this description, then the pain is probably not just physical. Acupuncture, acupressure, flower essences and Chinese herbs, as well as following the suggestions in this handbook, may be helpful.

The four signs are:

1. There is chronic pain that does not respond to standard treatment.

2. Structural imbalances, recent trauma and serious medical problems have been ruled out.

3. There is chronic emotional stress or a deep unresolved psychological issue in patient's history.

4. Part of the patient seems to be dormant. This may manifest as a depressed

affect, a lack of connectedness, a mist over the eyes, cloudiness in the person's aura and/or a feeling that the mind is not at ease.

Possible Causes:

- maternal vitamin and nutrient deficiencies during gestation
- insufficient touch and tactile stimulation during infancy
- restrictive child-raising practices that did not allow freedom of bodily movement and expression
- ancestral and familial issues that have been "swept under the rug"
- early childhood abuse forgotten by the conscious mind but "remembered" by the soma, resulting in disturbances of the po in later years
- refusal to face one's own "shadow"; trying to be "all goodness and light" while denying deeper layers of emotions
- resistance to life changes crucial to one's karmic development and destiny
- a break between the upper and lower spirits, a split between what is consciously thought should be done and the wisdom of the body

THE FROZEN MUSIC OF THE STONES

When the light of heaven is carried to earth by the gentle penetrating wind of the hun, the ephemeral markings of spirit can be seen in the ripples of the sand dunes and the waves of the seas. Psychologically, these ephemeral ripples mark themselves on our lives as the visions and plans we make for our future and the ways that we begin to organize random events into coherent patterns. The yi gives us the capacity to commit to our visions and our attempts at organization, to plant and cultivate them in the rich soil of embodied purpose. Through the yi, the windy breaths of the hun are transformed into vibrations of sound, the words through which we express our promises and intentions, and the muscle power of our bodies through which we begin to manifest our words.

But when these ripples of the wind soul are permanently fixed in the underlying structures of the world, they have passed through the celestial pivot of the earth to descend to the realm of the po, the stone soul, the element of metal. Here the crystallized vibrations of spirit become mineralized and hardened by their burial in matter. In the metal element, the celestial music is frozen in the patterns and forms of the natural world: the precious gems, the hidden shimmering alloys, the minerals that form the structures of the physical body, the forgotten memories of our bodies, and the innate patterns of our true nature that are crystallized in our genetic codes.

Psychologically, the po is the realm of the body unconscious, the sensations, emotions, talents, strengths and passions that are part of our innate neurological responses to life. At the level of the po, the light of the shen becomes a star seed hidden in the matrix of our physical being. The po represent the potent unconscious psychic forces, the habits, sensual proclivities and emotional responses that fix our identities and influence the course of our destinies and yet may remain hidden for a lifetime from the light of the conscious mind.

PO AS SOMA

In terms of Western psychology, we can draw parallels between the hun and the psyche (the human mind, imagination and dreaming function) and between the po and the soma (the human body, senses, emotions and unconscious physiological responses). Both are centers of awareness, with the soma embodying a complement to the psyche, the material, physical aspect of consciousness. Because human beings are often cut off from the wisdom of the body, the soma becomes a reservoir of memories, feelings and instinctual drives that can be entirely hidden from the light of conscious awareness. This hidden material is stored in the tissue memory, in the muscles, fascia, nerves and organs of the physical body. Some is stored because it is not relevant to a person's current situation, while some is kept hidden because it is too frightening or overwhelming to the conscious personality and threatens to disturb the current equilibrium of a person's life.

The soma is nonverbal and nonlinear in its organization, and its workings generally occur below the level of ordinary awareness. Problems at this level are expressed through dream images, irrational longings and obsessions, feelings of depression and anxiety, and especially bodily problems such as eating disorders, chronic tension and psychosomatic distress. Arnie Mindell refers to events that take place at this level of the bodymind as "secondary process" and emphasizes that these experiences "happen outside my control and are unconscious."

Each time we descend to the level of the soma and consciously interact with the po, we shine light on previously darkened parts of our awareness. We are presented with a sort of identity crisis, a fundamental reevaluation of who we thought we were and where we thought we were going. Jungian psychology refers to this as getting in touch with the shadow. As we reincorporate these unfamiliar, shadow parts of the self, we ultimately broaden the parameters of the self and free up previously unavailable psychic energy. This is a crucial stage in the journey of healing, the return to wholeness.

Many Western acupuncture patients with chronic pain are actually "somatizing" a threatening psychological issue by expressing it through a body symptom. Beneath many acupuncture channel blockages there is a po disturbance, a problem at the level of the corporeal soul. Disturbances of the shen or spirit result in symptoms we in the West more commonly label as "psychological distress." Anxiety, panic, mania, hyperactivity, emotional agitation, confusion and insomnia are some typical examples. When psychological and emotional issues affect the po, the qi tends to slow down and sink, to congeal into lumps of discomfort buried like stones in the living tissues of the body, and the po loses its vital connection to the hun and shen and sinks toward earth.

The yang vitality of conscious awareness can greatly enhance the work of moxa and needles in bringing movement and life back to these stuck, painful places in the bodymind. Although it is not always necessary to know the underlying emotional issues in order for a symptom to disappear, healing that goes beyond the physical to the level of the Spirit sometimes does require this kind of expanded awareness. The process of consciously bringing the awareness or shen back into contact with the instinctual body or po may open the door to a patient's recovery. By illuminating the po with the light of the shen and recoupling it with the lifting energies of the hun, movement and health can return to chronically stuck places in a person's body, and meaning, direction and vitality can return to his or her life.

AWARENESS AS RESTORATION OF MOVEMENT

One of Chinese medicine's most basic principles—if there is free flow, there is no pain—reminds us that life in harmony is a process of continual transformation. When an organism no longer responds and changes, it is a sign of a disease, disintegration and, ultimately, death. When ways of being become repetitive habits or when muscle tension becomes chronic holding patterns, vitality diminishes. While this concept is most often applied to pain at the level of the physical body, it is equally applicable to emotional, psychological and spiritual distress.

Problems begin when the endless oscillations of the hun and the po are arrested. When the transformational whirlwind of the souls no longer promotes easy movement between above and below, spirit and matter, the bodymind begins to spin uselessly, expending energy but going nowhere. The souls become gui, psychic complexes or psychosomatic blockages that rob the organism of vitality, and the organic processes—the rhythms of the breath and heartbeat; the taking in of nourishment and the letting go of waste; the movement from vision to action; the alternation of activity and rest, waking and sleep; and the transition between life and death—become blocked and pathologically disturbed. When emotional stuckness manifests on the level of the somatic unconscious, chronic physical pain may be the result. Such pain, which in the West is often labeled "psychosomatic," is a concretized expression of the soul's distress. It is a place where the life force has slowed down to a death sleep and the animating energy of emotion has crystallized into an inert stone that is buried deep in the unconscious strata of the psyche.

However, like the element of metal with which it is associated, the po not only relates to the underworld, death and disintegration but also to renewal, replenishment and resurrection. The po is raised up from the lower depths toward life by the airy breaths that come from heaven. The yin po is bound to the processes of life through its relationship to the yang spirits, the hun and shen, the psychological functions of imagination and conscious awareness. The po has a special relationship to each. "The hun and po live as a couple; their union is life, their separation is our death."[11] The po's relationship to the shen is equally important. Like the other spirits, there are many ways to begin to bring vitality back to the po. Qi moving and blood de-congealing herbs and tonifying acupuncture can be used to restore free flow to the channels. Breath and touch can be used as needles to bring oxygen, circulation and warmth back to these areas. Rhythmic exercise such as tai ch'i, dance and walking meditation can also be very useful.

But when these forms of standard treatment fail, patients may need to develop some kind of conscious relationship to their own body in order for their symptoms to subside and their personal development to continue. Their physical pain may be the way that the deepest self is calling out for a profound life change. In these cases, self-awareness and imagery can actually be used like needles to move the qi. The shen or light of conscious awareness can reawaken the po, while the hun or visionary imagination can redirect and animate it. By focusing the light and energy of these yang spirits on the hidden pockets of darkness in the psyche, psychological movement is restored and the stuck po lifted back in the cycle of life. In this way, the heavy lead of unconscious suffering can be transformed into a "living" metal, the gold of illuminated matter.

THE PO AS AGENTS OF TRANSFORMATION

When we arrive at the realm of the po, we enter uncharted territory, a shadowy place away from sunlight that cannot be navigated by the conscious mind but only by the lunar light of embodied knowing and animal wit. For this phase of the healing process, it is necessary to enter the unexplored parts of the psyche, the depths of body where the memories of forgotten traumas and wounds are stored in our neurological responses, our muscular holding patterns and the configuration of our cells.

This is the part of the healing process when old ways of being die so that new ways can come to life. Just as the lungs function to take in the air we need to live and the intestines to let go of what is not useful to our life, the po guide us in letting go of ways of being that are no longer efficient and opening to new, more efficient possibilities. In mythologies the world over, this phase of the healing journey is known as a descent to the underworld. In alchemical terms, it is the time when we enter the alchemical cauldron of matter and the body, the phase of the healing process when real transformation begins.

Case Study: Listening to the Body

By bringing the light of consciousness to the shadows of the somatic self, we engage in an alchemical process that melds the soul substances of the shen and the po. This can sometimes open the door to embodied realizations and insights that turns the tide of a person's healing process.

The following case study is an example of how the unconscious symbolic murmurings of the body can be brought to the level of conscious awareness. It is a story that leaves many questions unanswered but shows some of the ways that the energy of difficult emotions can be buried in the po of the somatic unconscious. It also gives an idea of how they can be gently brought back to life by the warmth and light of consciousness.

Renie arrived at my office wearing a green washed silk suit and a string of pearls. She had come directly from work, where she was a partner in a law firm. Renie was forty-four, professionally successful and married to a man ten years older who had two grown children from a previous marriage.

Renie's chief complaint was a pain in her left elbow that had begun without warning about a year earlier. Over time it had grown steadily worse. Like most of my patients, she had tried a number of other modalities and had been seen by several Western doctors. X-rays revealed nothing, and she had been given a Western diagnosis of tendonitis. When Renie came to see me, the pain was so bad she could barely use her left arm or bend her elbow to pick up a cup of tea. She was taking anti-inflammatory drugs to relieve the pain, but they were not helping. She described the pain as achy, unmoving and unresponsive to any treatment.

"I don't understand it," she said. "I'm right-handed. I don't use my left arm to write or lift things and I don't play tennis. But the pain is always there and now it's keeping me up at night. It bothers me all the time."

Before I began treating Renie, I inquired about the rest of her life. She said her health was good. She enjoyed her work and was happy in her marriage. She exercised regularly and ate well. I felt that she was holding back, and after further questioning she told me that for a long time she had very much wanted a child. Her husband, however, had been reluctant to begin the process of parenting all over again. This had been a point of contention between them for the first years of their marriage. By the time he agreed, Renie was over forty. When she finally conceived, she miscarried after six weeks. After trying unsuccessfully for three years to become pregnant again, she had given up.

"After that," she said, "I must have gone numb. There's nothing that seems to matter much anymore."

From a Five Element perspective, Renie was a classic metal constitution. There was a pale white tone to the skin around her eyes and a weeping sound to her voice, but the "giveaway" was the poignancy and grief that emanated from her, as if there was a lost waif hiding underneath the shiny attractiveness of her outer appearance. I was struck by the sense of a mist hovering at the edges of her body, especially around her upper body, chest, eyes and the sides of her face. As previous case histories have shown, the sense of patient's "not being all there" suggests a Spirit level problem, and mistiness in the aura often points me in the direction of the po. This was an early clue that I made note of, although I was not immediately sure what it meant.

Treatment #1

I began with standard Five Element acupuncture treatment, needling Lung 9 and Large Intestine 4, acupuncture points connected to the metal element. I felt that these constitutional points on the lung and colon meridian would begin to harmonize her energy and bring vitality back to her life force. Coincidentally, they were also points recommended for pain in the hand and elbow.

Treatment #2

Renie reported no change in her arm pain after the first treatment, but during the week she began to be aware of a strange sensation. "It's like there's a cloud around me. Nothing can get through to really touch me. I guess, all these years, I've been depressed without knowing it."

I inserted acupuncture needles at Large Intestine 9 to harmonize the metal, relieve pain and activate the channel. Lung 9 was repeated. After I needled these points, I noticed that there was a bit of pink coming into Renie's cheeks, and she looked as if she were trying not to cry. I burned three rice grain moxa on Dove Tail (C.V. 15), which I think of as the meeting point of the energies of the upper *jiao*, the lungs and the heart. After this her color further improved and she said that she felt calm and centered. For the next two weeks, I suggested that she take five drops of Jade Pharmacy Meridian Passage in the morning and evening[12] as a way to support the clearing that the needles had already begun. While this particular formula is often used for stubborn physical pain, it is less well known that it can also soften and clear deeply held emotional pain.

Treatment #3

Renie reported a slight improvement in her elbow after the last treatment but said that she was feeling increasingly depressed, as if a dark cloud hung between her and the world. "I feel cut off. I never used to be this way, but now I don't care about anything." I asked Renie to close her eyes and relax, to feel her feet on the floor and just breathe. Then I invited her to turn her attention inward and describe what she saw.

"It's like a wasteland," she said. "I see a barren landscape, potholes and dirt. Nothing is growing." As Renee turned her awareness inward, I did the same. I scanned my emotions and the sensations in my own body. I also allowed my imagination to drift and began to sense a lost child standing behind Renie. A deep grief swept over me, and my mind went to the miscarriage. I asked Renie if any of this made sense. At this, she began to sob deeply. "I've been feeling so hopeless," she said.

I shared with Renie imagery from Chinese medicine regarding the metal element, how death and loss were a way to prepare the ground for something new. I performed acupuncture treatment on Large Intestine 7 to calm the spirit and continue to work with blockage in the channel. I then had Renie turn over and needled Bladder 42, The Door of the Corporeal Soul. Although this point is generally recommended for nourishing and tonifying the lung, in Five Element acupuncture it is used to touch the spirit or soul level of metal. According to classical texts, it was used to clear people of possession. My purpose in using this point was to assist Renie is letting go of the baby she had lost (who had in a sense taken possession of her soul) and moving forward to the next chapter of her life.

Treatment #4

Renie came in and said that the pain was getting "incrementally better." She said she was feeling a bit less depressed and that she had kept returning to the visualization she had had of the barren field. "It's a relief," she said, "just to acknowledge that I've been living in a wasteland, to let it be without trying to change it." I asked her if she would like to revisit the place inside and she agreed. When she went back to the field, she saw the same muddy expanse of ground, but a shoot of green grass had appeared in the center.

At that point, I discussed with Renie the nature of the wood element and its relationship to spring, anger and renewal. The green shoot became symbolic of returning life. She began to speak about her rage at not having a child, her fear that her husband really would abandon her if she decided to adopt a child, and her anger at his lack of support. This time, I needled Liver 3 to spread qi and help further release constrained emotion as well as to support movement in the elbow. I supported the treatment with points on the lung and large intestine meridian.

Two Months Later

I continued to treat Renie with points on the lung, large intestine and liver meridians. When difficult emotions surfaced, I sometimes added the *mu, shu* and source points of heart and pericardium. As the physical pain improved she stopped using the Chinese herbs but found that Bach Flower Rescue Remedy was helpful between sessions when she experienced emotional upset.

Two months later, Renie reported that her elbow pain was "ninety-three percent better" with only slight twinges during the day. At this point I decided to do a point on the lung meridian called "Broken Sequence," located just above the wrist, a point that is used to balance the yin and yang aspects of the metal element. It is specifically recommended for pain along the large intestine meridian but it is also a point known to have effects on a psycho-emotional level. Before I needled the point, I told Renie its name and explained that although it was useful for arm pain, it was also known to have psychological effects, such as the recovering and letting go of painful memories.

The point had a very powerful and immediate effect on Renie, but it was not the effect either of us had been expecting. What she experienced when I needled this point on her wrist was light shooting through hand and arm and up into her body. "It's as if this light is breaking through the clouds from my center upward through my chest to my face," she said. "I keep seeing this image of the spirit of the baby I couldn't have. I'm afraid if I let go of that image, I'll have nothing to hang on to."

I suggested that Renie bring her awareness to her body, especially to the pain in her elbow. "What's going on in your elbow right now?" I asked her.

"It's throbbing," she said, "and I want to just shake the pain out of me."

I told her to just go ahead and follow the impulse to shake her hand, but she said that it made her feel "like a silly kid" and she didn't want to do it. So I suggested that she relax and allow the feelings and images to move through her. I reminded her to stay with the rhythm of her own breath moving in and out through her lungs. I told her that no matter what, she would always have her own emotions and the rhythms and cycles of her own body to come back to.

Over the next few weeks, we focused on acupuncture points that would assist Renie in letting go of the child she couldn't have. Many of these points were also useful for elbow pain. But in addition to the acupuncture points we used, I focused on helping Renie reconnect to her po, the steady, reliable rhythms of her own body, her weight, her solidity, her breathing, and most of all her own emotions, especially her grief and her returning sense of the preciousness of life.

One day she came in and said she had realized that she was feeling better. "I still might try to get pregnant," she said. "Or maybe I'll adopt. I actually made a call last week to an adoption agency. Somehow, though, I don't feel so desperate. The other morning before I left for work, I looked outside and noticed the light falling on a patch of ferns in the garden. I actually felt happy. I never noticed how beautiful that spot was before."

During one of these sessions, Renie came up with an important image. She felt that she had been like a traveler walking aimlessly through a deserted landscape that had a mountain in the distance. Now she saw that at the top of the mountain was a hut. That hut was her destination. The emergence of this image marked a turning point in her treatment. The hut symbolized the realignment of her visions and goals with the pathway of her life, the recoupling of her hun and po. Over time, it became clear that the goal of this part of her journey was indeed to adopt a child.

Renie's elbow continued to improve. Several months after she had first come to see me, she reached over and picked up a glass of water with her left hand. She took a drink and put the glass down without thinking about it. Then she realized what she'd done. "That's pretty good," she said. "I couldn't have done that a few weeks ago."

Six Months Later

By this time, Renie's elbow pain had completely faded. Her treatments focused on her emotional state, her marriage and her decision about adopting a child. Her biggest conflict was the pull she felt between her husband's desires and her own deep need to be a mother. She spoke about a darkness around her heart, as if light and color could not penetrate. I focused on spirit level points that would help to open her heart and rejoin her fire and metal. She began an imaginary dialogue with the baby girl whose presence she imaginatively felt hovering around her. Meanwhile, we worked to differentiate whether the child was her own young wounded self, the sage within her who was struggling to be born, or in fact a presentiment of a child who "was meant" to come to her. Gradually, it became clear that all were true.

At this point, Renie began to experience a string of startling coincidences. On a business trip, she walked into a room where she was going to lecture and was met by a man holding a radiant Chinese baby girl in his arms. On the return airplane trip, she sat down to find a book on infant development lying on the seat next to her. She had recurrent dreams of holding small animals in her arms and of finding young children waiting for her in abandoned houses. These all had a powerful effect on her, and she began to feel that she needed to trust the voice of her deepest self and that her marriage would ultimately support the development of her true self.

One Year Later

A year after Renie first came in for treatment, she was free of pain and in the midst of the adoption process for a baby girl from China. She often refers to the process as a journey and says, "I just keep my eye on that little hut on the mountaintop, and one step at a time I know I'll get there."

At her last treatment, we wondered what the child's name would be. Renie looked at me and said, "I can't believe all this is happening. Honestly, this is the most amazing process I've ever been a part of!"

Was Renie's elbow pain connected to her depression and her miscarriage? From a Western medical point of view, perhaps not, but from the point of view of the po, these seemingly unrelated symptoms were connected in the underground matrix of Renie's somatic soul. Until the poetry and music of her own body could once again be heard, Renie wandered through life in a daze, cut off from the beauty and preciousness of her own life.

Statistics indicate that Renie's elbow would have gotten better from acupuncture even if she and I had never exchanged a word. But the truth is that no one definitively knows. True healing, despite all the advances of modern science, still remains a mystery.

THE GUI

It is said that the po, because of their yin nature, do not rise to heaven with the hun and the shen after death but sink back toward the earth to become gui, "white ghosts" who come and go with the mists until these spirits finally disintegrate along with the shell of the physical body. As the flesh and bones dissolve back into the stones and minerals, the po also sink back into the soil, but before the body completely decomposes, the gui tend to linger at the doorway between the upper and lower realms.

The po, being related to the yin and the earth, are also related to the forces of entropy, negative magnetic attraction and gravitational pull. "This faculty of grasping sometimes makes the po danger-ous,"[13] as it may allow them to take possession of other living souls and drag them into the underworld. If after death or during a per-son's life the gui separate from the physical structures of the body, they become starved and desperate for physical nourishment. Then their grasping at life is especially dangerous and they are sometimes spoken of as "hungry ghosts." In order to not attract the attention of the gui, the ancient Chinese were very respectful when they walked past the resting places of the dead. As an extra precaution, they sometimes inserted a jade plug into the anus of a corpse to try to keep the po trapped until it grew weak and disintegrated within the container of the body.

In Chinese folklore, the gui are related to the ghosts of dead ancestors who were not properly mourned or people racked with guilt over harmful deeds for which they never made amends. The gui are stuck in a limbo space between spirit and matter. They cannot move on so they linger at their grave sites while their ephemeral forms haunt the living. These gui are the earthbound remnants of the soul, mists contaminated with matter. They are too heavy to rise up with the shen to the bright pure light of the heavens, yet for one reason or another they still grasp at life. They cannot let go and dis-integrate back into the sheng cycle, the great round of life, death and transformation. "Unfinished business" keeps them stuck between realms. When rituals that in former times were used to help them move on are forgotten and lost, the gui congregate in damp, dark, forgotten places: dumps and marshes, bogs, drowned caves and abandoned houses.

From a psychological perspective, the gui represent the shadowy parts of the psyche that pose a threat to the conscious personality. They are the mythical parallel to the psychological complexes, the stuck areas in the psyche where we are not able to be present and respond freely to our environment. They are the emotions, impulses, bodily needs and desires that have been ignored and denigrated. Like the gui, psychic complexes are heavy, damp, stuck and disassociated from the nourishing essences of organic life. They hide at the shadowy edges, hovering outside the circle of life. Like the gui, the complexes draw nourishment from the vital parts of our being. They pull us away from life and consciousness, down into regressive states of denial, fantasy and inertia.

Many of the strange, undiagnosable psychosomatic symptoms that plague our society today are like the jade plug, used to keep the yearnings, instincts and wisdom of the somatic soul held in, separated from consciousness, in the underworld of our psyches. In Taoist terms, in order for human beings to become sages and walk the path of Tao, they must dare to know the wholeness of the self, including the ghosts and demons that linger around the dark places in the psyche. Healing at this deep level means shining the light of awareness on the shadow. It means expanding the boundaries of the self to include disowned parts. It means letting go of things that need to die and allowing new things to come to life.

When the po are cut off from the light and air of the shen and the hun, the yang light of conscious awareness—which in Western terms is known as disassociation, a split between the body and the mind—the po are deprived of the yang, lifting, negentropic energies they require in order to fulfill their function. When this occurs, the yin, grasping, gravitational nature of the po is no longer tempered by the yang and the gui take over. Rather than assisting us in the process of transforming outworn patterns and moving on with our lives, these disenfranchised psychic entities suck vitality from living organisms and interrupt the graceful flow of unfolding life.

The gui torment us with fears of death, violence, disease and dissolution. They drag us into compulsive behaviors, eating disorders and sexual addiction, or haunt our lives in the form of psychosomatic symptoms that seem to make no sense, digestive disturbances, panic disorders, allergies, hormonal problems, depression, and vague but debilitating aches and pains. In modern psychological ter-minology, we refer to these as personality disorders, phobias, addic-tion and neurosis. Modern psychology describes them as conditions in which the ego has lost its centering function and healthy instinc-tual impulses have become distorted. The ancient Chinese would say that the Spirits are in disarray, the integrity between the po and the hun has been lost, and the person has become possessed by the gui.

The gui appear when we ignore the authentic needs of our bodies. They are the externalization of our personal and collective hatred and fear of the yin, dark gestational powers of the body, the yearnings and hungers of emotional life, and the embodied wisdom of the somatic unconscious. This attitude of deep antipathy toward the lower spirits, the yin wisdom of the body, is found in every civilization that has emerged from Neolithic to modern times. When we refuse to honor and surrender to the power of the lower spirits, the transformational yin potency of the underworld and the needs and wisdom of the body, the po become weak. When we cannot let go of what needs to die and insist on accumulating much more than we need, the vital forces of life become perverted and the gui gain in power.

Psychologically, the fear and contempt of the somatic soul man-ifest in an unwillingness to look at the shadow side of our selves, a refusal to deal with our emotions, our authentic body needs and the parts of ourselves that do not fit in with collective norms. More than half of the patients I treat are suffering from symptoms that origi-nate in emotions, needs and embodied understandings that have been shoved out of the sight of consciousness. The strange, incurable psychosomatic symptoms that plague us are the jade plugs we use to keep the po held in, separated from consciousness, buried in the body, hidden in the underworld of our psyches.

Healing involves much more than simply needling points in order to move energy through the body. True healing requires bring-ing the light of the shen down into the body and illuminating somat-ic symptoms with consciousness and meaning. It means celebrating the marriage of yin and yang, matter and spirit. It means holding fast to the power of the one as the joining of the hun and po restores wholeness to the soul.

THE GUI AND THE COLLECTIVE MODERN PSYCHE

The disenfranchisement of the po is reflected in the collective psyche of our society. As a culture, we seek to deny the voice of the "feminine," the voice of the body and the intuition. The voices of mothers, artists, mystics and poets are too often ignored by those in power, as are the needs of the physical body and the reality of death. Our collective approach is to try to push our poor, our "different" and our aging away to the edges of our communities where they will not be seen, rather than include them as part of the "circle around the fire." These members of our society are treated as refuse and deprived of the light and air of conscious cultural awareness. They are the shadows who come back to haunt us in our fears and our dreams.

We find the disenfranchised gui or "white ghosts" wandering in the halls of old age homes, senior centers and nursing facilities where our elderly, the potential sages and wise ones of our society, exist in a limbo state between the world of the living and the dead. We see the gui wandering the streets of our cities with the homeless and the drug-addicted, the "cast-off" and despised members of our society, whose physical and emotional needs have been buried along with the potential gold of their gifts and wisdom. We see the gui in the depression and emptiness of isolated, exhausted mothers and unloved children who are shifted from one foster home to another. We do not want to look too hard at the faces of these forgotten ones. Theirs are the faces of the stone soul we try desperately to forget in our cultural denial of the sacred wisdom of the body.

Though the Chinese language is rooted in the images of the earth, we still must wade through layers of patriarchal misogyny, the disrespect and terror of the feminine body and the organic life/death processes of nature, to find the essential kernel of ancient somatic awareness that hides in the concept and Chinese character of the po, the yin embodied aspect of the soul. But it is in this kernel that we find one of the keys to our deepest healing.

SPIRIT POINT: STONE GATE

The acupuncture point on the Conception Vessel called *Shimen* or Stone Gate is located below the umbilicus at the center of the lower tantian, the lower cauldron or "cinnabar field." This is the area of the body that is metaphorically underground since it is located below the "horizon line," Stomach 25, Celestial Pivot, at the line of the waist. In the lower cauldron, we find the large intestine, the bladder and kidneys as well as the uterus and the reproductive organs. This lower cauldron is the mixing bowl of life and death. Here the dead cells of our body and the unusable parts of our food are excreted through the large intestine to rejoin the Great Round. And here, in the uterus, beneath the sacred Stone Gate, the jing of mother and father meld and the fetus passes from the void of nothingness into life. Here, living water spills from inert stones.

The acupuncture point Stone Gate is located approximately three inches above the pubic bone, just at the level of the upper edge of the uterus when the gestating fetus is about three and a half months of age. This is the age when the placenta is fully developed and the life support of the infant switches from a direct interchange with the mother's blood to its own filtering system. At this point the infant makes a crucial step away from the maternal matrix, the realm of the great mother, into individuated existence.

In classical texts, it is said that needling this point can turn a woman into a "stone woman," meaning that she becomes infertile for life, but there is no mention of this in modern texts and no evidence to indicate that this point should have been accorded this dangerous power. I believe this interpretation derives from a misunderstanding of alchemical language and that the name of this point alludes to the alchemical *lapis*, the cinnabar stone of the tantian. Cinnabar stone, composed of mercury and sulfur, marries the opposites of yang and yin, white and crimson. It is the sacred stone of immortality that resolves the alchemical paradoxes of spirit and matter, life and death.

The Stone Gate represents the entranceway to the pelvic basin, where the mystery of the huntun takes place. The huntun is the primordial chaos, the mixing together of all opposites and the domain of the dark goddess. It is the furnace where form is melted down to a liquid state and reformed in the shape of a new being. It is the place where opposites unite in the sacred container: the metal cauldron of the great mother, the white bones of the pelvic bowl. This domain is represented by the caves and labyrinths deep beneath Kunlun Mountain, the dark pathways that lead down to the liquid fire at the heart of matter.

This secret is held in the deep somatic unconscious of us all, for each of us has passed as infants through the portals of the Stone Gate of death and nonbeing. We have all passed through the whirlwind, the primordial state of swirling chaos where the miracle of creative transformation occurs. And when the great stone is at last rolled away from the doorway of the dark cave, we have passed out of the chthonian chaos into life.

Ming men, Gate of Life, is the portal that leads out of the labyrinthian caves into life. It is represented by the acupuncture point Governing Vessel 4, ming men, located on the lumbar spine exactly opposite to the *shi men*, just above the rim of the pelvic basin. Each of us, as we pass through the Gate of Destiny, carries with us the sacred soul of the po that comes directly from the goddess. This stone carries the imprint of our destiny, the stamp of our innate nature, the frozen music of our Tao.

The greatest gift that the po spirits offer us is this recognition of the mirroring nature of life and death. When we live with the understanding that the Stone Gate is the opposite side of the Gate of Life, we realize that endings and beginnings are with us each moment, with every breath we take.

ALCHEMY: THE LIGHT THAT RISES TWICE

As the messengers who come and go between the yi and the zhi, the po are the connecting link between the middle world of life and the underworld of death, transformation and rebirth. Like the lungs that regulate the rhythm of the breath, the po regulate the rhythms of the psyche, the passages between one moment and the next, between birth and death, death and rebirth. Like the minerals that solidify the structures of the physical body, the po solidify the intentions and actions of the yi into structure and form and then support the letting go and decomposition of these forms at the end of our days. And at death, when the po sink down from the lungs and exit the body through the anus, they bring our essences with them as gifts to Xi Wang Mu, the dark goddess of the underworld. These life-building substances, the precious minerals that formed the matrix of our living bodies that they carry back to the underworld, are used to support the generation of other living forms.

Through our lives, as the po interact with the hun, the light of conscious understanding transforms them. Through the insight of the hun, the po begin to understand the ephemeral nature of their own being and the essentially ungraspable nature of life. Gradually, as we age and our essences dwindle, our bodies come to understand that life is a precious gift that cannot be held onto. If the alchemy of the spirits is successful, this understanding transforms the po's grasping, animal hunger into a poignant appreciation of the moment, an appreciation for life as it passes, moment by moment, each moment like a snowflake melting in the sun, like a meteor burning into darkness.

The radical for "white," a picture of the rising sun, that is part of the Chinese character for *po* is symbolically tied to the bright light of conscious awareness. But white is also the color of the moon that rises at night, the color of bones buried in the darkness beneath the earth. The white light of the po reflects the golden light of the sun and stars, the yang light that pours down from heaven. This light also rises up from the luminous fire of the essences, the yin light of life that shines upward from the earth. The po souls combine the light and the darkness in the realm of the shadows. The paradoxical whiteness of the po represents the paradox of life and death and the mystery of transformation.

In order to resolve the paradox of the po, however, and return to our original wholeness, we must pass through the Stone Gate into an even deeper darkness. We must dive deep into water, into the shimmering ocean of the essences, the realm of the Mysterious Feminine, the boundless, collective realm of the archetypes, cell memories, instincts, genetic codes, primal symbols and luminous threads of destiny that are the yin reflection of the Tao.

In the darkest cavern of the psyche, we come to the cinnabar throne of Xi Wang Mu, Queen Mother of West, Earth Goddess of the instinctual body. Here we come to the center of the mystery, the fiery spring at the core of the dark stones, the realm of the zhi and the spirit of instinctual power, aligned will, courage and wisdom. Here in the hot, dark center of the earth, inert stone comes back to life and the alchemical waters of life pour forth, rivers of liquid light gushing up from the heart of darkness.

> And if we are baptized in the fountain of gold and silver, and the spirit of our body ascends to heaven with the father and the son, and descends again, our souls will revive, and my animal body will remain white.
>
> —HERMES TRISMEGISTUS, TABULA SMARAGDINA[14]

WAYS TO CULTIVATE THE PO SPIRIT

The po is responsible for the five senses, the limbs and the somatic emotional responses. In order to cultivate this spirit, all these areas should be addressed.

- Feed the senses!

  Listen to beautiful music.
  Eat fresh, beautifully prepared food.
  Wear colors that nourish you and complement your mood.
  Keep fragrant flowers in your home and if possible in a garden or window box.
  Use aromatherapy; find scents that relax and calm your body.
  Take walks in places where you can feast your eyes on the landscape.
  Touch and be touched by people you feel close to.
  Bring your body into contact with the natural world—air, water, sunlight, earth.

- Spend time with animals. Let your pet teach you about the animal soul. Watch how your cat or dog observes and reacts to the world. Notice the life around you. Watch fish swim and birds fly. Watch foxes, deer, mice, rabbits. Animals reflect a part of our own wild nature, our unconscious visceral responses to the world around us.

  Next time you face a difficult situation, imagine how the animal part of you would react. Stay in communication with that animal as you deal with the situation. Ask questions of your animal: Should I sign this contract? Should I date this person? Notice your reactions on a body level. Are your muscles tightening or relaxing? Are you sweating or feeling agitated? Is your skin crawling? Do you feel a sense of well-being or are you ill at ease?

  You may discover that your po, your animal soul, wants very different things than does your shen or conscious mind. It is imperative for our health and for the successful completion of life projects that these spirits come into some kind of alignment. Even if you cannot react to life purely from your animal soul, make sure to pay attention to its messages, feelings and responses. Acknowledge its gifts. Be deeply respectful of the body's wisdom and desires. If you cannot immediately satisfy the needs of the somatic soul, let the po know that you are listening and that you will try your best to respond to it as soon as possible. In this way, there is less likelihood that the po spirits will turn to malcontented gui who produce depression, stress-related illness and psychosomatic pain.

• Nourish your limbs.

Stretch. Move. Dance to music.
Get massages or massage your own body with almond oil.
Swim in the ocean.
Take moon baths: lie under the night sky in the summer.
Use natural bristle brushes to stimulate the skin of your arms and legs.
Brush your skin regularly to slough off dead skin and to nourish and activate your nervous system.
Practice yoga, tai ch'i and qi gong.

• Develop a meditation or conscious breathing practice. During life, the po reside in the lungs. When we meditate or focus on quieting the breath, the po also becomes calm. From this place of relaxation, you can check in with your body and hear the voice of the somatic soul more clearly.

• Notice where strong emotions go in your body. Is your heart beating faster? Are you beginning to tremble or feel warm? Is your stomach tight? All the physiological responses to emotion are governed by the po. As you become familiar with your body's reactions, you are connecting to your po spirit. Rather than trying to do anything about these visceral reactions, practice wuwei, doing by not doing! Don't do anything. Just be. Just breathe. You will find that the po usually responds to your gentle awareness by calming down. Once you are calm, ask yourself what your body needs in this moment.

Do I need to take a walk outside alone for a few minutes?
Do I need a glass of water?
Do I need to stretch?

If you create this space around your emotions, you may find that an image or message emerges from your own body. You may be surprised by what comes up.

WHAT TO EXPECT AS YOU HEAL
AND CULTIVATE YOUR PO SPIRIT

As you heal your po spirit you will notice changes in your life, including

- a sense of enlivenment and a zest for life as the energies of the lower body return

- a feeling of being "back on track," as if your life force is aligned with your goals

- increased desire to move and explore the world

- increased sensory acuity: music sounds are clearer, colors brighter, textures more pleasurable, scents more noticeable

- a feeling of relief as you let go of old patterns and move on

- more awareness of body needs and messages

- increased inner stability and sense of solidity: you have a body, and you cannot be pushed over!

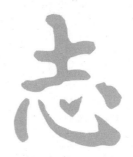

Chapter Ten

Zhi: The Spirit of Water—Instinctual Power, Aligned Will, Courage and Wisdom

> The highest form of goodness is like water.
> Water knows how to benefit all things without striving with them.
> It stays in places loathed by all men.
> Therefore, it comes near the Tao.
>
> —LAO TZU, TAO TEH CHING, CHAPTER 8[1]

WATER

Last summer there was a drought and our well ran dry. I went to get water at the spring outside of town where water flows continually from a tap set into an old carved granite basin, but the tap had been closed off due to bacteria in the water supply and the granite basin was empty. Then I went to a friend's house. We loaded his pickup truck with five-gallon drums filled from a hose. My friend was worried about his vegetable garden and drying up his own well so I didn't want to take too much.

I ordered drinking water from a supplier but we went through it in a few days and the cost began to add up.

The flowers in the garden withered. The green faded from the leaves. I carried water into the house from the drums, pouring it, pitcher by pitcher, into the sink. Each time I washed a cup or plate, I watched water disappear like quicksilver down the drain.

The plumber came and didn't say much. He stuck a long pole into the well and went down to the cellar to check out the pump. He said they'd been swamped with calls. Wells all over the county were drying up. "Water table's way down," he said. "Way down."

Neighbors told me how much it cost to dig a new well. I heard how the last guy had to dig five hundred feet down before he hit anything. "Do you know how far down five hundred feet is?" someone asked. I had never seen a hole that deep.

When it finally started to rain after the long dry spell, my daughter and I stood in the middle of the road and danced. The wilted, dusty trees shook themselves in the wind and reached their branches to the sky. The ditches filled and the springs began to run again. And when I looked down our well, the darkness shimmered with light as fresh water rose up from the stones.

THE ZHI

Water is the first element on the Wheel of Life and also the last. Water is the turning point, the end that is also the beginning. When the water wheel turns, the cycle begins—and without water, there is no turning. Zhi is the spirit of water. As water is the first and last element on the horizontal wheel of the Five Elements, zhi is the first and last of the spirits on the vertical axle of the Five Spirits. We meet the zhi at the bottom that is also the top.

In the macrocosm of the mountain, the realm of the zhi is the dark cavern of the underworld, the home of the goddess Xi Wang

Mu and the source of the mythical rivers of fire that flow from the core of the earth. In the microcosm of the psyche, the zhi reside in the most hidden parts of body unconscious, in the instinctual responses of the sex organs, the biochemical intelligence of the endocrine system and the knowing of our bones. The zhi connect us to the collective unconscious, the part of our psyche that draws us out of, and back into, the infinite.

In the macrocosm, the power of the zhi can be likened to the power of a hot spring, a geyser or the steaming vents of sulfurous fire that shoots up from the trenches of the deep ocean floor. This energy cannot be argued with. It emerges and bursts upward in a fantastic display of negentropic potency. In the human microcosm, it is related to the power of the life force, the instincts, the will and the driving urgency of ambition. Zhi is the will to live, the unknowable mystery of quickening life. Zhi rises from the wellspring of our being and imbues us with the desire to grow, thrive and live fully. We encounter this mystery each time a child is conceived, a seed sprouts or a new creative impulse is engendered.

Zhi is the spontaneously arising will of *spanda*, the mysterious potency of matter. It is not the ego-driven control of Western "willpower" or the initiatory energy of abstract ideas and visions. Rather, it is yin fire, the pilot light that ignites the flame of organic processes.

The light of the zhi spirit can be seen in the shimmering moisture of mineral-laden caves, roots and creatures that crawl beneath the earth. It can be seen in the luminous algae and phosphorescent plankton that shine from the darkness of the ocean. It is the iridescent blue-green chlorophyll, the gleaming hemoglobin, the rich red marrow of the bones, the green essences of life that slither like snakes through the spring grass.

The realm of the zhi spirits is the realm of what Vedic philosophers called karma, the realm of the unconscious forces and collective energy threads that determine the course of our lives. Here the light of consciousness is buried in darkness and the spirits bathe in the underworld waters of the unconscious. Here the lights of the spirits wait, like the nutrients and minerals waiting in the soil, until the goddess releases them back into the life cycle to nourish new psychic structures.

A Look at the Chinese Character

In the *Neijing* we read, "When Intent becomes permanent, we speak of Will." The character for *zhi* shows us the picture of the open bowl of the heart. Above it is the radical indicating a new green plant ascending upward from the depths of the dark earth toward the sunlight of heaven.

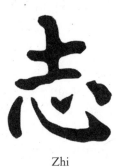

Zhi

This character emphasizes the connection between the zhi—the will—and the yin essences of life, symbolized by the green plant ascending from the soil. The upper radical is *shi*, which is a shortened version of *sheng*, the sprouting green of life, but is also used to represent the potency of wisdom and was originally used as a phallic symbol.

Shi is a shorthand sign that points to the alchemical mystery of this spirit. Shi is the moment when yin reaches its extremity and spontaneously transforms into yang. It is the turning point at the bottom of the taiji symbol when the tail of the black swirls into the white. It represents the creative yang potency of the feminine, personified by Xi Wang Mu, the underworld goddess of manifestation and creative power who also personifies the zhi. She embodies androgynous wholeness and is related to the spontaneous arising of life, to the forceful, expulsive pushing of the womb at the end of labor, and to the vigorous phallic force of sprouting bulbs and seeds in spring.

There is a graphic parallel between the characters for the spirits yi and zhi, as there is between the characters for the two souls, hun and po. Both the yi and the zhi contain the radical for heart, which points to their relationship to the shen or spirit.

In yi we see a picture of vibrating sound rising from the empty bowl of the heart. The vibratory frequency of the shen is slowed until the light of spirit manifests as sound: the words, poetry, songs and prayers we use to voice our intentions and commitments to the world. Over time, as these sound vibrations are subjected further to the entropic influences of the earth, they are slowed and solidified, impressed and crystallized into the matrix of matter. With time they are swallowed into the underworld, where they become the frozen music of the po.

And as we descend down, deeper even than the realm of the po soul, the sound and light of spirit drowns in the endless water of the underworld. The character zhi represents the turning point, the crux or enantiodromia, the moment when the vibration of spirit approaches the absolute stillness, darkness and silence of death . . . and then come back to life. In the dark and silent womb of the yin, yang spirit is reborn, this time not as shen—light birds from above—but as golden light materialized, a green plant rising up from below.

ASSOCIATIONS AND CORRELATIONS

Zhi is related to:

Element: water
Organ: kidneys
Emotion: fear
Psychological functions: instinctual power, aligned will and courage
Psychospiritual issues: surrendering to Tao, returning to origin
Chakra: first/second—Root: illuminated body
Virtue: wisdom

SIGNS AND SYMPTOMS OF ZHI DISTURBANCES

When the zhi is disturbed, people continually push themselves to the point of total exhaustion or have no initiative at all. They use chemical stimulants, emotional excitement, ambition and desire to whip themselves forward. Results include rebound exhaustion, insomnia, hormonal conditions such as hyper- and hypothyroidism, high blood pressure, anxiety, chronic fatigue and back pain. Other common symptoms are:

- general forgetfulness
- inability to memorize data
- lack of drive, motivation and initiative
- inability to stay steady in pursuit of goals
- addictive patterns, lack of willpower
- depression
- fear
- sleep disturbances
- sexual disturbances
- over-controlling nature

Spirit Level Signs
- lack of heroism
- absolute despair, lack of hope of ever healing or changing
- inability to face fears, which interferes with expression of true self
- "con artist" mentality—rather than taking on our own lives, we try to wriggle around obstacles and ultimately short-circuit the evolution of our own soul
- "identifying with God"—using will to try to try to control others and situations around us

- complete disintegration of the nervous system, which is one form of zhi disturbance (in earlier times this was labeled neurasthenia or a "nervous breakdown"). The person's "roots" are completely dry and there is no ability to hold steady or even to face the day-to-day challenges of living. This may be the result of years of addictive behavior or drug abuse, extreme stress or the long-term repression of instinctual impulses.
- spiritual paralysis, an inability to move on or take on life. Our English expression "cold feet" is coincidentally apt, as in Chinese medicine, this psychological problem is often associated with a physical sensation of cold hands and feet!

Possible Causes

Any time the will is employed to push the body beyond its own limits, the zhi are affected. The following list includes some of the most common causes of zhi disturbances in our culture.

- overwork
- excessive physical activity, i.e., excess marathon running, biking, weight lifting
- use of substances that impinge on adrenal function, such as caffeine, amphetamines and steroids (the herb ephedra can also cause problems in this area)
- chronic disease
- addictive behavior of any kind, including excess sexual activity
- chronic fear and anxiety, particularly during childhood
- shock, trauma and guilt
- multiple births and excess blood loss during periods
- a lack of discipline and encouragement during childhood

RETURN TO WHOLENESS: THE NIGHT SEA JOURNEY OF HEALING

Water has a dual nature, containing within itself the polarities of yin and yang. It is a shape shifter—existing as a vapor, a liquid and a solid—that endlessly gives birth to its own opposite. In Chinese medicine, the dual nature of water is represented by the kidneys that flank GV4—ming men, Gate of Life. The left kidney contains the energy of kidney yin and the right contains the energy of kidney yang. This duality is significant on a psychological level in terms of our relationship to zhi and the way we use and direct the energy of ambition and will.

In the healing process, the transformation that is a prerequisite for the return to wholeness and health takes place in the underground realm of the zhi. Here in the realm of Xi Wang Mu, the parts of us that need to die can die, and something truly new can come to life.

The mystery that takes place "in the water" has two parts, which reflect the two aspects of the alchemical mystery, the sulfur and the mercury of the cinnabar, the yin within the yang and the yang within the yin. They also reflect the stages of the actual birth process, the stage of gestation and the stage of labor. The first part takes place while the person is still going down into the disintegration of a disease process or psychological crisis. The second takes place after the turning point has been passed and the person is beginning to reintegrate, to come to a new wholeness and to heal. Between the two parts of the water journey is a third mystery, which in the birth process is called "transition." In Taoist alchemy, the turning point or time of transition is a moment of divine mystery they called the huntun, the realm of chaos.

Stage One: The Emergence—Holding Steady in the Darkness

. . . when one stays in darkness long enough, one begins to see.

— C. G. JUNG, ALCHEMICAL STUDIES

In the first phase we rely on the wisdom of yin within yang, the wisdom of wuwei. This is the phase where we wait and actively do nothing. Phase one takes place when, after long struggle and resistance, we finally let go; we find the point of active stillness in our confusion and despair. This is the time when we begin to use our will to not do, even as every part of us is screaming to take action, to fix the problem, to make everything okay. In the first phase we surrender, at long last, the light of consciousness, the light of the ego or small self. We sacrifice our rational knowing and plunge headlong into the unknown. At this point we do not know if we will live or die but realize the choice is not ours to make. Whether or not we survive to tell the tales of our journey is in the hands of some greater power. All we can do at this stage is to follow the left-hand path, the path of the yin. We trust, we wait and we surrender to the unknown.

The *I Ching*, Hexagram #3—"Difficulty at the Beginning"— refers to the moment before the buried seed sprouts spontaneously from darkness and the life force once again rises up toward the light. The hexagram symbolizes a blade of grass, the first shoot of new life, encountering an obstacle as it sprouts from the earth and pushes upward toward the sky. The commentary to the hexagram gives us important clues about the nature of psychosomatic illness and about how to proceed at this crucial time.

> When it is a man's fate to undertake such new beginnings, everything is still unformed, dark. Hence, he must hold back, because any premature move might bring disaster.[2]

This is the pivotal moment Carl Jung refers to in his Commentary on *The Secret of the Golden Flower,* when he speaks of staying long enough in the darkness. We must stay still while we hold the tension between two opposing polarities.

In this moment, a new way of being is struggling to come to life, and it is necessary to actively and with great intentionality do nothing to life. However, when we encounter an obstacle that may manifest as a body symptom or chronic pain, we are distracted from the need to drastically revision our life. It may be an anxiety, phobia or muscular armoring that locks in psychic energy and blocks emotional discharge. Or it may be a holding pattern such as chronic rage, drug or alcohol addiction or habitual self-sabotage that needs to be addressed through changes at the level of the physical body. But whatever the real problem is, at this point in the healing process the solution is unclear. We must call upon the yin wisdom of the water, the wisdom of receptivity and patient stillness. Like water, we must do nothing. Like water, we must wait until the next step rises spontaneously up from a deeper part of our nature.

At this time, there is often a sense of great desperation. In clinical practice, this is the time when patients are besieged by choices, none of which seem exactly right. There is a tremendous desire to break out of one's situation. People may attempt to make radical, impulsive changes in their lives, break off relationships, undergo surgery, change healing modalities or give up trying to get better. But this is the time when, according to ancient wisdom, we must follow the left-hand path of the yin and wait in unknowing.

Stage Two: Stabilizing Zhi—Becoming the Mountain

If we survive the first initiation of the water, we pass through the dark gate of chaos and enter phase two, the yang within yin. This second phase is the return. In Taoist tradition it is said that the stabilizing of will is the first step of inner alchemy. This is how a human being becomes like a mountain. This is how mercury and sulfur combine to form the fixed, non-reactive stability of cinnabar. This is how the divine child, the wholeness of the self, is reborn.

In order to give birth to this divine child, the goal of all alchemical psychology, we must stabilize the instinctual life force, the zhi, as it emerges spontaneously from the lower depths. We do this by sacrificing the conscious knowing of the shen and the conscious doing of the ego. In the words of Lao Tzu, "the sage goes about doing nothing . . . waiting quietly until the mud settles."[3] As we consciously extinguish the light of our shen, we become aware of another light shining from the darkness. This is the light from below, the light of the essences, of embodiment and matter.

The appearance of this lower light marks the rebirth of spirit, when the light of the original nature appears again after its burial in the darkness. Through the emergence of this lower light, the tables are turned and yang shines from below rather than from above. Now zhi is no longer the agent of our individual will driving us to make our way through the world. Through an alchemical marriage, fire joins water, zhi joins with shen. A new illumination enlightens us and leads the way back to our right path. We return to our self but in a new way. In phase two, we align our individual will with Tao and attain wisdom.

We see this understanding expressed graphically in the character *zhi* where the heart, the vessel containing the light of the shen, is pictured below the up-shooting sprout of the zhi. The hidden wisdom of this character tells us that in order to stabilize the will and achieve wisdom, the yang light of the shen must go below the yin. The light of the spirit becomes the root or foundation. Here, conscious awareness does not direct us from above or force the instincts or ways of nature. Rather, it lowers itself down to support our original nature as we walk through the world. The power and potency of our instincts is stabilized and guided by the knowing of our hearts. In this way, wisdom is attained.

By aligning zhi with shen and shen with zhi, we become our own ridge pole. We become the mountain. We become one with the way of Tao. When we infuse our experience of illness or emotional crisis with the light of conscious awareness, then we have gained wisdom through our journey and we are twice-born, like the sage.

Encountering the Dark Mother: Facing Fear

The last and possibly most important aspect of our work with the zhi entails facing fear. This is when we descend to the bottom of the labyrinths of Kunlun Mountain and face Xi Wang Mu. Here we release the parts of us that need to die and wait to see what, if anything, comes to life. In this part of the journey, there are no definite answers, no certain outcomes. We must be willing to let our own will go and trust that a larger wisdom will emerge to support and guide us.

Ideally, this part of the journey should not be attempted until we have healed and strengthened all of the spirits, particularly the zhi. However, sometimes life brings us to this phase before we are completely ready. When it does, it is particularly important to find a helper or guide to support you, to hold steady as you move through the fear and chaos of transformation.

In addition to the support of a counselor, therapist or acupuncturist, the wisdom of ancient myths offers a great deal of support and guidance. For example, the Sumerian myth of Innana, the goddess of above and below, is a wonderful story to meditate on during a time of life crisis and transformation. It also helps to find a symbol or image of power that calms and centers you.

MAKING FRIENDS WITH FEAR

The first thing to do when encountering our fear is to stop resisting it. When presented with a frightening situation, the body's natural response is to activate the adrenal glands' fight or flight response. But now, in the alchemical healing process, rather than taking action on these instinctual responses, we pause and follow the wisdom of wuwei. . . . We breathe and we wait and do nothing.

Get familiar with your fear. Sit next to it. Ingest it in small doses. For example, if you discover that you are afraid to speak your truth, find opportunities to speak in public. Tell the truth about yourself. Gradually, you will become familiar with the water. You will begin to learn how to swim. In the words of the Taoist sage Chuang Tzu,

A good swimmer has forgotten the water. If a man can swim under water, he may never have seen a boat before and still he'll know how to handle it. That's because he sees the water as so much dry land, and regards the

> capsizing of a boat as he would the overturning of a cart. The ten thousand things may all be capsizing and turning over at the same time right in front of him and it can't get at him and affect what's inside.[4]

Becoming familiar with fear and being willing to live near the unknown on a daily basis is like learning to swim in the river. Once we are used to swimming in these currents, we no longer resist them. Once we become used to this place of surrender, then we no longer expend energy in trying to control the outcome of our lives. As we surrender our will, another power enters our lives and we discover a wisdom we never knew we had. Like the ferryman, we intuitively know "how to handle the cart" and we continue on our journey despite the setbacks and challenges of life.

PUTTING IT INTO PRACTICE: DISHARMONIES OF THE WILL

Disharmonies of the will are rampant in our culture. Rather than carefully nourishing the tender shoot of the zhi as it rises up with the life force, we tend to drive ourselves relentlessly, rarely if ever stopping to consider the voices of our hearts, the guiding messages of the spirit or the music of the soul. Darkness, quiet, sleep and dreams, the passage of time, the void of the unknown . . . these are qualities that are not highly valued in our culture, yet they are exactly what the lower spirit needs. Clarity of purpose, direction and a strong sense of identity . . . these are qualities that are difficult to develop in a culture bereft of spirit and moral depth, yet they are the things that are needed in order for the zhi to unfold along its destined path.

The light of self-awareness is crucial for the healthy functioning of the zhi. Without this light, the zhi is like a plant that does not receive adequate sunlight. Its growth will be stunted, or the plant will shoot up wildly searching for light but there will be no strength in its roots. We each must come to know how much we really can do and what it is that we are truly willing to accomplish. Cultivating the will through the appropriate alternation of rest and activity gradually leads to the development of truly strong character and ability.

On the deepest level, the person whose zhi is out of balance is out of touch with the mystery of life. Such a person will either be caught up in compulsive yang activity or be stagnating in yin lethargy. Making room for the return of spontaneity, quiet and the voices of the deep self are crucial to helping this person heal.

CASE STUDY

Being with Aloneness: Healing from Sex Addiction

Claude is a forty-two-year-old New York graphic artist who first came to me for help with anxiety and stress-related muscle tension. He said that these symptoms had begun after his breakup with James, his partner of seven years, a man ten years younger than himself. At first Claude claimed that he had never experienced anxiety until the relationship with James ended; however, he readily admitted that in the past he had used alcohol, pot and prescription anti-anxiety medication to help get through stressful situations. He had also occasionally used club drugs, such as MDMA (ecstasy) and "special K,"[5] at parties or all-night dance clubs.

During the early phase of treatment, our work focused on Claude's muscle tension. I needled local and distal points to relax the muscles of his neck, shoulders and lower back, and used my hands to do gentle acupressure on points on his occipital region and jaw. Claude responded well to treatment, usually falling asleep on the table once the needles were inserted. He said his body felt more relaxed between sessions but that the anxiety continued, especially when he was alone at night. Gradually, rapport and trust developed between us and Claude began to tell me more about his personal life.

Claude described his father as an emotionally distant family court judge and his mother as a "whirlwind," a charming and dedicated board member of a host of charitable organizations. His mother had dropped out of law school to take care of her children but she had always been more interested in being a fundraiser than in being a mother. Claude loved his parents but he did not feel seen by them. Both parents had been disappointed in his choice of profession. And, after initially refusing to accept his sexual orientation, they dealt with his gay identity by ignoring it.

After a few weeks of treatment, Claude began to describe a kind of emptiness, a "dark hole," in his solar plexus that he associated with his anxiety, a feeling he had first noticed when he was very young. As a child, when he felt this emptiness, he was so frightened he would sweat and tremble. He had had no one he could talk to about this, and at a young age he began to self-medicate by blotting out the emptiness with sexual fantasies.

"When I get that feeling, I immediately think about sex, about having something to fill me up, about feeling someone's skin against mine. Having sex or even fantasizing about it makes the feeling go away. Of course, it comes back, so I have to get turned on again.

"When I met James [Claude's former partner], he was young, curious about life, and innocent. Taking care of him was like another full-time job. It filled me in a way sex never had. I never had to feel alone. When he left, my world fell apart. It was like the dark hole was going to swallow me up again, and the only thing I could think of doing was to go back to my old habit of casual quick sex. I started going online to meet guys for one-night stands. The fear and anxiety I feel when I go out to meet these guys takes my mind off the dark hole. At first, it's an exciting adventure, but afterwards it's totally dissatisfying. I can't stay away from it even though it makes the anxiety worse in the long run."

I began by offering some cognitive information. I told Claude that from a traditional Chinese medical perspective, the human instinctual and survival drives are under the jurisdiction of the water element. The delicate balance of the water and fire elements regulates our sexual energy as well as our capacity to respond to danger and to love. Thus our sexual desire lives very close to our fight or flight response. The sweating, trembling and hypersensitivity of sexual excitement is neurologically connected to the sweating, trembling and hypersensitivity we experience when we feel that our lives are threatened.

Our sexual energies as well as our other instinctual energies of survival emerge from ming men, Gate of Life, the balance point of yin and yang located between the second and third lumbar vertebrae at the base of the spinal cord. This is the balance point between stillness and action, death and life, entropy and negentropy, passive surrender and active response. The spirit that regulates this delicate balance is the zhi, the spirit of water, the spirit of instinctual power, aligned will, courage and wisdom. Healthy sexuality as well as appropriate reactivity to danger and to love depend on the harmonious communication between the zhi and shen, between our instinctual drives and our insight, awareness and compassion.

Restating this ancient Chinese wisdom in more modern medical terms, we can say that the sympathetic nervous system and adrenal glands that are located just above the kidneys at the base of the spine play an important role in normal sexual response, but they are also involved in the fight or flight response that is part of our instinct for survival. When water and fire lose their delicate balance, it is common to see a yang hyperactivity of the nervous system and adrenals followed by yin collapse and exhaustion.

From a Taoist perspective, casual, unconscious sex is yang and overly fiery, and it drains the water element and the kidneys' reservoir of yin cooling essences. With this in mind, it is easy to see why Claude's bandage of quick, casual sex ended up aggravating his anxiety. The use of anti-anxiety medication and recreational drugs exacerbated it by allowing him to override the wisdom of the zhi, the embodied wisdom of the autonomic nervous system, ultimately resulting in more kidney and adrenal depletion and a vicious cycle of fiery over-activity and exhaustion.

This cognitive information was very comforting to Claude and helped reassure him that there was nothing essentially wrong with him. It also allowed him to stop trying to use his will to stay away from casual sex and shift his focus towards cultivating his sexual energy in a gentler and more accepting way. In addition, it helped him understand how the use of recreational drugs, especially club drugs like MDMA that overexcite and subsequently drain the adrenal glands, are especially dangerous for people with anxiety disorders.

As we continued with his acupuncture treatments, I encouraged Claude to bring his awareness into his body, to notice the first signs of anxiety such as muscle tightness and shallow breathing. He began to realize that he had options, that he could respond to anxiety by stretching, breathing and visualizing himself in a safe place like the beach or resting after his acupuncture treatments rather than going online or out to bars. By consciously calming his nervous system rather than revving himself up with sexual fantasies, Claude practiced neidan or inner alchemy. He was bringing the light of his shen down to calm his watery zhi and in this way began a process of transformation and gradually stabilizing his will so that the Five Spirits could act in harmony.

By not acting on his impulse to go out looking for quick sex, Claude entered the first stage of his healing process: the stage of "Emergence, Holding Steady in the Darkness." At this stage, the key is to wait, to not do. By holding steady and waiting, he opened himself to the possibility of change. He had begun his descent, the first initiation of the water.

Today Claude's healing is far from complete. It may take several more years of treatment for him to truly free himself from his sexual compulsion, or he may simply come to accept his compulsion and learn to live alongside his fiery sexuality in a new way. To heal completely will mean reorganizing his nervous system, a kind of essential rewiring of his responses to eros and intimacy. Over time, acupuncture treatment on a regular basis will support this neurological rewiring and Claude's bodymind will actually learn to respond differently to stress. Retraining the nervous system is much like training a young puppy. It takes consistency, patience, and repetition, but eventually the new way of being and reacting to stimulus stabilizes and becomes integral to the organism.

Eventually Claude will have to face his own darkness, the hole of terror and uncertainty at the center of his being. Very likely, he will need to go back in time to reconnect with the very young boy who had no one to support him through his bouts of anxiety. Even earlier wounds—the wounds of the Dark Mother, of birth trauma and early maternal abandonment and loss—may surface as his healing work continues.

There are many acupuncture points that will be allies for Claude as he moves more deeply into his healing process. Points such as Kidney 24 (Spirit Burial Ground) and Kidney 25 (Spirit Storehouse) will help him recover lost parts of himself, particularly the innocence, curiosity and vitality he recognized in his younger lover, James. Bladder 52 (Chamber of the Zhi) will assist him in finding his own center point, his own inner mountain, the point of balance from which he can hold steady when the high winds of fear and erotic attraction threaten to blow him off his course.

Claude's healing process will take time and will contain moments of loneliness, dark despair and terror, but gradually a new light will emerge from the depths of his body. As the essences flow back through the Gate of Life into the reservoirs of his bladder and kidneys, he will experience a steady flame of serenity and vitality that will eventually supplant his driving need for the quick fix of casual sex. And as he gains the capacity to be alone with his own darkness, he will gain the capacity to relate to others out of true desire and vital curiosity rather than from compulsion and need. Although the process will be challenging, it will be deeply rewarding.

In Claude's words, "I might as well just sit down and see what's under there, get to know who I really am. Every time I don't act out on the impulses, I feel a little stronger, a little more whole. Some day, I hope to be a partner in another committed relationship, but until then I'm okay with this, with being alone. There are moments when I'm actually starting to enjoy having my own life."

ALCHEMY: TRANSFORMING WILL TO WISDOM

In seeking Tao, the sage follows the way of water, the path of least resistance, the path of wuwei. The sage understands the mystery of matter, the pull of the yin. She gives up the struggle to make things go her way but, like the Shaman Wu, she waits and watches until she can see the way of the rivers, of the land and sea. And then she flows. Through the understanding of the yin, the sage, like the river flowing to the sea, returns to origin. She becomes like a mother carrying a child in her womb. She gives up personal striving and opens her self to the world. In this way she aligns her personal will with a greater power, the way of Tao.

The child of the sage is not an ordinary child. It is a divine child, a living stone, a concretized bit of light or consciousness. The child of the sage is wisdom, born like a child from her own body after enduring the weight of embodiment, the pull of gravity and the passage of time.

This alchemical mystery is encoded in the point names of the Upper Kidney Points. Kidney 21, *you men*, is the Dark Gate, located just above the midline of the body. It is the entryway and resurrection point, the point through which spirit passes on its way down and back from the underworld. As the spirit returns, it moves upward to the Upper Burner, the cauldron of the ribcage, and passes from yin inner darkness to yang outer light as it "Walks on the Verandah" at *bu land*, Kidney 22. *Ling xu*, Spirit Burial Ground, Kidney 24 is the point of resurrection, located at the level of the heart, two inches either side of the midline. In stimulating this point, the healer calls the spirit back from its sleep in the underworld.

WAYS TO CULTIVATE THE ZHI SPIRIT

The zhi is related to the water element and is connected to the organs of the kidney and bladder as well as the adrenal glands. It is also closely connected to the reproductive organs housed in the pelvic cauldron. Any physical disturbances that affect these organs will have an effect on the zhi. In Taoist alchemy, the connection between the jing of the sexual fluids and the zhi of the will is particularly stressed. This connection is reflected in tantric practices where the male sexual fluids are contained during ejaculation so that they can circulate back into the body to nourish the essences and the will.

Healing the zhi must include learning to listen to the voices of the po and the shen, the wisdom of the body and of the heart, rather than acting solely out of our own will. In this way, we can learn to bring the will into alignment with our true strengths and capabilities. It also brings the strength of the will into the service of a higher purpose: the manifestation of personal destiny that is our mandate from heaven.

If you have a history of addictive drug use—especially excess caffeine, amphetamines, or steroids—consult with a traditional acupuncturist or Chinese herbalist who can support the healing of your water element and adrenal glands.

In general, the zhi spirit will respond well to the following practices:

- nourishing food, rest, meditation and natural beauty

- calming physical exercise, such as yoga, tai ch'i and qi gong, which strengthen the spinal column and align the posture. Find a practice and stick to it! Finding a practice and doing it on a regular basis is one of the best ways to strengthen and stabilize the zhi.

- avoidance of excess thinking, working and craving. Maintain as much as possible a reasonable schedule and make special time each day to do nothing!

- time spent with water. Watch how water moves. Drink plenty of water. Keep a bowl of water with flowers or just some special stones on your desk or by your bedside. Watch rivers, oceans, ponds. Let water be your teacher.

- foot massage. The kidney meridian begins at a point called Bubbling Spring located on the bottom of the foot (see diagram in Appendix i). Acupressure massage on this point will relax the body while it stimulates the kidney qi and revitalizes the zhi.

- meditation and guided imagery. These are especially important for the zhi as a quiet mind and subdued ego will allow the lower light to shine forth.

WHAT TO EXPECT AS YOU HEAL
AND CULTIVATE YOUR ZHI

As you become familiar with your zhi and learn to recognize and understand its messages, you will feel empowered instead of drained by life. Other changes may include:

- a sense of power and equilibrium

- increased serenity as you stop trying to control the world around you

- an increased sense of trust

- the ability to know and speak your authentic feelings and to stay with projects until they are complete

- less fear and anxiety, more excitement and curiosity

- courage to face the unknown

- less wobbling; a more definite sense of what matters to you

- increased initiative, motivation, and perseverance

- regard by others as someone to trust

Part III:

Transformation and Return

師曰此經乃九天八會

道元始天尊昔經歷千

偏生死五運遷變萬

居景雲之上上清之境

羣生火慈不舍吾古

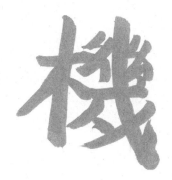

Introduction to Part III

The movement of Tao is to return

The way of Tao is to yield

—LAO TZU, TAO TEH CHING, CHAPTER 40[1]

The last phase of the alchemical journey takes place beyond the bounds of ordinary reality and everyday consciousness. Ancient mythology refers to this realm as the underworld. In Taoist cosmology, it is regarded as the domain of the dark goddess Xi Wang Mu and the watery cavern at the bottom of Kunlun Mountain, where the light of the spirits dies and is reborn. In traditional Chinese medicine, this final phase is related to the elements of metal and water and the time between the dying of late fall and the first quickening of life in early spring.

This final phase is the time of transformation when an old structure disintegrates and a new possibility of higher complexity and value emerges from its reorganized fragmented parts. In inner alchemy, it is the time when we finally let go of an old, outmoded way of being and surrender to the unknown, trusting that some new, more efficient possibility will arise.

The new possibility cannot be planned or predicted. Its emergence is independent of human desire or will. Our actions and attitudes, however, can either impede or support its arising. Through the wisdom and tools of alchemy, we can learn how to catalyze transformational processes and then how to weather the storms that accompany these cataclysmic shifts of structure and form.

In Part III, we approach the turning point or time of return, the final phase of transformation. In the following chapters, we will explore the attitudes and skills that can help us move through this part of the healing process. Included in these chapters are

- an in-depth look at transformation from a mythological, alchemical and clinical perspective
- an exploration of the shifts in attitude that allow us to work with transformational energies
- clinical methods that support the emergence of new psychological structures and psychosomatic patterns
- case studies that demonstrate how theories and tools can be used in practice
- a look at the archetypal meaning of key Chinese characters and how these archetypes directly impact our everyday experiences

In Chapter Eleven, "Chaos," we look at the relationship between personal transformation and the mysteries of birth and death. We examine the crucial role of chaos and entropy at these pivotal moments, exploring why alchemists counseled treasuring rather than avoiding chaotic states. A case study illustrates the intrinsic role of chaos in personal transformation and how it can be successfully worked with as part of the healing process.

The focus of Chapter Twelve, "Lead," is the resistance and avoidance of chaos on both a cultural and personal level. We look at the negative effects of this avoidance and explore how the energy trapped in resistance—like the potential energy contained in the alchemical lead—can be freed and used to potentiate transformational processes.

Chapter Thirteen, "The Golden Flower," is a meditation on rising light, the new possibility that is born from the heart of darkness. Taoist alchemists referred to this new birth as *jin hua*, the Golden Flower, which is a symbolic description of the illuminated soul.

Chapter Eleven

Chaos: Transformation at the Turning Point

> The clouds gather to spit forth thunder and rain. . . . In the chaos of
> difficulty at the beginning, order is already implicit. . . . [I]n order to
> find one's place in the infinity of being, one must be able both to sep-
> arate and unite.
>
> —THE I CHING, HEXAGRAM #3, "DIFFICULTY AT THE BEGINNING"[1]

THE TURNING POINT

The contractions began in the middle of the night.
Awakened from sleep, I looked out the window to see
an icy crescent moon. Then came the first twinge, a
shudder in the belly and a deep breath.

December 21, 1987. Three-thirty in the early morning. After
nine months of gestation, my baby was ready to be born.

All day the contractions came and went. I walked around the
house, lay on the couch, took a bath. My senses were acute.
Everything was very clear: the gray light on the blue spruce tree, the
flavor of the tea, the sound of the sparrows picking at pine cones on
the lawn. At 2:00 p.m. I knew it was time to go.

When I got to the birthing center, the midwife guided me quickly into a quiet room. I lay back on the bed and relaxed. Almost immediately the contractions began again, only this time stronger. Breathing my way deeper and deeper, I let the waves take me out to sea and then wash me back. Breathe, I heard a voice say from far away. The velocity of the waves increased. Faster and faster, they came in floods. Cold on my lips, a piece of ice, hands rubbing my feet. For a moment, I surfaced and saw the light dissolving as afternoon ebbed into early evening. Then I was gone as another contraction broke on the shore of my awareness.

Hours passed. Or days. Or lifetimes. I washed back and forth in a blur of breathing and sleep, riding the dragon's back as she took me farther out to sea, deeper and deeper into the ocean of the birthing process.

At 5:00 p.m., my water broke. Standing up, I saw something clear, like egg whites, running down my legs. And then the ground collapsed. The earth opened and all hell broke loose. From every orifice of my body, fluids poured. I whirled upward into a violent gale of rain, then down into dark rivers of molten fire. I heard a voice in my head saying, I can't go on. And another voice saying, This is it.

Then everything stopped, and for a moment I was gone. Deep inside I saw an archway opening, and through it poured a galaxy of stars. I had come to the source, the narrow gate, the spaceless space where nothingness enters the world of form. I had come to the point of no return, the place from which life springs into time and being.

A woman's voice called to me from the darkness. From deep in my belly, I heard her voice. "From this point on, there's no turning back. Now, there's no way out but through." I had nothing left. No hope. No understanding. No ability to think or plan. I could barely stand or even breathe. Even my body was no longer my own. All I had was this voice from deep in my belly, the voice of a woman who had done this journey many times before and would do it again and again, a woman who was me and who was not me. . . . I had nothing left but her voice and a tiny thread to which I clung. "Let go," she said.

And then I dived. Headlong into the waves. Push! I heard voices from another universe calling me but I didn't care. It was the waves, only the waves that were left to guide me. I was drowning and all I could do was trust that these powerful currents would bring me to the other side of this sea.

At 7:00 p.m., I reached down between my legs and felt something round and solid emerging from my body. It was the crowning of my daughter's head. Another human being was coming to life on our planet. At 7:07 p.m. on the winter solstice of 1987, my daughter, Nina, was born and the girl I had been transformed into a mother.

THE DARK GATE

Birth is the prototype for all transformational processes. It is a universal archetype that transcends time, culture, gender and geography. At the core of the deep unconscious, every human being holds a buried body memory of this cataclysmic event when the dark gates opened and we were pulled by an irresistible tide from the dreaming darkness of the womb into the world. Birth is the time when living beings come closest to the dark gate, the turning point of being and non-being. It is the moment when the unity of Tao divides into the ten thousand things, when the Mysterious Feminine, the yin hidden creator, does her work of manifesting the divine.

Not only birth but all transformational processes begin and end in the underworld with the mythical dark mother who is the origin and ground of being. Transformation happens in places hidden from the light, deep in the belly, under the sea or in labyrinthine caves far below the surface of the earth. Seeds, embryos, tadpoles . . . "the seeds of things have mysterious workings," wrote the Chinese sage Chuang Tzu; "all things come out of the mysterious workings and go back into them again."[2] It is only in matter, in the body, in the soil or beneath dark waters, where things die and come to life, that the mystery of transformation can occur. Transformation happens in a realm outside our everyday awareness. Its outcome can never be certain, and it occurs independent of our will.

According to traditional Taoist wisdom, the flickering of new life and possibility can only come from the darkness down below, from the place of unknowable mystery where life and death swirl in the womb of the Mysterious Feminine. "Endlessly creating / Endlessly pulsating," Lao Tzu writes of this mystery, "Although She becomes the whole universe / Her immaculate purity is never lost."[3]

THE HUNTUN: CHAOS

Authentic transformations always entail an encounter with Tao in the form of the "endlessly creating, endlessly pulsating" Mysterious Feminine. Like birth and death, these encounters are cataclysmic shocks that result in the dissolution of old, outmoded structures or ways of being in order to make way for some new possibility. When they occur, transformations of this magnitude obliterate the boundaries of the individual ego, turn our lives upside down and flood us with overwhelming emotion. Whether they take an outer form, such as the rupture of a relationship, the death of someone close to us or a natural disaster, or an inner form, such as an illness or the reorganization of a psychic structure, authentic transformations smash to smithereens the foundation of our lives.

The time after an old form dissolves and before a new structure constellates is described in Hexagram #3 of the *I Ching*, entitled "Difficulty at the Beginning." In Richard Wilhelm's translation of the commentary, we read that "the situation points to teeming chaotic profusion; thunder and rain fill the air. . . . [These] times of growth are beset with difficulties. They resemble a first birth. But these difficulties arise from the very profusion of all that is struggling to attain form. Everything is in motion."[4]

Floods, tidal waves, tornadoes, earthquakes and thunderstorms are metaphors used to capture the numinous power of transformational processes. The force that drives these meteorological events is most often referred to as a whirlwind, a "violent, mad wind that rises up 'like a ram's horn,' a bird-wind, the great phoenix . . . at once the means of flight and the one who flies, both the divine chariot and the spirit who rides in it."⁵ This wind destroys pre-existing structures and states of order and has no regard for cultural values or individual human preferences. This cosmic force is primeval, transpersonal and morally ambiguous. Taoists referred to it as the huntun, the whirling wind of chaos, a wind that sweeps through our lives as the Queen Mother of the West, the dark goddess, passes by.

The huntun marks the beginning and end of organic and psychic processes. It is present at conception and birth, when the hun and po souls join to initiate the flickering of life in the infant. And it is present at death, when the po decays back into matter with the zhi and the hun prepares for its flight back to the stars with the shen. Chaos is also present at transitions and transformations that occur in the course of life—at weaning, puberty, menopause and other significant moments of change, such as marriage, divorce, illness and recovery.⁶

While Western philosophy turned away from the disorder and dissolution of the dark goddess in its quest for a rational understanding of the cosmos, alchemy treasured chaotic states as the fertile ground from which new possibilities could arise. In the words of Nathan Scwhartz-Salant, a Jungian analyst and authority on European alchemy, "In alchemy, created disorder is called *our chaos* and is embraced for its power to change or dissolve rigid structures into more spiritual and related forms."⁷ Although there is no way to control or contain this powerful, high-grade energy, a proper attitude toward our chaos is a prerequisite for neidan, the inner work of alchemical transformation.

Modern scientists and mathematicians use the word "chaotic" to describe apparently irregular, unpredictable systems such as cloud turbulence or the erratic shifts of decline and growth in biological populations. Chaos theory emerged as a dominant trend in science in the early 1970s when high-powered computers revealed regularly repeating cycles in the apparently random disorder of certain natural phenomenon. Chaos theory opened the way for science to identify repeating, predictable patterns in what had previously seemed impossible to predict. It is a rational method of understanding apparently irrational, erratic fluctuations in nature, of discovering reliability in something that appears to be ruled by chance.

Chaos theory dovetails with the Taoist concept of the huntun when it speaks of changing degrees of form and formlessness in the creation of biological organizations, of islands of order constellating spontaneously from flux. Chaos theory also dovetails with Taoist ideas when it acknowledges the creativity inherent in disorder and refutes the absolute inevitability of entropy and the Second Law of Thermodynamics—the law that states that the universe and all systems in it are headed down a one-way street from complexity and potency "to final equilibrium in a featureless heat bath."[8] How is it, chaos theory asks, that we find complexity, order and new, interesting structures continually being created if the cosmos is on a one-way downhill ride?

While Taoist alchemists searched for a way to transform the forces of decline and death into the potent energies of renewal, scientists now seek to discover how it is that systems return spontaneously from random disorder to complex organization. However, scientist Joseph Ford inadvertently sums up the crucial difference between the modern scientific view of chaos and the creative mystery of the Taoist huntun when he says, "God plays dice with the universe. But they are loaded dice. And the main objective of physics now is to find out by what rules were they loaded and how can we use them for our own ends."[9] Here the modern scientific concept of chaos, born of the rational mind, massive computers and highly sophisticated technology, parts ways with the Taoist notion of the huntun. The huntun has no rules and can never be used "for our own ends." When Taoist alchemists spoke of chaos, they spoke of a divine mystery that exists beyond any kind of inner rhythm, regularity or rule. The huntun precedes any possibility of order or predictability because it is the mother from which order is born. The huntun is the unknowable One, "a Unity that admits and permits the diversity for which it is the crucible, the womb of all possibility."[10] Webster's defines this kind of chaos as the "confused, unorganized state of primordial matter before the creation of distinct forms; the state of things in which chance is supreme." It is the primordial sea, the mythical realm of the dark goddess—the primal mother—and the origin of life, death and transformation. Order, structure and predictability have nothing to do with this realm, and the rational mind is swallowed up in it like a speck of salt dropped into the ocean.

Creation myths the world over describe a state of undifferentiated unity that existed long before the beginning of history, before the separation of heaven and earth, before the land rose from beneath the windswept waters. The ancient Greeks believed that chaos existed from the beginning, together with Nyx, Nothingness or Night. The gods and goddesses of madness, of destruction and creation, of inebriation and the dance—the Hindu Kali, the Sumerian Ereshkigal, the Greek Dionysus—dwell at the edges of this realm. The Taoist goddess of the huntun is Xi Wang Mu, the goddess of the pelvic basin, the labyrinths, the volcanic steam vents beneath the sea.

From a Taoist perspective, attempting to control the energy of the huntun or to use its energies to implement individual human values and goals is not only incomprehensible but dangerous, as it leads inevitably to grandiosity and madness. Honoring chaos, holding it with awe and maintaining one's faith while surrendering to its power—these are the attitudes that allow the Taoist sage to ride the waves of the huntun, to die and be reborn from the dark whirlwind of Tao. These same attitudes allow the alchemical healer to use the potent energies of chaos to move through the wildly destabilizing energies of the healing processes, to bring vitality to deadened places and to transform outmoded, inefficient mindsets, habitual behaviors and values into new, more efficient and more potent ways of being.

A Look at the Chinese Character

The Chinese character for the word "chaos" is *huntun*.

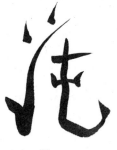

Huntun

This character can also be used to mean "innocent as a child," referring to the infant's proximity to the unbroken perfection of origin, the state that exists before the opposites of self and other, good and bad, have been separated by the conscious mind. The character is described as a picture of a wave of water almost completely covering a village. It is made up of two parts. The graphic on the left—*shui*—is a stylized picture of a breaking wave, with flecks of foam flying from the top. The graphic on the right—*tun*—depicts a sprouting seed shooting up through the earth, two first leaves or cotyledons forming at the tip of the stem just below the point where the plant rises up through the surface of the earth from darkness to light. The character for "village"—*tun*—is a graphic depiction of the "one" of origin unfolding from undifferentiated unity into the "two," the creative polarity that is the prerequisite of life. *Tun* means "a town or village" and refers especially to the uncertain and difficult stages of early development when the ground must be broken and organized structures formed.

The character as a whole does not tell us whether the inundating wave is approaching the village or receding from it. In this way it communicates the ambiguity and uncertainty inherent in the early stages of any truly new, creative endeavor. The sprouting seed, like the village, represents the difficult beginning of a new establishment when risk is supreme and the outcome is still unknown. Uncertainty is also expressed in the wave's ambiguous creative/destructive aspect. It is clear that the water has the capacity to destroy the newly established structure if the wave crashes down on it. However, as they recede, the floodwaters of the river will leave behind a layer of nutrient-rich silt that will nourish the new crops in the village fields. So floodwater, like original chaos, precedes differentiation and combines the opposites of destruction and creation.

According to James Legge's version of the commentary to Hexagram #3, "Difficulty at the Beginning," this hexagram is "intended to show how a plant struggles with difficulty as it rises gradually above the surface. This difficulty, marking the first stages in the growth of the plant, is used to symbolize the struggles that mark the rise of a state out of a condition of disorder, consequent on a great revolution."[11]

The sprouting plant represents a cosmos arising from chaos—the transformation of the divine "one" as it unfolds from primordial unity into the "two" that is the basis of life on earth. The character tells us that in order for the divine to manifest in form and matter, it must rise up from the earth rather than descend from the distant heavens. True transformation, the character reminds us, emerges not from intellectual understanding, personal desire or will, but from the depths of our organic nature, from our ability to feel and to withstand the suffering and the ecstasy of embodiment. It depends upon our willingness to not know, to tolerate chaos and to trust that something shining with the green of new life will germinate in the darkness of our unconscious being. As the commentary to Hexagram #3 reminds us, we must hold steady and have faith that, "in the chaos of difficulty at the beginning, order is already implicit."

ORIGINAL NATURE

"Show your original face before your parents were born." This is a well-known Japanese Zen koan, a paradoxical statement or question that is essentially unanswerable from the viewpoint of the rational mind. The koan is the focus of a Zen student's long and arduous meditation. After turning the question over in the mind for days, weeks and years, the meditator at last surrenders to inner confusion. The repeated questions "Who am I?" and "Where do I come from?" gradually break open the gate that encloses the limited, personal mind, and the small self is inundated by the floodwaters of Tao—the original undifferentiated chaos of the divine.

The solution to the koan comes without warning, like the green shoot of the crocus sprouting up from the ground in early spring, or the fertile banks that are revealed after the floodwaters recede. The face that the Zen practitioner eventually sees appears like a sudden clapping of hands, after he has completely given up trying.

In a state of total exhaustion, the student's limited individual identity drowns in a flood of conflicting concepts and ideas. In a clashing together of opposites,[12] "I" and "not I" converge and a new possibility emerges spontaneously from chaos. In Western theology, this new possibility is known as *homoousia*—the discovery of the face of the unfathomable divine in the small mirror of the self. It is the direct encounter with the vastness of Tao in the small but perfect reflection of tao within.

The concept of the original face precedes Japanese Zen. The roots of this idea are found in the concept of original nature, which is a crucial concept of Chinese Chan Buddhism and Taoist philosophy[13] as well as Taoist psychology. Original nature is the state of archaic wholeness, of undifferentiated unity between self and cosmos, referred to in the *Neijing Suwen* as the "ancient time when people understood the way of Tao."[14]

Original nature is the ground of being. It exists in me before I know myself as I. It existed before the world was broken into the opposites of subject and object, good and bad, dark and light. According to the *Neijing*, the people of ancient times lived constantly in this state of wholeness. They were "tranquilly content in nothingness and the true vital force accompanied them always. . . . [T]o them it did not matter whether a man held a high or low position in life. These men can be called pure at heart . . . . [T]hey are without fear of anything; they are in harmony with Tao, the Right Way."[15]

In Chinese, the word for "origin" is *yuan*. The character is a picture of a spring gushing out from a cliff, the origin of the water.

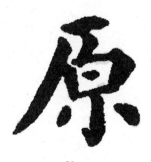

Yuan

The picture gives us insight into the concept. Just as a spring gushes spontaneously from the unknown darkness below the earth or water floods from the river, original nature gushes from the huntun, the undifferentiated chaos of Tao. Like a spring, original nature rises upward into the light, brimming with vitality and potency. Unfettered by moral considerations of good and bad, right and wrong, original nature follows its own course, nourishing plants, flooding fields, wandering freely back to its beginnings in the sea.[16] Parallel to the Chinese character, our word "origin" derives from the Latin root *origo*, which also means to "rise up from a source, to become visible."[17] Both the Chinese and English words contain the same implicit reference to an abrupt emergence of being from the dark mystery of nonbeing.

In Chinese medicine, original nature is associated with the spark of yang that is hidden in the yin. It is related to the bit of alchemical fire that illuminates and warms the element of water, and to the zhi, or will, and the jing, or vital essences that come to us at conception. Our original nature is related to our pure instinctual nature, to the deeper and lower parts of the body, the genitals, knees, feet, bones and sexual secretions. It is related to what we in the West call the unconscious. In Vedic traditions, it is related to Shakti, the life and death potency of the great mother. In esoteric alchemical texts, this aspect of the divine is called the lower spirit.

Like a spring that gushes from the stones or the molten fire that pours from the black recesses of a volcanic cauldron, original nature wells up from the darkness of matter, from the underworld realms of Xi Wang Mu. The sprouting sunflower seed, the cracking serpent's egg, the developing human embryo all represent the power of original nature, the spontaneous differentiation of chaotic potential into manifest form. From the moment of conception, original nature springs forward into life. It rushes from the Tao, propelled by its own powerful will to become and an irresistible impulse to manifest its own destiny and follow its own tao.

Original nature is the unfolding of Tao into form: the original nature of the acorn is the oak; the original nature of the spark is the fire; the original nature of the black seed is the golden sunflower. This drive to manifest the truest and fullest expression of Tao can be found in every living thing. It is as innate and powerful as the instincts of survival and procreation, and it is the most potent manifestation of qi, the life force.[18]

But for human beings, the situation is more complex than for an acorn or a flower! In order to live in society, we deny, hide or tame the pure spontaneity[19] of our original nature. A woman, for example, may suppress the strong urgings of her ambition, adventurousness and creativity in order to fulfill her role as mother and wife. A child may hide his curiosity and excitement in order to please a parent whose own innate excitement has been suppressed. A man may resolutely maintain an expressionless stone face in order to mask emotions he fears are unacceptable.

When human beings deny or suppress the spontaneous unfolding of their true nature or when conditions do not allow the original nature to be expressed, the force of life turns back on itself and sickens. We see the perversion of original nature in the stunted form of an acorn kept in a small flower pot, the impoverished quality of trout grown in a trout farm, or the snarling nastiness or chronic timidity of a poorly treated young animal. In human beings, we see the pathological expression of original nature in the form of uncontrollable obsessions, addictions, eating disorders, anxiety, neurosis and psychosomatic symptoms as well as cancer and environmental pollution. It is, in fact, the primary cause of disease in modern culture.

Human beings deny their own nature for many reasons. The pressures of family or culture or even the fear of our own greatness may initiate the abandonment of our own authenticity. But as the ancient Chinese texts clearly tell us, when the spontaneous expression of original nature is resisted or blocked, the alignment between the small tao in me and the great Tao of the cosmos is lost.

Acupuncture's primary purpose is the clearing away of impediments so that our qi can flow, our original nature unfold, and tao reconnect with Tao. Yet the process is not simple. It is too late for human beings to return to a state of unbroken unity with nature and the instinctual energies of the great mother. We can no longer exist in a state of identity with the endless, invariable organic cycles of life and death, birth and decay. A world without distinctions and preferences is no longer an option. Attempts by modern humans to live in utopian communities free of moral restraints seem inevitably to end in ridiculous and sometimes tragic failure. So how is it possible for human beings to return to Tao?

Over two thousand years ago, Chinese healers, the authors of the *Neijing Suwen* and the earliest Taoist philosophers grappled with the knowledge that a simple return to original nature was not enough to heal the suffering of human beings and restore wholeness to their broken cosmos. Something else was needed in order to heal the world, something that could stand apart from the primordial vitality of the instincts, that could act as a guiding principle as our original nature unfolded into life. The Taoist solution to this problem was alchemy, specifically the shattering and reintegration of the self and the upgrading of the instinctual will into the healing light of wisdom.

Taoists referred to the special individuals who had endured the arduous experience of shattering and reintegration as sages or masters. But anyone who has endured illness, loss, pain and humiliation—in short, anyone who has endured the disappointments, challenges and suffering of life—has experienced the shattering of the original golden wholeness of infancy. A person who has endured this shattering without succumbing to bitterness, hopelessness and despair, who has transformed pain and suffering into compassion and an abiding, spontaneous joy and gratitude for the experiences of life, has been involved in an inner alchemical mystery.

In the words of Taoist alchemist Liu I-ming, "If people can be flexible and yielding, humble, with self-control, entirely free of agitation . . . not angered by criticism, ignoring insult, docilely accepting all hardships, illnesses, and natural disasters, utterly without anxiety or resentment when faced with danger or adversity, then people can be companions of earth"[20]—that is, truly at one with the receptive.

Such a person has given up the implacable and insatiable wanting of the ego and surrendered the limited will to the infinitely more potent and unknowable will of Tao. Such a person has experienced the breaking down of wholeness and the descent into chaos and has not only survived but been reorganized by the energies of the dark goddess. The gift of the underworld is not a life free of suffering and challenge but a profound shift in attitude and values. Entropy, disintegration and breakdown have resulted in an increase, not of outer gold but of inner illumination. The outcome of this kind of transformation is an inner freedom and joy that is not dependent on the outer vicissitudes of life but rather rises from our own original nature as water gushes up from a spring. Through this return to origin, to the chaos of the underworld, we rediscover our own true nature. The secret to this reversal is found at the lowest place, at the very bottom of the alchemical cauldron, at the dark gate, the point of no return that is actually the doorway to new possibilities.

THE *WEIJI:* TRANSFORMATION AT THE CRUX POINT

At the heart of the transformational process is a point of breakdown, dissolution and uncertainty when we do not know if the light will be reborn from the darkness. The ancient Chinese spoke of this time as the *weiji,* the crux or crisis point.

The character for *weiji* has two parts. On the left is a picture of a man standing at the edge of a cliff, which represents danger or crisis, and on the right is a picture of many trees, which represent the many opportunities inherent in the wood, the unlimited possibilities of choice. When combined, the two parts express the idea of a dangerous crisis that is also a time of potential opportunity.

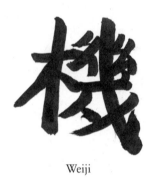

Weiji

The weiji is the time when we truly do not know if the healing process will succeed, if the birth process will complete, if the new possibility will come to life or turn back to the dark death womb of the goddess. It is the time of the impasse or seemingly impossible dilemma. It is the time that Taoist alchemists referred to as the Far Journey, the time when we leave behind the world we know and risk a descent into completely unfamiliar territory. It is a time very much like our own time, when we do not know if the planet as we know it will survive. Because they understood that the weiji was an inevitable and even necessary part of the transformational process, ancient Taoist alchemists developed a way to move through the impasse. They discovered that the weiji was the turning point, the time of the alchemical reversal when the yin becomes yang, yang becomes yin and crisis becomes opportunity. In the words of Taoist scholar Isabelle Robinet,

> The first task of the alchemist consists in finding the "true Lead" and the "true Mercury," which are the Yin and the Yang, and conversely, the kernel inside the fruit. . . . [T]he alchemical task is carried out not on the obvious Yin and Yang, the upper Yang in Heaven and the lower Yin on Earth, but on the rising Yang that is below, grounded in Earth, and the descending Yin, that is above, coiled in the Yang. This is one of the features of the principle of "inversion," of the "inverted world," that controls alchemical practice. Unlike the usual observations among mortals, where the Yang rises to form Heaven and the Yin descends to form Earth, here the Yang is below and rises, and the Yin is above and descends.[21]

In *The Secret of the Golden Flower*, Lu Tung Ping, the ancient author of the text and founder of The Completely Real School of Taoism, receives the following magic spell for this journey through the most treacherous part of the transformational process. This spell or poetic incantation reveals the central importance of paradox and reversal at the time of transformation.

> Jadelike purity has left a secret of freedom
> In the lower world:
> Congeal the spirit in the lair of energy,
> And you'll suddenly see
> White snow flying in midsummer,
> The sun blazing in the water at midnight,
> Going along harmoniously,
> You roam in the heavens
> Then return to absorb
> The virtues of the receptive. . . .
> The homeland of nothing whatsoever is the true abode.[22]

Thomas Cleary, a translator and authority on Taoist alchemy, believes that "[w]hite snow symbolizes the primordial unity [the huntun] . . . that this white snow flies in 'midsummer' means that it is manifested in the 'fire of consciousness'." Further, he says that "The 'sun blazing' symbolizes positive energy, 'water' stands for real knowledge hidden within, and 'midnight' represents profound stillness. Therefore 'the sun blazing at midnight' means the emergence of the positive energy of real knowledge (wisdom) from the depths of quietude."[23]

The crux point is the time of reversal when we must surrender our most cherished ideas about our selves and the world. It is the time when the yin leads and the yang follows; when action must become the agent of stillness and stillness must become the agent of activity; and when pain, suffering, limitation and uncertainty may in fact be the agents of growth and creativity. At such times of crisis, of illness, loss and betrayal, often we hear people say, "I feel as if my world just turned upside down." From the perspective of alchemy, this may be good news in disguise because the upside-down world, the world where the light rises up from below, is the world where transformation happens.

Holding Back: Wuwei Reconsidered

At the time of the weiji, the alchemist follows a counterintuitive path. He uses the traditionally active and unlimited light of the shen—the light of consciousness—to limit and still the incessant activity of the instinctual will. He makes a conscious decision to move from activity to inactivity, to turn his back to the light and walk toward the darkness.

Hexagram #64 of the *I Ching* refers to this time of crisis as "Before Completion." In the commentary we read, "In times of disorder there is a temptation to advance oneself as rapidly as possible in order to accomplish something tangible. But this enthusiasm leads only to failure and humiliation if the time for achievement has not yet arrived. In such a time it is wise to spare ourselves the opprobrium of failure by holding back."[24]

At the crux of the transformation process, a person must reverse the natural yang impulse to do something. At this time, all instinctual responses—to attack or flee, to run, fix, figure things out or take decisive action—are useless. We must willingly allow ourselves to enter the dark waters of chaos with nothing but the light of faith to guide us. At the time of the weiji, the only hope is to surrender to the yin and to allow the powerful tides of change to carry us to the next stage of our lives. By doing nothing, by waiting and by faith, the energies of individual will and the limited self are submitted to the transforming energies of chaos.

We see this situation in clinical practice when a patient reaches a crisis point in his or her healing process. This may occur due to external circumstances such as a job change or a severed relationship, or it may come from internal shifts such a giving up of cherished ideals or the revelation of the underlying causes of a chronic symptom. These moments often have a sense of tremendous urgency when both patient and practitioner feel compelled to do something, to take charge, to make the situation better. But if the practitioner is able to resist the urge to act and is willing to suffer the anxiety induced by chaotic states without rushing into words or action, an empty space is created in the field. Through this empty space, something other, something beyond the limited ego, may be able to enter the healing process.

We discover Tao in our own lives when we are willing to allow change to occur without interfering, by actively and intentionally surrendering the control of the conscious ego. While this attitude of active surrender goes against the grain of Western consciousness, my own personal and clinical experience has been that this is often the only viable way to move through the chaos of important life transitions.

The patients in my practice who have resolved insoluble conflicts and healed chronic psychosomatic and emotional symptoms have had to discover a new attitude toward chaos. Solutions to insoluble dilemmas—such as whether or not to leave an unsatisfactory but long-standing marriage or how to live with terminal illness—cannot be arrived at solely through conversation, intellectual struggle or rational analysis. Rather, solutions to these problems come after we have tolerated the discomfort of breakdown, after we have surrendered the limited activity of the ego and the will and allowed the structures of our lives to fragment and dissolve.

An acupuncture needle placed in an appropriate point will sometimes facilitate this process. A needle in the hands of a centered practitioner with a clear intention can function as an organizing principle that catalyzes the constellation of a new order. After such a treatment, a new possibility may appear as a dream image or while a person is in nature, walking in the countryside or watching waves crash on rocks besides the sea. The solution arises effortlessly from the chaos and once recognized it seems obvious, as if it had been there all along. In the words of a patient whose life had been shattered by a life-threatening illness, "I realized that my worst fear had already happened. I could relax. I was finally free."

REVERSING THE LIGHT

Taoist alchemists referred to the process of turning the outer-directed light of consciousness inward and using it to consciously still the incessant movement of the instinctual will as "reversing the light." The following is an adaptation of a traditional Taoist meditation that can be safely used to experience this alchemical reversal in an embodied way. The only requirement is a compassionate attitude toward the self and patience in regard to the will, which like a rambunctious puppy constantly wants to follow its own curiosities, desires and ever-moving nature.

Find a quiet place to sit or lie down comfortably. Scan your body with your mind's eye and invite any tense areas to relax. Breathe normally and allow your awareness to rest on the breath.

Now reverse "the handle of the stars" by turning the two eyes inward. Turn away from the outer world by closing your eyes. Drop the light of the eyes, the fiery spark of awareness that is the shen, downward to the zhi, the vital movements and energies of the lower cauldron, the part of the abdomen just below the umbilicus.

"Lower the eyelids and gaze inward at the chamber of water," writes Master Lu Tung Ping. Bring the fire of consciousness down to the point of origin at the umbilicus. When you have found this dark, empty place in your center, simply breathe. As thoughts appear, do not get attached to them but let them come and go like flickering shadows on a pond. You may experience resistance, anxiety or even physical distress such as palpitations. Do nothing. Simply breathe.

As your resistance and anxiety increase, keep breathing. Each day, increase the amount of time you practice by one or two minutes. Remind yourself as you practice, that you are facing the greatest fear of all: the fear of the self. As the churning of resistance increases, you will know that you are approaching the "turning point," the moment when you will pass through the dark gate and discover the light from down below, the light from within, the light of the inner self.

As you continue to practice, I do not know what you will discover, but at a certain point your conscious mind will let go. It may happen in a moment or it may take days or weeks. Each time you do this meditation, you will be increasing the potency of your zhi spirit. You will be aligning your will with your shen and learning to hold a point of stillness in the storm of your own emotions and desires. Eventually, from the place of darkness that is both inside and outside of you, a light or warmth will emerge and a deep sense of relaxation will flow through your body.

Now you can begin to get to know this light. With your inner imagination, walk around it. What color is it? What is its texture? As you become familiar with the energies of the lower cauldron, you can use them for your own healing. It is especially good to circulate this light or warmth around the area of your kidneys, the lower part of your back. You may find that if you breathe down into the lower cauldron, imagining that you have an extra pair of lungs all the way down in your genitals, the light get brighter and even moves up towards the area of your heart. Now listen carefully, for at this moment you may hear a message or voice that comes from deep within you. This message is the gift of your meditation journey.

Allow the light or warmth to sink back down to the pelvis. Acknowledge your body for supporting your practice. Slowly open your eyes and take in the world around you. When you have completed your meditation, make a note of any images or messages you have received. Join the zhi with the shen by consciously articulating and recording the messages of the body.[25]

WISDOM

The journey of alchemical healing follows the path of Tao. Like Tao, the journey goes here and there, this way and that. We can never know its outcome as it wanders back and forth between between zhi and shen, body and mind, instinct and spirit. The journey "goes everywhere, left and right. . . . It resolves all paradoxes and unties all knots and yet, it does not boast. It accomplishes its work, yet makes no claim."[26]

The early Taoists and Chinese healers regarded the new possibility that was created through the healing journey as a real, vital substance, a mediating psychic substance that formed a bridge between the instinctual will and conscious awareness. This mediating substance combined both human and divine qualities. It tempered the raw potency of the will and brought compassion to the pure, uncompromising light of the shen.

The Taoists called this special psychic substance wisdom and used obscure, esoteric symbols such as the phoenix, the pearl or the blossom-

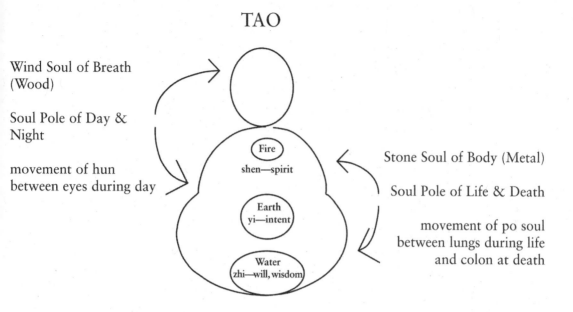

TAO

Wind Soul of Breath
(Wood)

Soul Pole of Day &
Night

movement of hun
between eyes during day

Fire
shen—spirit

Earth
yi—intent

Water
zhi—will, wisdom

Stone Soul of Body (Metal)

Soul Pole of Life & Death

movement of po soul
between lungs during life
and colon at death

FIGURE 12: MEDITATION MOUNTAIN
*The Three Cauldrons of the Spirits
and the Two Transmuting Souls*

ing of the secret golden flower to refer to it. They considered wisdom
an invisible light, a liquid fire that was cultivated through an alchemical process that transformed chaos, pain and suffering into inner illumination. Its appearance marked the resolution of the paradox of
spirit and matter, of consciousness and instinctual will, and heralded
a new wholeness, the rebirth of the self as Self or Tao and the transformation of ordinary life into an embodied reflection of the divine.

The ceaselessly active striving of the instinctual will is the alchemical mystery of the yang within the yin. It is yin fire as it rises from the watery darkness of matter and the alchemical cauldron of the pelvis.

Wuwei represents a compensatory mystery, the yin within the yang. It is the quiet, receptive stillness at the center of the fire. It is yang water, the rain that falls from the spirit and shimmers in the alchemical cauldron of the heart. At the point of greatest yin, yang rises from below. At the point of greatest darkness, light appears. At times of dissolution and death, new life rises like a phoenix from the ashes of fire. This mystery can be seen in the taiji, where the tiny dot of light appears at the center of the darkness. At every point of change, at every turning of the tide, there is a swirling reversal when opposites mix and meld, and for a time the world dissolves into chaos as we return to the awesome, unknowable unity of our origin.

In our lives, this is the moment when after a long gestation the quickening of birth begins, or when after a long impasse the way forward is revealed. In the healing process, it is the time an old way of being dies and a new possibility comes to life.

CASE STUDY: HOLDING STEADY UNTIL THE LIGHT RETURNS

Mark came in for treatment six months after he had injured himself cross-country skiing in the Colorado Rocky Mountains. He had a sprained right ankle, but although he had not broken any bones, he had had several previous injuries to the leg and foot. Even though his sprained ankle had healed, he had searing pain in his calf that extended down his Achilles tendon into the heel.

Mark was forty-five, an avid athlete who relied on jogging, tennis, skiing and rock climbing to release the tremendous tension he accumulated at his job managing a large mutual fund. When he found himself unable to go back to his usual physical activities after the accident, he felt he was going crazy as he vacillated between depression and pent-up anger. When he came to me, he had already tried lidocaine trigger point injections and physical therapy. His orthopedic doctor had told him that the next step was surgery on the scar tissue around the tendon, but even his doctor was not sure the surgery would help. Mark decided to try acupuncture after his doctor suggested it and said he would "give me a month," but if needles didn't help he would schedule the surgery. I suggested waiting a bit longer and we finally settled on ten sessions.

I began stimulating points in the Bladder and Kidney meridian. I also suggested that he take a low-potency (6X) homeopathic dose of St. John's Wort to support healing the injured tissue. After three sessions, there had been no improvement—Mark said that if anything the pain was worse and he really didn't see any point in continuing. But I reminded him about our agreement and said that I thought it might help to look at what was going on in the rest of his life.

Mark did not want to talk about his life and said all he wanted was to get back on his feet so he could run again. When I told him that I believed lingering pain from an injury can be an important message from the body, he looked at me skeptically. But after I explained the relationship between the area of his pain (along the Bladder and Kidney meridians of the water element) and the emotions of fear and anxiety, adrenal stress and burnout, he became interested and said he was "desperate enough to try anything."

That was the point when Mark began to express the real desperation underlying his compulsive athletic activity. He was sick of managing other people's money but was financially strapped taking care of his ex-wife and two children. He had been living alone for two years in a small house he didn't like, seeing his children every other weekend. Although he was considering moving in with his current girlfriend, it didn't really feel right. He was sick of living alone but wasn't sure about the relationship. He was tired of his job but had no idea what else he could do. He worked ten hours a day yet had no real savings. And now the pain in his leg was depriving him of his greatest enjoyment, his intense athletic activity. He told me he was at the end of his rope.

Mark was at an impasse he was hoping to get out of through orthopedic surgery, but I believed what he needed to do was follow the wisdom of wuwei and wait until the chaos of his life resolved. I chose Water points on the Kidney and Bladder meridian not only to bring qi and blood to the area of the injury but also to bring Mark's energy down to the yin aspects of his being and reduce his enervated hyperactivity. I suggested he try a yoga class as an alternative way of moving his body.

After six sessions there still was no change, and I noticed I was beginning to take on some of Mark's desperation, as I felt that I had failed. When he came in for the seventh session, he said he'd had it. He was fighting with his girlfriend, he was too busy to see his kids, the stock market had crashed and his life was crashing with it. He said if he didn't do something right away to get rid of the pain in his foot, he was going to lose it.

I felt tremendous pressure to act and was madly trying to figure out which point would take away his pain when a voice inside me reminded me to breathe. Mark's driving will to achieve and succeed was taking me over. I realized what I needed to do was just the opposite. I needed to go to what Lao Tzu refers to as the loathed place, the place of failure.

Instead of taking out a needle, I just sat down and let myself feel Mark's terror, the icy fear of failure that rose up from his kidneys and drove him to constant activity. I could feel the fear in my own body, and as I did, the wisdom of water came into the room and settled down between us. I began to talk to Mark about wuwei, doing by doing nothing. I admitted that I wasn't sure what to do for him next and asked him what it might feel like to wait, to stop and do nothing except make breathing room for a new possibility to emerge.

Slowly, I could see this strange idea sink in. Mark's body relaxed a bit and the tension in his body began to subside. He sat back in his chair. "It's been a long time since I trusted in anything outside of myself," he said. "I feel that if I stop, the whole thing will just fall apart." The "whole thing" was Mark's psyche. And the truth was that his current psychic structures needed desperately to crumble. The pain in his leg that was the support of his body was symptomatic of his inability to support the weight of his current way of life.

Now I felt I could needle a point without pushing or forcing Mark's healing process. He had come to his own crux point—his own weiji—and the qi was beginning to turn. I knew I could now use acupuncture to support a process that was already underway. I could "get lower" than the river, since I could now see how the water naturally wanted to flow.

The point I chose to do that day was Bladder 57, *cheng shan,* Support the Mountain. This point functions to relax the tendons and alleviate pain and brings energy to the calf and heel. On a spirit level, cheng shan stabilizes the backbone and brings stability to the yin. It stabilizes the alignment between heaven and earth as it supports the mountain or the inner psychic ridge pole of the spine. This is a point that can help us to hold a steady center during times of chaos and change.

Mark's pain did not go away quickly. It took several months of acupuncture and herbs as well as yoga and massage before he said he "barely felt it any more." But he never needed surgery. When he was ready to return to jogging, I suggested he try walking for a while rather than pushing to run and asked him to really try to listen to what his body needed. He agreed but assured me he did it "just to humor" me.

Mark didn't quit his job or move in with his girlfriend. He said he decided to just wait a while, make time to get to know his kids again and to get to know himself better.

CONCLUSION

This case is an example of how important it is for the practitioner to understand the Taoist idea of wuwei. The forceful use of the needle to move the qi at a time when nothing should be done can wreck the possibility of transformation.

There are several important clues that can let us know that a process has reached a crisis, weiji or crux point. One marker is a sense of desperation and compulsiveness. Both practitioner and patient feel that something must be done to make things better. This need to do has an urgent and desperate quality and is extremely difficult to resist, but it is exactly at this moment that one must relax and surrender. In this way we create a space for something new to arise from another level of the psyche. As we make space, frozen structures melt, old pattern decrystallize or, to paraphrase Lao Tzu, the knots untangle of themselves. In the process, potent energies locked in the rigid structures are liberated to fuel the healing process.

Another sign that we are at the weiji is a feeling of hopelessness, the certainty that nothing will work, or a sense of failure. This is the time for faith. This is the time to wait until an authentic, non-compulsive action or word arises, not from the yang energies of the mind or imagination, but from the yin energies of the body. Sometimes it is necessary to tolerate silence and non-action. Sometimes it is necessary to speak a difficult truth. At these times, the needle must be placed with great awareness. The qi should neither be pushed nor drawn forth but should come at the needle of its own accord. It is in the space of the gestating silence and emptiness of wuwei that something completely new is born.

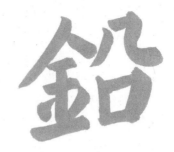

Chapter Twelve

Lead

All flesh that is derived from the earth must be decomposed and again reduced to the earth which it formerly was; then the earthy salt produces a new generation by celestial resuscitation. For where there was not first earth, there can be no resurrection in our majesty.

—Basil Valentine[1]

The lead in the homeland of water has just one flavor.

—Master Lu Tung Ping[2]

THE TREASURE IN THE TRASH

When China became a republic in 1914, traditional Chinese medicine, including acupuncture, herbs, massage and breathing techniques, as well as all forms of embodied spiritual practice such as tai ch'i and qi gong, were officially outlawed. Chinese Marxists regarded traditional Chinese medicine as a conglomeration of delusional superstitions and useless folk remedies, a garbage heap of several thousand years of misdirected theories and practices.

Now that acupuncture is reinstated in China and flourishing in the West, we may wonder at the negative attitude of the early Chinese republic towards its own rich and complex medical system—yet the Taoist sages and alchemists of the past would probably have been mischievously delighted by it. According to these adepts of transformation, the greatest treasures are to be found in the lowest places, and in the ashes and collected garbage of the past we discover the gold of resurrection. In states of putrefaction and lifeless, corrupted substances, alchemists recognized the backward glance of the dark goddess—spirit buried in the tomb of the earth. A medieval European alchemist expressed this basic principle when he said, "Out of the gross impure One there cometh an exceeding pure and subtile One."[3]

In their laboratories, alchemists made healing tinctures from urine, spit, feces, menstrual blood and bile as part of their attempt to harness the potential vitality—the new life and possibility—hidden in decomposing matter. Alchemists the world over secretly treasured these substances and regarded them as prerequisite ingredients for all creative and transformational work. While the alchemist's obsession with these taboo substances has often been used to support the view of them as weird, slightly lunatic eccentrics, there was a rationale behind their passion for decay and putrefaction. In the inverted world of alchemy, decaying and inert, lifeless matter is close to the divine. Having been drained of all their animating, negentropic energies, these substances are heading back down to the goddess, to the primordial state of undifferentiated unity, back to the earth, to the compost, to the original chaos out of which the world was formed. There, deep in the belly of the goddess, through the mystery of the lower spirits, corrupted matter is rejuvenated and assimilated back into the life cycle. So in European alchemy, base, apparently worthless substances were spoken of as the *prima materia* or primary material because they were the building blocks or raw material of new organic forms.

The alchemist's reversal of attitude toward disintegration, waste and corruption was based on the idea that the powerful, downgrading forces of entropy are crucial to the reorganization and renewal of organic systems as well as to the transformation of the human soul. Negentropic growth and expansion was seen as only one half of a two-sided equation. Without the complementary effects of entropic inertia, decomposition and contraction, processes of growth eventually deplete their own potency. In the words of an ancient Gnostic philosopher, "The worlds of darkness and the worlds of light complement one another . . . moreover, each deriveth strength from the other."[4] Just as a seed needs its time of dormancy in the dark underground before shooting upward in the spring, the human soul must bear the dark in order to fully open to the light. From this perspective, our times of confusion, disintegration, depression, illness, aging and despair are as valuable, if not more valuable, than our times of clarity, integration, joy, health and hope.

In his writing on the energetic processes of the psyche, Nathan Schwartz-Salant expresses this same idea from a psychological perspective:

> . . . without the "dark" entropic movement, negentropic processes do not have stability: the upgrading process reaches quick heights, say in abstraction, but then falls just as quickly . . . [we see] the coupling of entropic and negentropic processes, say, in the emergence of the negentropic functions out of an experience of depression or dissociation. That is, the negentropic potential is often released through an entropic process.[5]

Like a skillful swimmer in an undertow who allows himself to be carried out to sea and then brought safely back to another part of the shore by the incoming tide, alchemists counseled going with the powerful forces of decay and decomposition rather than struggling against them, trusting that these disorganizing energies will ultimately bring us back to ourselves in some completely new way. Alchemists believed it was possible for a system to gain, rather than lose, potency and value as energetic processes occurred over time if one consciously surrendered to the energies of entropy and allowed reorganization to constellate spontaneously from chaos.

THE RESISTANCE TO CHAOS AND THE STALLING OF TRANSFORMATIONAL PROCESSES

According to the sages of Taoism, it is in the garbage heaps of our own pain and shadowy rejected parts that we will discover our greatest virtues and gifts. It is in the formless chaos of mud, sexual fluids and exploding nebula that new life forms constellate. The low and marshy places are the most fertile. Lao Tzu, for example, advises us to be "like water and go to the places loathed by men,"[6] to "welcome disgrace as a pleasant surprise" and "prize calamities as your own body."[7] He tells us to avoid publicity, pride and fame, to remain humble and stay close to the ground. The Taoist sage Chuang Tzu tells a story of a great strong oak tree felled by a woodsman's ax while a useless gnarled pine that grew nearby lived on to venerable old age.

But as cultures became increasingly dualistic and masculine in orientation, a strong preference for the yang, expansive, upward-oriented energies of the mind and spirit replaced the appreciation of the yin, contractive, gestating, descending energies of the body and matter. In the Western philosophical and religious traditions, the realm of the mind and the upper spirits became the focus of intellectual and religious investigation while the realm of the body and matter—that which is dark and gnarled, wet and fertile, hidden and low—was rejected. The yin, embodied, instinctual aspect of our lives was split off, relegated to the shadows of the unconscious and dreams. With this shift in orientation, the recognition of the yin, embodied aspect of the divine was lost almost completely. And as the world split between above and below, the Way of Tao—that rambling path that leads us back to original wholeness, to our embodied connection to the divine—disappeared from view.

Another important factor in the ever-increasing resistance to entropy and the yin has been the development of human self-awareness and the subsequent emergence of a sense of discreet individual identity. Taoists related this kind of awareness to the shen spirit—bright, yang, illuminating, and immaterial—that tiny speck of the golden sparks of sunlight and starlight that rain down on us from the sky. This spirit endows us with the capacity to experience ourselves as unique individuals whose identity endures over time.

In psychological terms, the capacity for conscious self-awareness and the formation of a unique self-structure are a crucial part of the development of human consciousness. It is in the nature of this self-structure to strive to maintain and increase its own uniqueness and to preserve its organization. The yin, entropic, fusing energies of the underworld and the dark goddess threaten the very existence of a unique self. Yet when divorced from the revitalizing transformational energies of the Mysterious Feminine, the underworld of the "endlessly creating endlessly pulsating . . . hidden creator,"[8] the individual self becomes an isolated ego, a rigidified, lifeless structure without the capacity to change and grow. This is the great dilemma of modern Western consciousness: How can we preserve our hard-won individual identity while still maintaining a connection to our origin in the primordial sea of the deep unconscious, to the fertile waters of chaos, to the yin wisdom of the earth and of the body?

The hyper-organized, rigid self that refuses to surrender to dissolution is the greatest stumbling block to healing and transformation. Just as women may seek to stay in control and block out the powerful waves that are a natural part of the last, most intense transition phase of childbirth, patients and practitioners often seek to hang on to familiar structures and avoid the uncertainty, chaos and awe that are a crucial part of truly transformational healing. As a culture, we seek to "numb out." We avoid going "too deep." We have forgotten the value of the yin, the rich fertility of darkness, the nurturing gestational energy of silence, the power of surrender and the vast creative potential of chaos and uncertainty. Yet when we learn how to work with it, the resistance of consciousness to its own dissolution can become the prima materia from which a completely new possibility can form.

Lead

Alchemists recognized parallels to their own inner experience in the nature and behavior of metals. When they spoke of a particular metal, they were using it not as a metaphor but rather as a direct expression of psychic experience. For the alchemist, a metal does not personify a certain kind of psychological state; it *is* that state in an extroverted form.

Because of its lifeless, opaque and unresponsive nature, the substance most commonly associated with the rigid, resistant, stagnant or hyper-organized states that often precede the descent into chaos and transformation was lead. Inertia, depression, introversion, entrenched resentment and melancholy were psychologically equivalent to this heavy metal. The alchemist's real affinity to this metal came not from the recognition of its obvious dark, inert nature but from the belief that a great treasure, a gleaming nugget of gold, was hidden at its core. Lead, in fact, was often viewed as the true prima materia and an expression of original chaos, since it was thought to contain both the darkness and the light. In European alchemy, lead was said to "contain the radiant white dove."[9] It was hatched in the womb of the earth but nourished by the light of the stars.

"Within the Mystery there is another Mystery," says the sage Lao Tzu,[10] and we see this wisdom graphically portrayed in the Chinese character for "lead," *qian,* which is made up of two elements. The graphic on the right, *yan*, denotes a gully or drainage marsh, which reminds us of the low, yin, dark nature of lead. But it is combined with the radical on the left, *jin*, which is a picture of a nugget of gold hidden beneath the cover of the earth. So lead, which is opaque and without apparent value, contains within itself that which is shining and precious.

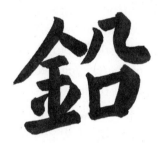

Qian

Lead represents matter, weight, entropy and darkness. But, even more importantly, lead represents the power of resistance—the potential golden light hidden deep in opaque silence and inertia.

The Leftover Chaos

An alchemical attitude that values dissolution and chaos is found in the Chinese creation myth of Pan Gu that was introduced in Chapter Two. In the myth, as the muscles, bones and blood of the giant's body dissolved and disintegrated, Pan Gu's corrupted flesh became the prima materia out of which the entire cosmos was formed.

Returning to the myth, we find that after the creation of the world from Pan Gu's body, there was a new problem. As the cosmos formed from the disintegrating parts of the giant's body, a bit of extra disorder was left out of the new wholeness. In the myth, this leftover disorder, the dregs of the creative process, is represented by the insects and lice that crawl on the giant's body.

In the story of the Zen cook or tenzo, who turns everything in the kitchen into ingredients for his soup, the tiny roach that falls into the pot represents the extra disorder. No matter how mindfully the tenzo combines the ingredients and stirs the pot, there is still a bit of mess, a bit of imperfection in the mix. This messy bit of imperfection is a defining characteristic of our humanity. While the tenzo's roach may not be part of the original recipe, it becomes part of the final meal. It is this extra bit of disorder that the head monk or sensei deliberately places in his bowl.

In practice, the dregs are the irritating symptoms we want to get rid of, our obsessions, worries, allergies, resentments, secret habits, addictions, warts, lumps, muscular holding patterns and chronic aches and pains. They are the crises and catastrophes we hadn't planned for, the life-threatening illnesses, financial setbacks, emotional betrayals and failures. They are the bits of stuff left over after we complete the creation of our egos and our orderly, socially acceptable identities. These irritating, seemingly meaningless symptoms are the visible signs of the hyper-rigidity of our ego structures, of our resistance to the ongoing, ever-changing processes of organic life and the disorganizing yet vitalizing effects of our emotions and instincts. They are ever-present signs that remind us of our limited state as physically embodied beings. The dregs are the bugs in the psychic system, everything that doesn't fit into the neat package of who we think we are.

But if we alchemically reverse our attitude toward these irritating symptoms, we discover that hidden in their seemingly meaningless disorder is a great treasure. Through their incessant gnawing at the edges of our ego structures, the bugs pull us back into the transformational vessel of the body. They return us to matter, to mater, to the yin, to our origin and our beginnings in the fertile, dissolving waters of chaos.

The leftover chaos is a remnant of the original chaos, a bit of the original prima materia out of which the universe was formed. Through the magical reversal of alchemy, this leftover chaos is no longer viewed as a problem but rather as our most valuable treasures. It is our Philosopher's Stone, the speck of sacred substance that will allow us to transform the lead of our physical and psychic resistances into the gold of illuminated awareness.

The myth of Pan Gu tells us that the return to Tao or constellation of new wholeness is not complete until this leftover chaos is somehow integrated into the system. The bugs are the glue that cements the new integrity. They are our legacy from the Tao and the secret of alchemical transformation.

INTEGRATING THE BUGS: ORGANIC CHANGE VERSUS ALCHEMICAL TRANSFORMATION

Organic Change

In Chinese medicine, the Law of the Five Elements represents the cycles of the natural world and of organic change. Organic change is repetitive. Its overall patterns follow circuits that are predictable. Water nourishes wood. Wood nourishes fire. Fire nourishes earth. Earth nourishes metal. And between metal and water, deep in the underworld, dead matter is devoured, decomposed and revitalized by the dark goddess, then sent back into the wheel of life. And so, through the infinite potency of the "Mysterious Feminine who never dies," the life cycle goes changelessly round and round.

This kind of change is an expression of the effortless movement of natural forces on the plane of the earth. It precedes the possibility of individual will, personal ego or resistance. Its perfect order relates to the time alluded to by Ch'i Po in the *Neijing Suwen*, when "man lived among birds, beasts and reptiles. . . . [W]ithin him were no family ties which bound him with love; on the outside there were no officials who could guide out and correct his physical appearance."[11] The Law of the Five Elements represents a perfectly balanced cosmos, a closed energetic system where both the quantity and quality of matter is conserved, where every bit of qi moves seemlessly through the five phases of transformation and nothing extra is lost or left over.

The Five Element cycle begins with a springing forth of natural potency. The qi moves from its origin in darkness and chaos toward expansion, differentiation and growth. The seed shoots forth from the dark earth to produce the flower. The infant struggles to turn over, to crawl and then to stand upright and walk. In organic change, the system uses the instinctual life force or jing to move against the force of entropy toward higher states of order. These elemental processes emerge from the darkness of origin and move toward expansion and light with a potency that gets used up as growth unfolds. Although there is a negentropic increase in complexity, organization and vitality during the initial stage of the process (represented by the upward thrusting energy on the left side of the wheel), the process ultimately surrenders to entropy as organic forms disintegrate and die (represented by the descending energy on the right side of the wheel).

In organic change, time is cyclical. There is no forward movement. There is gestation, birth, growth, disintegration, death and rebirth, but there is no transformation. When the qi runs down at the end of the life cycle, nothing is kept back from the dark goddess. At the end of the fall, winter comes; at the end of life comes death; after blossoming and harvest comes decay. When the negentropic energies of the yang are used up, all beings return to the womb of the goddess for recycling. This is the cyclic pattern of unconscious life, of the seasons, of organic systems directed by the forces of nature.

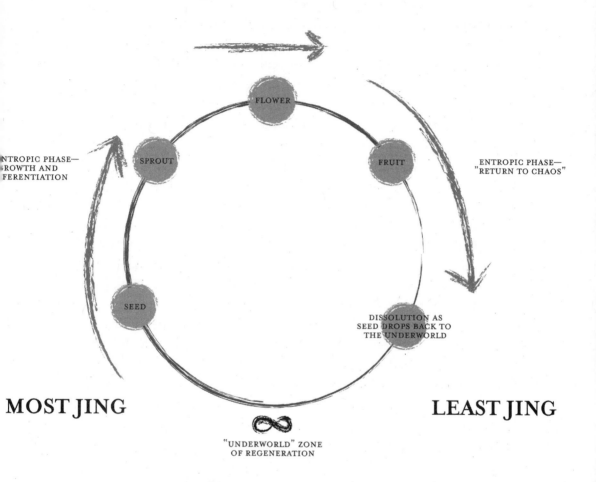

FIGURE 13: CYCLE OF ORGANIC CHANGE

FLOWER

SPROUT

FRUIT

NTROPIC PHASE—
ROWTH AND
FERENTIATION

ENTROPIC PHASE—
"RETURN TO CHAOS"

SEED

DISSOLUTION AS
SEED DROPS BACK TO
THE UNDERWORLD

MOST JING

LEAST JING

∞

"UNDERWORLD" ZONE
OF REGENERATION

While organic change is self-sustaining and continually regenerates its own power, it cannot produce anything truly new. At the bottom of the circle, the dark goddess takes everything into her womb, and nothing is left as natural entropy eventually pulls the entire system back into disintegration, chaos and the regeneration of repeating forms.

As long as human beings remained fused with nature and unaware of their individual identity, they lived in perfect harmony with this endlessly repeating cycle. But as the self became aware and attached to its own individuality, it began to resist its dissolution at the end of the cycle. For modern ego consciousness, there is nothing more terrifying than the descent back down—the return to the womb of the dark goddess. When we come to the last phase of the life cycle, when we come to the element of metal, we draw back from the abyss. We resist disintegration. We attempt to control the Mysterious Feminine and her rhythmic cycles of life and death. In this way, we disrupt natural law and we lose our connection to the Tao.

Alchemical Transformation

Ordinary change and development, propelled forward by the natural impulse of the jing, leaps propulsively toward an order and growth that inevitably deteriorates as the jing runs down. Organic change— as described by the Law of the Five Elements—first moves upward from disorder to order, then descends to a complete disintegration.

The Taoist alchemists understood that human consciousness had irrevocably disrupted the balance of the Five Elements and fragmented the perfect wholeness of the cosmos. They accepted this fall or fragmentation and realized that, for human beings, the original wholeness of the cosmos could not be restored. But they maintained faith in the infallible wisdom of Tao. They believed that human beings were born with a special bit of divine light, of shen or conscious identity, which gave them the divine capacity to create a new wholeness out of the fragments of the old. Alchemists discovered that the power of the conscious individual "I" to follow its own desires and resist its own disintegration could be used to ignite a new fire and to initiate the reorganization of a new integrity. The light of consciousness could be used to internally reverse natural processes of expansion and decay and liberate the instinctual potency of the jing for another "unnatural" purpose.

FIGURE 14: CYCLE OF ALCHEMICAL REVERSAL

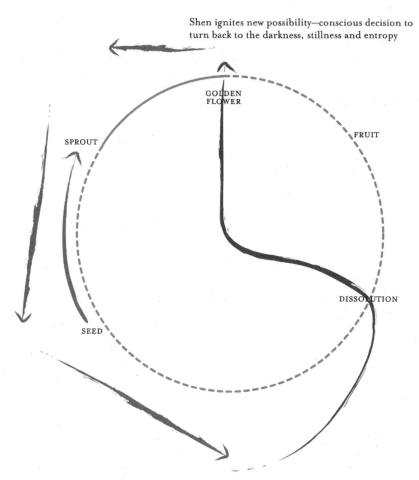

Shen ignites new possibility—conscious decision to turn back to the darkness, stillness and entropy

GOLDEN FLOWER

SPROUT

FRUIT

DISSOLUTION

SEED

Regeneration through burial of light in underworld—the spirit flower sprouts from down below

In alchemical transformation, the adept makes a conscious decision to turn back from order to disorder. He surrenders the outer brightness and illumination of yang spirit and reverses his gaze toward the inner yin darkness, making a conscious descent into matter and the body. As part of his neidan or inner work, the inner alchemist willingly suffers the pain, limitation and uncertainty of embodiment and uses the potency contained in his own resistance as fuel for his transformational process.

The inner alchemical process is not driven blindly by the instinctual potency of the jing but begins when the order is reversed, when there is a conscious reversal of the instinctual impulse to do, to expand and to move. Now the shen or light of conscious awareness is used to quiet and stabilize the jing and the individual will. Consciousness turns away from the outer world and looks inward as it follows the light of the descending spirit back downward into chaos.

Once consciousness drops into the realm of darkness, however, its light is extinguished. It only functions as an initiatory spark for a process that must be completely beyond its control. This conscious descent of the light into the darkness, of the knowing into the unknown, is the central mystery of alchemy. The turning around of the power of resistance so that we look directly down into our own chaos and disorder allows us to open ourselves to the transformational power of the dark goddess and the wisdom of matter and the physical body while maintaining a speck of our own unique integrity. This is what Taoists meant by the "true lead." In the words of alchemist Liu I-ming,

> Lead is dense and heavy, hard and strong, lasts long without disintegrating; what is called true lead is not ordinary material lead, but is the formless, immaterial true sense of real knowledge in the human body. This true sense is outwardly dark but inwardly bright, strong and unbending, able to ward off external afflictions, able to stop internal aberrations. It is symbolized by lead and so is called true lead. . . . Because its light illumines myriad existents, it is also called the golden flower. Because it is the pivot of creation, it is also called the North Star. Because it conceals light within darkness, it is also called metal within water.[12]

The transformation process itself happens independently of the yang conscious will or awareness. Human beings can only put themselves in a place where transformation can happen; after that, there is nothing more to do but hold steady and wait. At this stage, the yin qualities of faith, devotion and patience are most important.

Alchemical transformation requires the interception of some force that can redirect the power of instinctual drives and reverse the movement of natural energetic systems. It requires an initiatory impulse that can spark a new engine powerful enough to reverse the energies of the goddess. It needs a force that is not only able to face these potent energies, but also willing to sacrifice itself as it descends back down to the source, to the soup of creative chaos that swirls without beginning or end, in the belly of the underworld.

Paradoxically, the cure is in the poison and the only force potent enough to prepare the way for this reversal is conscious awareness, exactly the same force that caused human actions to diverge from natural law and caused the shamanic dilemma in the first place. This force is the spark of the upper spirit, the shen, the most formless, active, fiery, yang aspect of the qi.

For the Taoist alchemist, consciousness was the tool that allowed human beings to redirect the driving force of the instincts. The purpose of consciousness was to function as a spark that could ignite the fuel of the alchemical engine of reversal. Once this engine had been sparked, the alchemist could ride the dragon energies of the jing back down to the source from which they came. Once the instinct-driven will no longer pushed the system toward a flourishing that inevitably led to disintegration and death, the jing could be used to power the great work of reversal. In this way, alchemists learned to use the waters of the goddess to turn back her own tide.

Using consciousness to spark the alchemical engine opens the way back to the source of life. Once the engine begins to purr, once the way appears, once the alchemical opus has begun, the goal of the work is to surrender the will and let go the grip of consciousness.

Consciousness, the light of the upper spirit, must be sacrificed to the dark goddess so that something completely new can come to life from down below.

This "something new" is not consciousness, but it appears when the cycle of the life force reverses and the yang light of heaven descends downward toward matter. It appears when "I" turn inward, when I willingly submit to the limitations of my own flesh and wait until a new illumination comes up from below. This new illumination is the light of the soul or what Taoist alchemists spoke of as the light of the Five Spirits.

The Five Spirits add a new dimension to the endless round of the shamanic circle. Their appearance signals a shift from the horizontal limitations of the life cycle. The breath body's movements do not follow the cyclical rounds of the goddess but go "up and down" between the two poles of spirit and matter. In this way the energies of the soul initiate the spiraling motion that permits the upgrades of transformation.

But the appearance of the soul body is not the final stage of the transformational process. The soul is an intermediary form and is still susceptible to the pull of entropy and the forces of nature. With the appearance of the soul or vapor body, Taoists found a new way to bridge the broken gap between above and below. But they had not reunited the opposites of yin and yang, earth and heaven. They had not resolved the paradox of order and disorder or transcended the endless rounds of life and death. The secret of the One that is also Two, the unity that can shatter and still remain intact, has not yet been revealed.

REBIRTH: THE SECRET OF THE GOLDEN FLOWER

The last part of the Taoist alchemical journey is accomplished through a series of baths or reverse circulations as the soul body descends and dissolves in the watery yin darkness of matter and then rises up again to the light. Through these repeated baths, the soul shatters and reorganizes again and again until a new, more permanent body begins to form. This new body is unconstrained by time, space and the vicissitudes of desire, yet still it lives in the world of form.

Taoists spoke of this mystery as a pure spirit or light that crystallizes in the place of power, in matter and the body. This mystery is a light that comes not from the upper spirit, the sunlight and the stars, but from a luminosity that rises up from matter itself. It is a flourishing that comes from compression and death rather than expansion and life.

The lower light appears only after all other lights have gone dim, after the spirit has buried itself in the dark tomb of matter and the vaporous soul has dissolved again and again in the waters of chaos. It appears after the yang spirit that was once bright, active and initiating becomes yin, dark, inert and receptive. It appears only after the light of consciousness has willingly sacrificed itself to the darkness of matter. Then the ultimate mystery, the secret of immortality and freedom, is revealed. And the dark goddess who in the end takes all, at last gives something back.

While natural birth results in the creation of a new being in living material form, the alchemist has an unnatural birth that results in the creation of a being of living light.

When the yang becomes yin and the yin becomes yang, the lower light becomes the initiating fire as the goddess gives up a bit of her vital life-giving potency—the virtue of the receptive—to re-ignite the vitality of the fallen spirit. And through this alchemical union, a new light rises from down below as an eternal, ever-changing body of pure spirit is born from the darkness of matter. Taoist alchemists referred to this crystallized light body as the Golden Flower. This precious secret flower is a new kind of consciousness that rises up spontaneously from down below.

Whether or not this flower has ever actually blossomed on the earth is not the question modern Westerners need to ask. Rather, the important question is, can we imagine it? Can we once again open our vision to the luminosity and wisdom embedded in the lead of matter, embedded in our flesh and the physical world? In the words of the alchemical master, Lu Tung Ping:

> The light is neither inside nor outside the self. Mountains, rivers, sun, moon, and the whole earth are all this light, so it is not only in the self. All the operations of intelligence, knowledge, and wisdom are also this light, so it is not outside the self. The light of heaven and earth fill the universe; the light of one individual also naturally extends through the heavens and covers the earth. Therefore once you turn the light around, everything in the world is turned around.[13]

Jin Hua, The Golden Flower: A Look at the Chinese Character

The character for *jin hua* or golden flower is comprised of two parts.

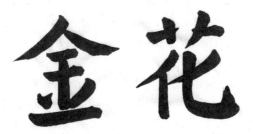

Jin Hua

The radical on the left, *jin*—gold—is a picture of two nuggets of gold buried under the canopy of the earth. In Taoist iconography, the buried gold represents the physical embodiment of sunlight or spiritual light. The character reminds us that in order to find this untarnishable, immortal luminosity, we must dig downward into the darkness of matter rather than reaching upward toward the stars.

The radical on the right, *hua*—flower—is formed of the composite of the characters for "plant" and "change." The lower part of the radical is a picture of a man turned upside down—a man in chaos, a man being tumbled, converted, reversed. The upper part of the radical is a picture of a plant. Like the tumbling man, the plant symbolizes transformation, the endless changes of vegetative life as seed turns to sprout turns to bud turns to flower turns to fruit and then turns back to seed.

Both gold and flower emerge from the darkness beneath the earth and thus remind us of the golden flower's symbolic connection to the Mysterious Feminine, to the underworld and to the treasures hidden in the darkness. But if we look more deeply at the words *jin* and *hua*, we find that the golden flower unfurls to reveal the secret mystery hidden in its heart. If we write the two characters one above the other so that they touch, the lower part of the upper character and the upper part of the lower character form a third word, the character *guang*, which means "light."[14] So the secret of the golden flower is light, the light that is born from the mingling of above and below.

First there is the light of the upper spirit, the fiery spark, the dazzling yang gold of heaven. And then there is the light of the lower spirit, the liquid flame, the shimmering yin luminosity of the earth. Joining these two lights into one unity results in a new possibility, a mysterious flower, an embodied spirit that both changes and endures. This flower is Lao Tzu, the old sage who is also the dancing child. This flower is the self, the ungraspable light, both mortal and divine, that glows at the empty center of our being.

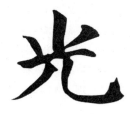

Guang

Case Study: Fire of the Phoenix

Jamie came to treatment two years after she had given birth to twins. Her main symptoms were fatigue, anxiety and depression. In addition to being exhausted from lack of sleep and overwhelmed by the needs of two babies, extreme food allergies made it nearly impossible for her to adequately nourish herself. But phobias were Jamie's most serious problem. She was incapacitated by fears of being alone, of aging, of swallowing pills, and especially of Western doctors and illness.

Although Jamie had been dealing with these symptoms for many years, they had gotten much worse after her children were born. The worsening of her symptoms along with the increasingly vicious cycle of malaise, malnutrition, inability to nourish herself and resulting anxiety about her health convinced her holistic doctor to suggest that she call me and try working with the tools of traditional Chinese medicine and Alchemical Acupuncture.

During the first stage of our work together, I diagnosed Jamie's problem as a case of postpartum depression exacerbated by a frail constitution. From a traditional Chinese medical perspective, the Earth element was weak and her problems related to spleen and kidney deficiency. I began by needling points to clear physical and emotional toxicity, then soon moved forward to tonification points on the spleen and stomach meridians.

Over time, with the help of acupuncture, herbs, flower essences, dietary changes, many hours resting on the treatment table and taking in my support, Jamie's state of mind improved and her energy returned. Gradually she became aware of a deeply felt connection to her children and began to enjoy the time she spent with them. She also discovered that eating simple meals and snacks with lots of fresh vegetables, high-quality protein combined with small servings of complex carbohydrates made a marked improvement in her digestion and energy level. I felt that the maternal feelings and better eating habits were signs that Jamie was reconnecting to the instinctual life-affirming energies of her body. From a traditional acupuncture perspective, I saw that her earth element was healing and that the energies of her spirits—especially her yi, po and zhi—were growing stronger. As hard as her life still was, both Jamie and I felt that she was making progress.

But Jamie's healing process did not proceed in the direction she or I had hoped for. Soon after Jamie's situation began to improve, her world once again shattered and she plummeted directly into the experience she had for years most feared and resisted. While on a weekend vacation with her children at a friend's home in the country, she discovered a small lump in her breast.

When Jamie told me about the lump, I couldn't quite believe it. I felt that surely her plate was full enough with her two young children, her phobias, exhaustion and depression. I expected her tests would reveal that the lump was benign. But this was not to be the case. All Jamie's worst fears became real when the lump turned out to be a quickly growing form of malignant cancer.

As an acupuncturist, I have been called on several occasions to support my patients through life-threatening illnesses. Although my scope of practice does not include the treatment of cancer or any other illness that requires immediate medical intervention, I am equipped to support my patients as they deal with the emotional as well as physical side effects of Western medical treatment. One of the most challenging aspects of this work is helping my patients deal with the difficult reactions they have to their diagnosis. Like many of my patients, Jamie's first response was to blame herself. "If only my state of mind had been better, then my immune system would have been stronger." "I must have brought this on with my own negative fears." "If only I hadn't take the fertility drugs." "If only I had eaten better . . . exercised more . . . taken the homeopathic remedies . . . had a better attitude."

There is a part of all human beings that wants desperately to find a rational way to explain the overwhelming irrationality of life-threatening illness. We resist being limited by the madness of illness, by the destabilizing experience of our body's betrayal and the inability of our mind to control the uncontrollable. As a practitioner, I watch my own rationalizing tendencies as I attempt to defend myself from the vast mystery of mortality and the realization of the infinite vulnerability of the human body. But the truth is that any rational explanation of a life-threatening disease like cancer is most often an attempt to contain our own terror of the unknown and to resist the overpowering energies of transformation that are part of these kinds of disease experiences. Generally, I have found that these explanations are clinically useless. They do not help people get better, nor do they reliably predict who will get sick or who will heal.

While some "New Age" healing modalities do overlay psychological meaning on somatic symptoms (i.e., tight shoulders equal carrying a burden you need to put down, dry eyes are the result of held-back tears), traditional Chinese medicine is not particularly concerned with cause and effect. Rather, the authentic Taoist physician engages in reveries and muses on conditions. The task is not to define precipitating causes but to discern patterns as they emerge from context and see how to best support the arising of Tao from the configuration of current events. In acupuncturist Ted Kaptchuk's words,

> Oriental diagnostic technique does not turn up a specific disease entity or a precise cause, but renders an almost poetic, yet workable description of a whole person. The question of cause and effect is always secondary to the overall pattern. One does not ask, "What X is causing Y?" but rather, "What is the relationship between X and Y?" The Chinese are interested in discerning the relationship among bodily events occurring at the same time.[15]

In working with Jamie, I felt that it would be a mistake to try and make a causal connection between her psychological issues, her eating problems, her depression and her cancer. And yet, at the same time, it would shortchange her to regard her life-threatening illness as a mere "coincidence" devoid of deeper meaning. I needed to support Jamie in becoming the meaning-maker of her own experience and to help her discover whatever wisdom could be found in her body's breakdown. The discovery she needed to make was not the psychological cause of her cancer but rather the acausal but nonetheless intrinsic relationship between her psychological and somatic life. In addition, she desperately needed to discover some bit of gold—some bit of wisdom and illumination—in the opacity of her depression, her phobias and the flesh of her body that seemed to betray her at every turn.

I treated Jamie with acupuncture and flower essences, including essences to calm her spirit and to help her move through change. With her doctor's permission, I also gave her low doses of herbal teas that are traditionally used to inhibit the growth of tumors. Acupuncture points such as Kidney 24 Spirit Burial Ground and Kidney 25 Spirit Storehouse calmed her anxieties and helped her to discover untapped reserves of patience and strength.

In addition, I used the stories and images of Chinese mythology to help Jamie to bring a larger, more transpersonal significance to her personal experience. It was helpful for her to revision her illness as a kind of mythical "descent" into a chaotic underworld where she could be reborn. She liked especially the story of the phoenix—the animal familiar and totem of the underworld goddess, Xi Wang Mu—who roasts in the flames and then rises up on crimson wings from the ashes of the transformational fire. As she mused on the meaning of the myth for her own life, Jamie began to organize a new way of thinking about her illness. The phoenix who was reborn from the ashes of the fire became an image of her own soul.

Gradually, she came to believe that she could be reborn from her illness as a stronger, wiser and more courageous woman.

For Jamie, an important turning point came when she had to decide whether or not to have a radical mastectomy. During this time, I saw a completely new side of her. When she first received her diagnosis, all her terror of Western doctors, hospitals and medication had come to the foreground, and for several weeks she had been racked with panic and tortured by nightmares. But as she moved further along through the challenges of her physical illness, a new strength emerged on the level of her spirit. With a newfound capacity for concentration and clear thought, she thoroughly researched her situation and then carefully assessed the information she gleaned from a multitude of medical journals. With amazing competence, she made appointments with doctors and oncologists and got second and even third opinions regarding her diagnosis and treatment.

But one day, Jamie came in to her session in a state of upset. She told me she couldn't make a decision, that the facts were contradictory and that her various doctors suggested completely different regimens. She told me she needed me to help her "go down into her body" to find the right path.

Using the tools of focusing, a gentle method of body awareness developed by philosopher and psychologist Gene Gendlin,[16] I invited Jamie to bring her awareness down into her body and see what was going on there. We had been working with focusing for several weeks and I had already shared some of the basic principles with Jamie, including the "focusing attitude," an attitude of gentle, friendly acceptance toward whatever comes up as we bring awareness inward. So, although she was upset, Jamie was able to bring her attention inward and notice what was there. When she did, she saw was something she hadn't expected. She saw something diseased in her breast that needed to come out. She also saw that she wanted the diseased part out of her and that her desire to live was much stronger than her fear of surgery.

She opened her eyes and said, "I want to live to see my children graduate college," and then she smiled.

With that insight, Jamie's attitude toward her doctors, medication, surgery and chemotherapy shifted. The very things that she had most feared and resisted became tools of her recovery. The strength of that fear and resistance became liberated into Jamie's healing process, and she came to a very clear place about her medical treatment. She realized that she could make use of both Western allopathic medicine and alternative methods, that she could bring many forms of healing into her recovery process. What was important was that her choices came from her own inner knowing. From that time forward, with each decision, each turn, she looked inside and came up with the next right step. The power of the shift came from her authentic desire to live, which rose up from the ground of her own being. In her words, "No one could have told me how to do this. I had to discover it myself. That made the experience completely different."

Jamie went through surgery and chemotherapy but did not opt for radiation treatment. Pathology tests confirm that the decisions she made about her treatment were on the mark. She has been cancer-free for over a year and her doctors are extremely pleased with her recovery.

Jamie is still plagued with depression and fatigue, and she still has to deal with her food allergies. We continue to work together on all the same issues, yet things are very different. She no longer talks about not wanting to live or resents the time she has to put into shopping and cooking the foods she needs to eat. Her love for her two children grows deeper with time, and over the past few months she has discovered that she has much to offer other women going through the experience of life-threatening illness. She is considering focusing her career in the area of cancer recovery. There is a new kind of fiber to her being. It's as if some new part of her emerged or was reborn through the process of illness and recovery. While she still struggles both physically and psychologically, there is a new and very different strength about her. In Jamie's words,

> It's too soon for me to say that I fully embrace this experience as a gift of transformation. I'm still not sure that it's all really over. But I can say that getting sick like this interrupted something that needed to be interrupted. It shocked me, shook me up. And now I find that I'm growing around it, like the bark of a tree grows around a severed branch. And you know, it's kind of cool. I'm not upset at the idea of growing old any more. I want to get old. Now, for me, every birthday is truly a celebration.

Although Jamie's treatment involved modalities that are outside the scope of traditional Chinese medicine, the underlying principles of my work with her come directly from Taoist alchemy. Without a sense of Tao as a containing and illuminating presence behind me as we worked, I would not have been able to lean back and trust Jamie's process. Without an understanding of emptiness and wuwei, doing by not doing, the responsibility of supporting her would have been too much for me. And without an appreciation of the hidden value of the lead, I would not have been able to help Jamie to discover her gold.

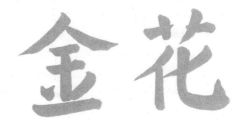

Chapter Thirteen

The Golden Flower

> The way to the goal seems chaotic and interminable. The way is not straight but appears to go round in circles. More accurate knowledge has proved it to go in spirals.
>
> —C. G. Jung[1]

> After a time of decay comes the turning point. The powerful light that has been banished returns.
>
> —The I Ching, Hexagram #24, "The Turning Point"[2]

THE POND

When I was eight years old, the state decided to widen the road that ran through the center of the small town I lived in. I remember the moment exactly when I heard about the coming change. I remember hearing the words, many of which I didn't understand: commuter traffic, six-lane expressway, four-leaf clover exit ramp. I remember especially the word "sump," that the plan was to fill in Brown's Pond to make a sump. I had no idea what a sump was, but when I heard the word I started to cry.

Brown's Pond was a small pond at the edge of the village. It was beautiful in every season, green with the reflections of willows in spring, cool with shadow and sunlight in summer and multicolored with the leaves of fall. But it was in winter that Brown's Pond came most alive, when the water froze and the orange flames of goldfish gleamed in the shining recesses of the dark ice. Winter was when the children of the town gathered to skate in endless circles around the pond. Our breath froze in the icy air, and at the water's edge, in the dry yellow forest of reeds, the older boys made small bonfires where we warmed our hands. I can still recall the clear crisp smell of the ice mingling with the smoky reed fires, the painful aching of my fingers and the call of the pucks against wooden hockey sticks. We skated after school while the gray sky darkened and the pond held us in her magic spell.

The traffic got worse. The highway came through town, and although they never built the four-leaf clover exit ramp, Brown's Pond was filled and became a drainage sump for a development of colonial-style houses. After the tractors left, there was still a hole in the ground filled with water, and by the next year some goldenrod and Queen Anne's lace grew up around the fence. But the pond was gone. And something else was gone too, something that knew about time and about the perfect hesitation of willow branches trembling just above the surface of the water . . . something difficult to name, something ineffable yet potent, something that took beauty with it when it went away.

BEGINNING THE HEALING JOURNEY

The destruction of Brown's Pond is my first memory of an irreparable tearing of my psychic wholeness, the end of my trust in the reliability of the natural world. It was my first remembered loss of innocence, the initial opening of a wound that would take many years to heal. But the destruction of Brown's Pond was also the beginning of my personal healing journey. It was part of the shattering of an original wholeness that would eventually allow a new, more complex wholeness to be born in me. Through this journey, I would eventually regain my child's sight as I began to see and work with the invisible rivers of light that are the acupuncture meridians and the radiant spirits that are the animating energies and resident deities of the human body/mind. Through this journey, I rediscovered my self and my world as interconnected living organisms in the process of great change.

The story of Brown's Pond is the story of my personal healing. It is also a mythological tale of transformation—of illumination, shattering, descent, impasse and renewal. In times of difficulty or transition, when I was filled with disassociation, numbness or despair, I was always in search of the other light, the illuminated knowing of my childhood. Eventually my healing journey led me back to my beginning—transformed—as I returned to my vision, my life, and my self with a new, more integrated wholeness. But the story also tells of an illness much larger than my own. The story of the death of this pond is the story of a collective shattering, a cosmic rift, a split in our culture between the realms of the divine and the mundane, between the mind and the body, between the timeless, ineffable realm of spirit and the temporal, sensible world of form and matter.

In the past five hundred years, Western culture has increasingly come to regard the physical world as a kind of a conglomeration of stuff, devoid of its own consciousness, spirit or integrity. We have tended to view the world as a predictable machine that can be manipulated, through mathematical calculation and technology, to suit our need for efficient productivity and economic growth. Spirits—the divine, unpredictable, autonomously enlivening energies of the universe—are viewed as something absolutely unknowable, something high up and far away from our lives down here on earth. While these divine energies may be acknowledged, they are not regarded as existing here and now, as an intrinsic part of our daily, embodied life. This dualism has allowed for huge advances in the realm of modern science and technology, but it has also resulted in grave losses in the quality of human life. It has led to a devaluing of the body and matter as well as the rejection of the feminine and the mother as cultural metaphors for embodied, instinctual life.

To human beings living in earlier times and different states of consciousness, the destruction of a living body of water would have been viewed as a serious action with multi-leveled consequences. Not only would it threaten the water sources as well as the lives of plants and animals on which human beings depend, but it would create a wound in the earth's integrity and a disruption of terrestri-al forces that would bring about other unpredictable problems such as disease, pestilence and fluctuations in weather patterns. To humans in more unified states of awareness, the disruption of terres-trial energies was obvious. It could be seen through a loss of quali-ty: the ugliness, stagnancy and sterility of the sump that replaced the beauty, vitality and creativity of the pond. The disruption was also recognized through a shift in atmosphere: the deadening sluggish-ness and emptiness that replaced the ever-shifting moods of the pond, which are the mark of a healthy living organism.

In traditional Chinese terms, this shift would be explained as a disharmony or blockage of the qi that circulated in and around the pond environment and extended far outward from the immediate area. But the blockage of qi was not the only problem. The qi became blocked because the spirits who had animated and enlivened it had been disturbed and scattered away. Without the animating, organizing effects of the spirits, the health and well-being of the pond collapsed.

Shamans and healers of earlier times, as well as modern arche-typal psychologists and ecopsychologists, refer to the departure of the spirits from the realm of matter and the body as a loss of soul. By this they mean a loss of the insubstantial yet crucial ethical, psychological, emotional and instinctual connections that support the integrity of life on our planet. They mean the loss of the capacity to recognize and honor the spiritual aspects of material life and to live on earth, side by side, with the mystery of the divine. In miniature, the story of Brown's Pond is the story of the loss of soul that, with the rise of dualistic science and modern technology, has spread like a virulent infection through every aspect of our lives.

In the late 1960s and '70s, Western culture saw the embryonic stirrings of a movement that sought to heal the wounds of dualism and to reweave connections between the realms of spirit and matter in modern consciousness. In America and Europe, there was a wave of interest in more unified worldviews such as Eastern philosophy and religion and tribal shamanism. In addition, various holistic philosophies including New Age medicine, astrology, feminist and earth-based spirituality, depth psychology and ecology became a visible part of popular culture. All these departed from the predominantly dualistic consciousness of the past five hundred years. Unlike Western philosophy and science, which separate spirit from matter and view the cosmos as a gargantuan mechanical system, these holistic philosophies view matter and spirit as intertwined. They all foster reconciliation between body, mind and spirit, and they all accept the reality of an immeasurable, immaterial integrating life force called variously qi, prana, the subtle body or soul.

In the late 1980s and '90s, however, this movement began to falter. The fantasy of a return to the simpler unified consciousness of earlier cultures quickly broke down in the face of the complexity of contemporary problems. The naïve, idealistic spirituality of the New Age movement was not a potent enough force to counter the relentless expansion of technological culture. It did not have the capacity to endure the suffering it takes to bring a new vision down into materialized form, to manifest change at the level of day-to-day life. European alchemists would speak of this as an inability to withstand the painful contracting forces of incarnation, the birth pangs that are a necessary part of bringing infinite, negentropic spirit into limited, material form. Taoist alchemists would describe it as a split between upper and lower spirits, a failure of communication between the shen and the zhi, the hun and the po—a disconjunct between inspiration, vision, intention, action and will.

The commitment to developing a new form of consciousness began to fade as people faced an increasingly challenging world. The difficulty of managing to survive in a world of ever-declining resources knocked the wind out of the sails of the youthful counterculture, and many people began to back down. They didn't have the tools, spiritual grit, mature wisdom or alchemical understanding to deal with the suffering, chaos and uncertainty involved in real, lasting personal and cultural transformation.

Nonetheless, the counterculture's dream of the reintegration of spirit into the material world and the emergence of a new, non-dualistic, multi-dimensional consciousness remains like the light seed of a golden flower planted in the dark unconsciousness of modern culture. As I complete this book, at the beginning of a new century, I believe we are at a turning point—a weiji—that is the moment of both great danger and rare opportunity. It is the moment when we stand undecided before a precipice: Should we turn back to the familiar but no longer efficient forms of dualistic consciousness; do we lull ourselves with regressive dreams of a lost fusion with the natural world or do we dare to take the leap into the unknown possibilities that lie ahead?

The weiji is the moment of greatest despair but also the greatest hope. It is a dark doorway that leads to the source, the doorway to death but also to new life. It is the time when the unknowable becomes known, the moment of faith when a mysterious light spontaneously rises from the darkness. It is the time of transition, the moment in the birth process when chaos reigns. And it is the only time that some truly new possibility can be born.

A New Consciousness

I believe that the surprising success of acupuncture in the Western world is part of a much larger phenomenon. As dualism, deductive reasoning and linear thought are no longer large enough to contain our current experience of reality, a new consciousness is already struggling to come to life. Some philosophers have called this new possibility "integral consciousness."[3] It is a consciousness that recognizes itself and the world as immanent light, as matter and spirit married in an endless dance of transformation. It is a consciousness that integrates the instinctual body knowing of the shaman, the psychic insight of the alchemist and the quantitative precision of the scientist. And it is a consciousness that honors the interconnectedness of the cosmos while recognizing the discreet uniqueness of the individuated self.

Philosopher and investigator of consciousness Jean Gebser refers to this new form of consciousness as integral consciousness because it reorganizes all the split parts of human awareness into a new wholeness. In the new consciousness, our past, our present and our future inform our immediate knowing. Inner and outer, past and present, self and other are reintegrated to form a multidimensional unity that both unifies them and maintains their individuality. Our organization of reality is informed by our instinctual sensing body, our dreaming imagination and our rational thinking mind. Integral consciousness allows us to be present to the unity of the cosmos as well as to all the ways we cut the world into parts . . . all at the same moment in time.

This new consciousness incorporates both ancient and modern forms of awareness. It recognizes but does not blindly follow the instinctual body wisdom of the shaman. It honors but does not get swept away by the psychic symbols and images of the alchemist. It maintains a capacity for self-reflective thought and analysis even as it recognizes the mystery of the unknown. In this way, the new consciousness calls the spirits back to the realm of matter, but rather than submitting to these potent energies as human consciousness did in earlier times, it begins to come into a self-reflecting, individuated relationship to the divine. It allows us not only to unite with the mystical light that flows through the material world but also to consciously see it.

Some mystics and philosophers say that this consciousness is dependent on the lighting up of previously dormant psychic structures or the opening of the chakras, especially the crown or seventh chakra located at the top of the head. Others say that it entails the reactivation or intensified activity of actual physical structures, such as the pineal gland located at the place at the center of the forehead referred to as the third eye. More recently, researchers in brain wave function have suggested that this mind state comes about through developing the ability to remain consciously aware of the delta wave state, the theta wave state, the alpha state and the beta state all at the same time, thus accessing our empathy and intuition, inspiration, spiritual connection, imagination and logical thinking processes simultaneously. I believe that this new consciousness is what the Taoist alchemists meant when they spoke about the mysterious golden flower. It is the crystallized light of a reborn consciousness that rises from the matrix of our bodies.

However it is named, certain characteristics of this new consciousness are key:

- It is a seed already present in us and waiting to awaken from dormancy. Just as gold is hidden but already present in lead, as order is implicit in chaos, this new consciousness is already in us as the ever-present origin of our being.[4]
- It allows us to live in awareness of the past, which is dormant, and of the future, which is latent, as well as of the present here and now. When we telescope our past and our future into one

ever-present moment, we leap into an entirely new dimension: the dimension of time.

- It maintains the autonomy of "I"—the individual self or ego—at the same time that it facilitates a reunion between I and thou, self and cosmos. Going in, we go out. Going out, we go in. Space collapses into a dream, an idea, and the center of the universe is everywhere.

- It makes the spiritual domain concrete and endows us with a new vision, an eye/I that allows us to see the immanence of spirit in the realm of matter. Thus it gives us a new relationship to light.

- It appears instantaneously as a burst of light, intuition, multidimensional insight or dramatically intensified perception. Although this momentous illumination may pass away and be replaced by ordinary consciousness, a person's life is changed permanently by the experience.

- It has been irrupting into human experience for many thousands of years. At the present time, however, these irruptions are increasing as the pressure of the new consciousness builds.

The new mutation waits like a light seed in the darkness of what is yet to become. It cannot be discovered solely by any form of return to the past or by forging straight ahead into a technocratic future. The new consciousness requires a completely new attitude toward time, space and transformation. It will constellate through a simultaneous integration of the wisdom of the past with the insights of the future, an integration of all the parts of our humanity: our darkness and our light, our chaos and our order, our bodies, our souls, our minds and our spirits.

The truly new requires that we take not only a leap but a plunge, that we are willing to keep breathing through the chaos until a new universe spontaneously arises out of uncertainty. In order to support the arising of this new kind of consciousness, we must surrender to chaos as we move through the weiji.

Moving Through the Weiji

At this critical point in human history, moving through the weiji means finding a way to reintegrate the realms that dualism split apart—not by turning back to an outmoded wholeness but by discovering a new, more complex integrity. It means developing a new way of honoring the spirits that animate the energies of life on our planet so that we can consciously recognize and relate to them, not as disembodied entities but as aspects of the divine that exist here and now, in our own being and in our daily lives.

Philosophers of consciousness have spoken of the shift from the dualistic worldview to a new, more integrated state as a mutation of human consciousness. They speak of the mutation as a quantum leap that arises from an energetic imperative of consciousness—something similar to the leap of an electron from one valence to a higher one.[5] However, I prefer to think of this shift from dualism to integral consciousness as an alchemical healing process through which a shattered, no longer efficient system reorganizes into a new, more potent and complex wholeness. In this way, human consciousness becomes an active and related participant in the process rather than something acted upon by an inner imperative.

We can bring the same tools we bring to bear on our own personal transformation to the transformation of planetary consciousness. In fact, as we work with human consciousness, we discover that the personal and planetary are intertwined. The inner and outer worlds reflect and affect each other. The same tools that support us as we move through the chaos of a personal healing crisis guide us through chaos and uncertainty as our planet shifts from a no longer viable world view to a new, more efficient consciousness.

Below is a summary of the principles of Alchemical Acupuncture presented in this book. These principles are universal; they can help us discover ways to move through our personal impasses and to weather the storms of the weiji as we collectively reorganize our shattering dualistic consciousness into a new, more integrated form of awareness. While the principles each relate to one particular stage of the transformational process, they are also synergistic and help give each other more power at any point in the journey.

The Eight Principles of Alchemical Acupuncture

1. Look for the opposites. Treasure the contradictions. Prize the paradoxes.
2. Consciously surrender the impulse to do. Hold the tension of the opposites until the "third" or new possibility emerges spontaneously from below—from the body and the unconscious.
3. Become familiar with the nature of the cosmos. Follow the life force. Let the heavy fall and the light rise but tether the yin to the yang and the yang to the yin.
4. Use skillful means. Don't block or push the river.
5. Like the tenzo, leave nothing out. The poison is the cure. The gold is in the dung heap!
6. Remember wuwei. Do by not doing. Be by being nothing.
7. At the crux point, go contra natura, reverse the light and face the darkness.
8. Be willing to not know. Remember that when the light comes back, it comes from below, from a source we cannot understand with the conscious mind—from the body, the earth, from mysterious, unknown parts of ourselves and from the deep sea of original chaos that connects us to Tao.

True healing is a mystery. It is the Far Journey, a movement away from what we know, a descent into the unknown, a radical transformation and then a return. The healing journey begins with a break or wound in our wholeness or integrity—a severe physical illness, for example, or an emotional or psychological crisis. The call that initiates the journey can be personal or it can come to an entire community or culture. The break or shattering of wholeness can come in the form of natural disaster, war or internal revolution. It can also come in the form of an outgrowing of accepted ways of organizing reality. When accepted ideas and customs no longer allow us to solve our problems and live harmoniously with ourselves and others, then our cultural container has grown too small and must shatter in order to be transformed! Although this kind of cultural reorganization is often frightening and overwhelming, ultimately it results in a renewal of creativity and possibility as well as drastic changes in the beliefs, practices, and rituals of the collective.

Whether it is personal, communal or even planetary, once the call to healing comes, it comes as an imperative. If the call is not heeded, there will be a backslide—gradual or sudden—into a swamp of decadence, devitalized putrefaction and disease. In psychological terms, this backslide is called a regression. It occurs, for example, when a traumatized adolescent returns to the behaviors of infancy, or when a patient's life process stagnates in depression or obsessive longing. In cultural terms, it can be seen in the adoption by modern Westerners of ancient traditions such as meditation, shamanism, healing touch, and even acupuncture without conscious critical analysis. In spiritual terms, it can be seen in the retreat to fundamentalism that has swept the world just as the birth process of the new form of integrated consciousness is beginning. But however it manifests, regression is the opposite of transformation! It is a wish or an active attempt to return to a previous, simpler form or way of being rather than take the risk of penetrating the unknown and face the challenges of a truly creative process of rebirth and renewal.

The call to healing is a call to transformation: the death and disintegration of outmoded forms, a descent into the dark unknown and then the reorganization and birth of something new. No matter how it begins, a true healing journey is alchemical, meaning that it results not in restoration or ordinary change but in a significant upgrading of the quality, order and complexity of an energetic system. At the end of the journey, there is a gift, an increase, an upgrade in understanding, insight and wisdom, and an augmentation of joy, spontaneity and compassion.

The authentic healing journey leads us away from our home and then returns us, but we are different. This journey is not a line or a circle. It is a spiral. In the language of the great sages of ancient China, it is a return to original nature, to the eternal, ever-changing Tao, to the instinctual, unpredictable urgings of the life force and to the guiding light of the divine.

We are living in the midst of transformation, a paradigm shift, a time of ending but also, potentially, of beginning. I believe it is possible to say that our entire planet is beginning a vast healing journey. According to the *I Ching*, such beginnings are times of clouds and thunder, confusion and chaos. They are times of possibility but also great danger when the new order, which is implicit, has not yet been revealed. At such times of beginning, it is necessary to sort the "threads from a knotted tangle and bind them into skeins . . . to separate and to unite."⁶

I have written this book as a way to sort the threads from the knotted tangle. It has been a way for me to distinguish what is truly useful about acupuncture and Chinese medicine, not only from the perspective of modern thought but from the perspective of the mythical reality of the soul and the magical instinctual knowing of the body. It has been a way for me to try to understand the ending and beginning that traditional Chinese medicine and acupuncture means to me and to my patients. But most of all, writing this book has been a way for me to discover what the wisdom of this ancient tradition can offer us as a planet at this time of shattering, transformation and tremendous potential for healing and renewal. In the process, I discovered that beneath a veneer of Confucian logic and modern rationalism, Chinese medicine remains the expression of an earth-centered, pre-patriarchal tradition that honors myth, magic, embodied spirituality and the potency of the Mysterious Feminine as essential aspects of the healing process.

The yin-affirming, earth-centered, body-positive spirituality of the Neolithic shamans and early Taoist alchemists precedes and radically contradicts the misogynist attitude that later resulted in the nightmarish atrocities committed against women and humanity in China. We will never know with absolute certainty whether the cult of the Mysterious Feminine, in its earliest and fullest expression, ever manifested as a true honoring and reverence of living women. It may have been no more than a reverential attitude or imaginal longing for connection with a divine, unfathomable goddess. But whether our integration of the Mysterious Feminine into our own consciousness is the restoration of a past harmony or the fulfillment of an as yet unfulfilled possibility, it is crucial, as we struggle to restore the connection between feminine and masculine, yin and yang, spirit and matter in our own lives, that we understand the concepts and practices developed in her name.

PUTTING IT INTO PRACTICE — WALKING MEDITATION: MOVING MINDFULLY ON THE EARTH

> You do not see the path, even as you walk on it.
> — THE HEART SUTRA

> *Bo bo thanh phong khoi.*
> (Each step will cause a breeze to rise.)
> — WORDS ABOVE THE DOOR
> OF A VIETNAMESE ZEN CENTER

What is it to follow a Way or path through life? Although these terms are used abstractly today to refer to various forms of spiritual practice, they are grounded in ancient traditions that are as old as recorded time. Labyrinths and spiral paths can be found in the myths and rituals of all cultures and civilizations. The basic laws of shamanic and alchemical traditions are universally based on circular patterns of endless transformation. Life itself, according to the Taoist sage Chuang Tzu, is nothing more or less than a "rambling walk directed by the Spirits." This Great Way is also the circle of life, the yang of light emerging from the yin of darkness, the *circulatio* of the breath between above and below, the wheel of the Five Phases that endlessly destroy and create each other.

In order to enter the sacred space where the ancient Taoist priests and shamans lived, we must find once again the sacred path that leads into it. To enter this place, the place where soulful healing work occurs, we must learn again to walk.

Thich Nhat Hanh, the beloved Vietnamese Zen teacher, teaches a special form of meditation he calls Walking Meditation. This is a completely practical and very down-to-earth application of Taoist ideas and a superb way to center ourselves in the Tao. Practicing this form of meditation allows us to use our breath and our steps to slow down the chatter of our rational minds and to enter the space of mindful relaxation. This allows us to experience in a simple, everyday way the spiritual alchemy that occurs when we bring our yang mind down to our yin feet, our consciousness to our walking. It is the perfect way to enter a state of alert receptivity before a day of healing work or to clear our selves afterwards. It is also a basic yet potent form of meditation that can be shared with patients and friends who need a way to get in touch with their deeper being and inner place of quiet.

My friend and teacher Claude Anshin Thomas, a Vietnam veteran, ordained Zen monk and student of Thich Nhat Hanh, who I fondly call a "neo-modern American Zen priest," takes this practice of walking the Way one step further. Anshin has reclaimed the vision of the ecstatic ramblers like Lao Tzu and other Taoist priests and Zen monks, who set off on spiritual pilgrimages into the hills and countryside carrying nothing more than their begging bowls and simple robes. In his book, *At Hell's Gate: A Soldier's Journey from War to Peace,* Anshin writes that he "walks just to walk. . . .[I]f I have an agenda, if I have a goal, then the unknown can't be my teacher, I can't really be in the present moment."[7] Alone, or accompanied by small groups of students, Anshin has walked across the United States and through war-torn parts of Europe and Asia, sharing his message of engaged Buddhism and inner and outer peace. Surely the dancing shamans were doing no more than this, putting one foot down in front of the other, as they journeyed from earth into the stars.

You yourself do not need to walk across the world to practice walking meditation. A path in a park or along a river or any relatively level, quiet road is fine. As Thich Nhat Hanh says, people have practiced this form of meditation in prison cells and crowded city streets.

To begin this practice, you simply walk a bit more slowly than usual and bring your attention inward. You concentrate on your breathing and the falling of your feet upon the ground. Each time a thought arises in your mind, notice it, and then let it go and bring your attention back to your breathing. Breathe normally and after you have found a comfortable rhythm, begin to count your breaths. Notice how many steps you take as you inhale. Then notice how many steps you take as you exhale. While filling and emptying your lungs, count your breaths. After a while, a repeating pattern will emerge.

Perhaps you will find that you take four steps with each inhalation and five with each exhalation. Whatever is most comfortable for your body is fine. It is only important that each inhalation and exhalation be equal, though sometimes you may extend your exhalation a bit longer to push any stale air out from the very bottom of your lungs. Continue to walk and breathe and count. After a while, you will feel your worries drop away. Your breathing will flow easily and your muscles will relax. The colors around you will brighten and you may notice, for example, the brief calling of a bird.

Walking this way over time will improve your circulation and filter your blood. It will also help you learn to relax your mind and listen to your body. Eventually the air around you will become quiet, and people will notice an aura of peace as you walk by. You will carry this space of stillness with you wherever you go, and even in the midst of chaos, confusion and noise, lotus flowers will seem to blossom beneath your feet. The earth will be healed by the little path of quiet your footsteps leave as you walk by.

> When you practice walking meditation, you go for a stroll. You have no purpose or direction in space or time. The purpose of walking meditation is walking meditation itself. . . . Each step is life; each step is peace and joy.
>
> —MASTER THICH NHAT HANH[8]

SILENCE

Amid all the commotion and noise of the material world, there is a silence. Beneath the talk and static of our televisions and radios, computers and cell phones, there is a lack of conversation. This silence is our aloneness as a species, our alienation from the natural world. It is the silence of our dying waters, our clear-cut forests and our infertile soil. One by one, plant and animal species die and the silence of their passing reverberates like thunder in the canyons of our unconsciousness. Even our language has become silent as the magical breath has evaporated from our words and we have forgotten that with each word we speak, we create and recreate the world.

When the acupuncture needle penetrates the surface of the skin, there is a moment of silence, an emptiness, a wondering and not knowing. When the metal needle meets the living body, there is a silence, a pause . . . before the tiny whirlwind spins and the qi redirects its course. For thousands of years, the intentions of healers and patients have met in that single breathless emptiness, that turning point of the soul that is the moment of transformation.

Perhaps, as we open to another form of consciousness, the present silence of our world will become that empty turning point, that breathless moment of change. Perhaps, if one by one we humans reclaim our vision of a living cosmos imbued with intention and intelligence and illuminated by wisdom, we will become like ten thousand silver needles penetrating and healing the body of the earth. Then perhaps, through healing our planet, we will heal ourselves and hear again the songs that the stones of the earth are singing to the clouds of heaven.

Glossary

༒

Active Imagination—A therapeutic process developed by C. G. Jung in which a person actively participates in a dialogue with images, fantasies and symbols drawn from the unconscious through dreams and meditation. The dialogue can take the form of an inner conversation or guided visualization and can be expressed through drawing, poetry, journal writing or spontaneous movement. Through this process, a connection develops between the conscious mind and the instinctual drives, desires and wisdom of the body and the unconscious. The connection between conscious and unconscious aspects supports the emergence of what Jung referred to as the "conscious life" of the self.

Acupuncture—Acupuncture originated in China more than 2,500 years ago. It involves stimulation of certain points on or under the skin with ultra-fine needles (manipulated manually or electrically) in order to adjust and balance the flow of qi through the meridians. Other acupuncture methods, used less often, involve the use of herbs and heat at various acupuncture points. Acupuncture originally involved only 361 points; however, there are now upward of 2,000 points recognized by licensed acupuncturists. Despite the fact that it requires no drugs or advanced technology of any kind, acupuncture has proven to be a remarkably powerful healing modality for a wide range of symptoms.

Alchemy—Alchemy is the organized investigation of the processes of transformation. It is an ancient spiritual discipline and natural science, rooted in the earth-centered spiritual traditions of prehistory, that was practiced the world over for thousands of years. As alchemy evolved over time, it incorporated the myths, symbols and unique characteristics of the cultures where it was practiced. Various schools evolved, including the Vedic alchemical tradition in India, the Hebrew Kabbalistic tradition, the European, Egyptian and Sufi traditions, as well as the Taoist tradition in China. The active development of alchemy continued until the mid-seventeenth century, when its intuitive methods were finally overshadowed by the rationalism of modern science. In the words of Johannes Fabricius, "[alchemy's] gospel of chemical faith combines a scientific investigation of nature's secrets with a religious quest aiming at an understanding of ultimate nature."

Amplification—Amplification is a therapeutic method developed by C. G. Jung in which a dream image or personal issue is elaborated and clarified through direct association and parallels with archetypal symbols, myths, folklore, natural phenomena and religious mysteries.

Archetype—Archetypes are ancient patterns of thought and behavior embedded in the human psyche over many thousands of years of evolutionary history. The term comes from ancient Latin and refers to a divine form that exists outside of time and space. However, at the turn of the twentieth century, C. G. Jung began to use the term to refer to a particular class of psychological phenomena he was observing in his clinical practice. Jung defined archetypes as universal images, patterns and symbols that have existed since remotest times and arise from the collective unconscious of humanity. Archetypes are timeless and universal. They are the result of the innate symbol-forming tendency of the human psyche and are similar to biological instincts in that they are innate and highly resistant to change. They form the basis of myths and religious symbols and appear in the individual as dream images and transcendent visions.

Bodymind—The expression "bodymind" or "body/mind/spirit" is commonly used in holistic medicine to describe the different aspects of a human being. It is a shorthand way to express the multifaceted complexity of a human being, the "all of who we are." This phrase parallels the Taoist idea that human beings are microcosmic reflections of the macrocosmic universe, which is made up of three intrinsically related parts: the yin aspect of matter or earth, the yang aspect of spirit or heaven, and the bipolar field of qi that connects them.

Body Unconscious—This is a term I use to refer to the body's function as a repository and container of forgotten experiences. The theory behind this term is that experiences that are threatening to the ego—such as early emotional or physical abuse, grave loss, overwhelming physical pain or mystical, transcendent experiences that occur during infancy and childhood—may be forgotten by the conscious mind and yet retained as memory traces in the muscular holding patterns and neurological patterns of the body. These memory traces may be brought to conscious awareness as holding patterns and rigidities are released through somatic healing processes such as acupuncture.

Collective Unconscious—"Collective unconscious" is a term developed by Carl Jung and now is an accepted part of modern depth psychology. It refers to the transpersonal, common substratum of the human psyche from which archetypal images, symbols and patterns emerge. The collective unconscious is universal in that its contents are the same irrespective of culture or geographic location, although the way it is expressed may vary from one culture to the next. In fact, the symbol-forming archetypal processes of the collective unconscious can be said to be an instinctive expression of our humanness. This aspect of the unconscious changes very slowly, in much the same way that the instinctual patterns of animals may shift only slightly over a period of many thousands of years. The archetype of wholeness is an example of an expression of the collective unconscious. This archetype is often symbolized by a circle and is found throughout space and time, on the walls of Neolithic caves, in Tibetan mandalas, Hopi woven baskets, Ukranian Easter eggs and world creation myths.

Dualism—A philosophical position that views the ultimate nature of the universe as twofold. From a dualistic perspective, the universe, as well as human beings, can be divided into two distinct and irreducible parts—i.e., spirit and matter, mind and body. In general, a dualistic approach leads to a preferential attitude toward one part over another, spirit generally being viewed as superior to matter, mind as superior to the body.

Enantiodromia—The compensatory function found in biological and psychic processes whereby some energetic event taken to its furthest extreme will spontaneously produce its opposite. C. G. Jung observed this phenomenon repeatedly in his work with patient's dreams and fantasies. The Taoist alchemists recognized this compensatory function in every aspect of the cosmos. They made it the centerpiece of their philosophy and symbolized it by the *taiji*, the graphic depiction of the swirling currents of yin and yang that, through the tension of their opposite polarities, create the vibrating field of life.

Entropy—The basic principle of modern science that states that as time passes, as work is performed, the quality and potency of the energy of a given system tends to deteriorate. The Laws of Entropy—stated as the First and Second Law of Thermodynamics—tell us that any process that converts energy from one form to another will never lose mass but will always lose some heat and potency. Or, in simpler terms, the universe is on a one-way ride downhill toward final equilibrium in a featureless heat bath of maximum disorganization.

Essences (*jing*)—The essences are the yin counterpart of the spirit. They are the ungraspable, quintessential substance that supports the vitality of all living organisms. The character is a picture of a grain of rice (qi) combined with the character for "greenery," the color of life. The essences are the evanescent juices of vitality that create the form, color and luminosity of living beings. The Essences of Anterior Heaven are received at conception from the mother and the father, while the Essences of Posterior Heaven come from the foods we eat and the air we breathe. The Essences of Anterior Heaven pass from one being to another through reproduction, while the Essences of Posterior Heaven pass from one being to another through the digestion and assimilation of food.

Focusing—Focusing is a simple yet very powerful technique developed by Eugene Gendlin in the early 1970s. It is a process of bringing conscious attention to the body in a gentle, accepting way and becoming aware of subtle sensory experiences and their meaning. Focusing can be used by patients and practitioners and is particularly compatible with body-oriented therapies such as acupuncture.

Gui—The Chinese word *gui* is often translated as "ghost" or "devil." The word is actually used to refer to any disembodied aspect of being that lingers after the physical body that supported it has disintegrated or has in some other way become untethered from its living matrix. The gui are generally associated with the po soul and are yin, murky, cold concentrations of vaporous qi that are stuck between the growth-oriented processes of life and the disintegrating processes of death. They are dangerous because they tend to steal yang qi from living organisms in order to maintain their existence. This is why we feel cold and damp when the gui pass by. They need to be supported in moving on to the next stage so that their qi can be reincorporated into the life cycle.

Heart—According to Taoist philosophy, the heart is not only a muscular organ that pumps blood through the body but also the center of consciousness and the organ that is responsible for organizing and maintaining individual identity.

Heartmind—The Chinese did not locate the organic matrix of mental function in the brain but rather in the heart. The character for "heart" is used to indicate the physical organ of the heart as well as the mental functions of the mind. "Heartmind" is a term used by both philosophers and practitioners of Chinese medicine in an attempt to convey the complexity of the Chinese concept of conscious awareness as a sensory-emotional and spiritual response of the human organism to the environment, as opposed to a strictly neurological function of the brain.

Heaven and Earth—When the ancient Chinese spoke of heaven and earth, they were not using the terms in a strictly religious sense but rather as designators of the two great realms of above and below, the two opposing polarities of yang and yin. Heaven was the realm of yang spirit, of subtle, nonmaterial, initiating energies, while earth was the realm of yin matter, of dense, materialized, manifest form. The dance of qi and organic life takes place in the field that constellates between these two opposing polarities.

Huang Di—The name given to the legendary Yellow Emperor, the first great ruler of China, who is said to have discovered Chinese medicine, founded agriculture, and invented the Chinese language when he received the Chinese characters as light scrollings from the stars. *Huang* means "yellow," the color the Chinese ascribe to the earth, and *di* means "emperor" or "deity." So Huang Di may refer as much to an original earth deity as to an actual historical figure.

Jing. See Essences.

Lao Tzu—A Chinese sage and poet who lived around 400 BCE, Lao Tzu wrote the *Tao Teh Ching*, a book of aphorisms and poems that form the philosophical core of the Taoist tradition. The name *Lao Tzu* means both "old master" and "old child." The name points up the Taoist belief that true mastery combined the authentic spontaneity, ease and joy of childhood with the wisdom and patience of the sage.

Mu—*Mu* is the Japanese word that is used as a focus for Zen meditation practice. It is related to the Chinese word *wu*, which means "nothingness" or "emptiness."

Moxibustion—Moxibustion has been widely used in China since at least the fourth century BCE. It entails the application of heat in the form of burning rice-sized grains of dried *Artemisia vulgaris* or mugwort to specific points on the surface of the skin. The grains are removed before the hot ember actually touches the skin, and the patient experiences only a sensation of warmth, relaxation and well-being.

Needles—No one can say precisely when the first healer inserted the first needle into an acupuncture point. From archeological evidence, we know that the Chinese people used needles in their rituals and healing ceremonies as far back as the late Stone Age. We also know from written evidence that the actual practice of acupuncture has continued without interruption for at least 2,500 years. Bone needles are often found in excavated Stone Age tombs, but most Neolithic Chinese shamans made their needles out of sharpened stones and jade. The Chinese word *pien* (stone probe) is one of the earliest words to refer to the acupuncture needle. In many early treatises, the word "stone" is used synonymously with "needle." The association between the Neolithic stone and bone probes and the origins of acupuncture reinforces the belief that the roots of this healing system go back to the spiritual practices and earth-centered rituals of prehistoric Chinese tribal healers. The needles used by these early acupuncturists were not mere medical instruments; they were "magical" tools the healer could use to banish demons and summon spirits.

Later, people during the Shang period (1500–1000 BCE) made needles out of thorns, bamboo slivers and animal horn, but these have disintegrated with time. However, bronze needles from the Zhou dynasty (1000 BCE) have been found, and it is likely that much older needles exist that have not been discovered. Copper, bronze, gold and silver have all been used in the making of acupuncture needles. However, by the time that the earliest Chinese medical texts were written, the most desirable materials were iron and steel carefully hammered to a fine point. Ancient Chinese historians claim that iron horse bits were a favorite source for acupuncture needles because the iron was tough, malleable and free from poison. The iron was melted and recast in the form of needles and was considered very valuable.

***Neijing Suwen*, The Yellow Emperor's Classic of Chinese Medicine—** The *Neijing Suwen* is considered the seminal text for students of acupuncture and Chinese medicine and is the oldest extant acupuncture text. Legend has it that the book was written by the culture hero *Huang Di,* the Yellow Emperor, around 2500 BCE. In fact, it was probably written around 350 BCE but is no doubt a compilation of earlier writings.

Prana—An Indian word for "life force" that is closely related to the Chinese word *qi.*

Prima Materia—Medieval European alchemists used this term to describe the basic, universal substance out of which the entire material world is formed. The individual elements—fire, earth, air, water and wood—arose from the swirling chaos of the *prima materia.* All phenomena were formed by the combining of these elements in different proportions. C. G. Jung and other depth psychologists associ-

ferent proportions. C. G. Jung and other depth psychologists associate the prima materia with the collective unconscious, the swirling ocean of symbols, instincts, images and archetypes that is universal to all human beings.

Psyche—*Psyche* is a word with etymological roots extending back to the Greek word *pneuma*, meaning "breath" or "soul." For the Greeks, the psyche was a subtle animating vapor that infused the physical body with life. Later the term was adopted by modern psychologists to refer to the nonphysical aspects of our being: the human mind as the center of thought, emotion and behavior. C. G. Jung used the term to refer to the totality of conscious and unconscious life in an individual.

Pulses—Acupuncturists and traditional Chinese herbalists rely strongly on pulse taking for diagnosis and treatment planning. The pulse can be felt at various places on the body but is generally read just above the radial artery. From the quality, speed and intensity of the pulse, the Chinese doctor can determine the state of the organs of the body as well as diagnose and locate areas of qi disturbance and imbalance. For example, from the pulse it is often possible to tell if a woman is pregnant, if the lungs are congested or if a patient has recently used drugs or alcohol. It is also possible to tell if a patient is tense or relaxed, where tension is located and how to best treat it.

Qi (also written Ch'i)—No single English word is equivalent to the word *qi*. Sometimes *qi* is translated as "energy" or "life force," but qi is not a noun, not a thing that can be pinned down and identified. Qi is the quickening, animation and transformation that occurs when the opposite polarities of yin and yang intermingle. Qi equals life, the mysterious desire of a living thing to become itself.

Radical—Chinese characters are often composed of more than one simpler character or element. In general, there are two or sometimes three graphic elements that join together to make a character, and a single element can be used as a building block to form many different characters. "Radical" is the term used to refer to one element of a character, in particular, the one that conveys the character's meaning.

Shaman—The term *shaman* is used to refer to the person who fulfils the role of healer/priest of earlier tribal cultures. Usually the person who takes on this role has some particular attribute or power that may manifest as telepathic ability, charisma or healing powers. In most tribes, the shaman is entrusted not only with the physical and psychological health of individuals but with the community and the integrity of its relationship to the environment. Catastrophes such as famine and drought fall within the shaman's sphere of influence. Shamanic healing focused on tending to the internal and external vital forces through ritual and various forms of natural healing practices.

Shen—*Shen,* usually translated from Chinese as "spirit," is a yang, ephemeral aspect of qi. It incorporates the functions of consciousness, vitality and awareness. When ancient acupuncturists and alchemists used the term "spirit," they were not referring to an abstract religious term or a disembodied aspect of human experience but rather to the finest, most ephemeral and yet most indestructible aspect of life itself. The spirits are indiscernible to human beings in ordinary states of modern Western consciousness, but they appear clearly to human beings in states of heightened forms of awareness, often as a kind of light, exquisite sound, presence or knowing. In Chinese medical terms, spirit is a form of qi. It is said to come to human beings from the stars. As it mixes with the slower, more structured vibrations of the earth, spirit illuminates matter and the energies of the soul appear. *See also* Spirit.

Soul—Every culture has its own way of describing and understanding the concept of the soul; however, the soul is almost universally regarded as the phenomenon that enables an individual living organism to initiate motion, to change or to develop from inner forces rather than being purely affected and moved by external stimuli. In the West, this word is often used synonymously with "spirit." The Western soul is generally conceived of as an abstraction, an animating principle that is separate in nature from the body and is often held to have a divine existence distinct from physical form. In contrast, the ancient Chinese conceived of the soul as arising from the mingling of matter and spirit. Both yin structure and yang function were viewed as expressions of the soul, and when these two aspects separated, the individual soul dispersed as the physical essences of the body dissolved back to the earth and the spiritual energies returned to heaven.

Spirit—In the West, the word "spirit" connotes the holy, the otherworldly. Spirit is a divine entity or energy that exists in and of itself in a dimension totally separate from the dimension of life on earth. *Shen*, the Chinese word that is usually translated into English as "spirit," refers to something else. *Shen* refers to the most yang, ephemeral, active and initiatory aspect of qi. Like the spirit of Western philosophy, shen is invisible, negentropic, and has a tendency to "rise upward." Like spirit, shen has a special relationship to light. However, shen as yang spirit does not exist in and of itself. It is contingent rather than self-existent. It can only exist in relationship to yin matter, as part of a larger wholeness: Tao. *Tao* is the Chinese word that is synonymous with "divine." It is the wholeness that divides into yang spirit and yin matter. *See also* Shen.

Spanda—*Spanda* is an Indian word that comes from same root as "spontaneity." Ancient Ayurvedic teachings describe spanda as a form of psychic energy that is expressed by an action or feeling of determination to carry out an action. This energy is experienced as a throb or vibration that is felt in the body. Action that comes from spanda is spontaneous and authentically powerful. Spanda is related to the Taoist concept of *ziran* and the spontaneous unfolding of original nature.

Sublimation—Freudian psychology uses the term "sublimation" to describe the process whereby the ego diverts the expression of an instinct, desire or impulse from its original form to one that is more culturally or socially acceptable, i.e., the sublimation of erotic desire into a work of art or athletic achievement.

Synchronicity—Synchronicity is a meaningful relationship between an inner subjective psychic experience and an objective event that occurs in the outer world at the same time. It is a meaningful coincidence that cannot be explained using the tools of logic and the rational mind.

Tantian—The literal translation of this word is "cinnabar field" and refers to the pelvic basin, the part of the abdomen below the umbilicus. It is the lowest of the three "cauldrons" or what Chinese healers call the "alchemical burning spaces" of the body. The tantian is thought of as a furnace that empowers alchemical transformation and is the power center of the body. The powerful energies of reproduction and vital heat of the tantian are considered the equivalent to fire that burns the planet's core. It is the place from which Chinese martial artists move and the area where the awareness is focused in Taoist, Chan and Zen Buddhist meditation.

Taiji—This is the familiar symbolic representation of the alchemical mystery of yin and yang, the primal opposites that come directly from the unity of Tao. In the taiji, we see how the yin contains a speck of yang and the yang contains a speck of yin.

Taoism—Taoism, along with Buddhism and Confucianism, is one of the three great philosophical and spiritual traditions of China. The system we now know as Chinese medicine was influenced by each of the three traditions, but the part of Chinese medicine explored in this book is based on the principles of Taoism and particularly Taoist alchemy. There is no precise date set for the beginning of Taoism. Unlike Confucianism, Taoism does not have a political, social status. It does not have a precise date of birth or a specific historical figure recognized as its originator. Some contend that Taoism is not a religion at all but rather a loose combination of teachings and philosophies based on the revelations of mystics, priests and sages over time.

Xi Wang Mu—The Taoist earth goddess, known as the Queen Mother of the West. Xi Wang Mu lives with her familiar, the fiery phoenix of resurrection, in a palace deep below Kunlun Mountain. Her throne sits just above the golden fountain, the waters of immortality that spring up from the earth's core. Xi Wang Mu is considered the goddess of life, death and resurrection. She is the keeper of the sacred Peaches of Immortality that grow only within the bounds of her secret mountain garden.

Yin and Yang—Yin and yang express the creative union of the opposites. Yin is related to the moon, cold, dark, water, moisture, quiescence and night. Yin is "reflective"—it receives and brings into form the impulses of the yang. Yang is related to the sun, heat, light, fire, dryness, activity and day. Yang is "initiatory"—it brings activity and possibility to the yin to be manifested in form.

Zangfu—*Zang* is the Chinese word used to refer to the fleshy or yin organs that preside over the purification and circulation of the blood: the heart, the spleen, the lungs, the kidneys and the liver. *Fu* is the word used to refer to the hollow organs that transform material received from outside the body into energy and blood: the small intestine, the stomach, the large intestine, the gallbladder and the bladder. *Zangfu* is the general term used to refer to all the viscera of the body.

A Chronology of Chinese History

～

Time of Origin
Before time, Pan Gu cracks the cosmic egg and gives rise to the cosmos.

500,000 BCE
Time of *Sinanthropus pekinensis*, or Peking man—tool-using hominids who inhabited the area southwest of what is now Beijing.

3000 BCE
Legendary Era; end of Neolithic Era. Mythological time of Huang Ti, the Yellow Emperor who, according to legend, "invented" writing, divination, agriculture and acupuncture. Bone needles, as well as instruments that may be acupuncture needles made of jade and stone, have been discovered dating back to this time.

2500–2000 BCE
Time of the Great Floods. According to Chinese mythology, this was the time when the great shaman Master Yu directed the building of canals to channel the waters of the Yellow River to the sea, opening the way for the development of cities along the riverbanks.

2000 BCE
Xia Dynasty. Development of bronze.

1700–1100 BCE
Shang Dynasty. Acupuncture needles probably made of thorns and slivers of bamboo.

1000–200 BCE
Zhou Dynasty.

475–222 BCE
Warring States Period. Time of Confucius, Lao Tzu and the codification of the *Neijing Suwen* or *Yellow Emperor's Classic of Traditional Chinese Medicine*.

200 BCE–220 CE
Han Dynasty. School of Yin-Yang and the Five Elements developed, building of the Great Wall, invention of paper, further codification of the *Neijing*.

300–589 CE
Six Dynasties. Introduction of Buddhism among intelligentsia, block printing, flourishing of iron and steel technology.

618–907 CE
Tang Dynasty.

960–1127 CE
Northern Song Dynasty. Development of rituals of *neidan* or inner alchemy.

1500 CE
Ming Dynasty.

1911 CE
The End of the Dynasty Era and the founding of the Republic of China.

1949–present
People's Republic of China.

A Brief History of Chinese Medicine

In the spring of 1921, a Swedish scholar and geologist named Johan Gunnar Andersson was engaged in excavation forty kilometers southwest of Beijing. Digging into the wall of an old limestone quarry, he and his assistant discovered some sharp bits of quartz alongside a pile of petrified animal bones. Andersson surmised that this discovery was evidence of the activities of ancient tool-using protohuman beings. Carefully digging deeper, the men made a startling discovery that confirmed Andersson's hypothesis: the molar and incisor of a human-like creature who had inhabited the area some 500,000 years ago. Later they discovered the bones of this ancient being and gave him the name *Sinanthropis pekinensis*— Peking man.

Andersson's find established the fact that the roots of Chinese civilization are in China and extend back at least half a million years into the Pleistocene Era. This confirms the fact that the numerous Neolithic settlements along the river were built upon the pathways and hunting grounds of even more ancient nomadic hunting and gathering tribes.[1]

For half a million years, people who lived along the banks of the great Chinese river were observing nature and developing ways to organize the world around them. Their culture, their myths, their religious traditions as well as their language, philosophies and medicine also developed gradually over a vast time period. Today, these ancient concepts continue to evolve as Chinese medicine and philosophy is assimilated into Western culture.

From archeological evidence, we know that the Chinese people were already practicing some form of acupuncture during the Neolithic Era. There is ample archeological evidence of the use of stone needles during the late Stone Age and the practice continued without interruption until modern times. Neolithic Chinese shamans (the healers of the earliest hunter/gatherer tribes) made needles out of sharpened stones and jade. In fact, the word *pien* or "stone probe" is actually one of the earliest words for "acupuncture needle."[2] In many early treatises, the word "stone" is used synonymously for "needle." The association of the Neolithic stone and bone probes with the origins of acupuncture reinforces our belief that roots of this healing system go back to the rituals and earth-centered wisdom of early Chinese tribal healers. The needles used by these early acupuncturists were not mere medical instruments. They were "magical" tools with which the healer could clear away demons and call up spirits.

Later, it seems probable that people during the Shang period (1500–1000 BCE) made their needles out of thorns, bamboo slivers and bones, which would have disintegrated with time. However, bronze needles from the Zhou Dynasty (1000 BCE) have been found, and it is highly likely that much older needles exist that have not been discovered.

The most important classic acupuncture text, the *Neijing Suwen* or *Yellow Emperor's Classic*, is said to have been written during the "Legendary Period" (2852–2205 BCE) by Huang Di, the culture hero who also discovered writing, pottery and agriculture. Actually, the *Neijing* is an anthology of theories and ideas that date back to the Neolithic times but the writing of the actual text dates back to the Warring States Period (approximately 350 BCE) around the same time that the great Taoist and Confucian texts were written.

From this point on, Chinese medicine continued to develop steadily. The basic principles spread to Japan, Vietnam and Korea, and these countries now have their own individual styles of acupuncture. In the second half of the seventeenth century, information about acupuncture—carried back by merchants and explorers along the Spice Route—began to attract the attention of European physicians. However, it was not until the 1800s that acupuncture actually began to be practiced in Europe. At that time, Western travelers and missionaries became aware of Chinese medicine and its efficacy. A great debt is due to the Jesuit missionaries who began the difficult task of seriously translating the classical Chinese texts.

In 1950, the People's Republic of China outlawed acupuncture as part of their attempt to eradicate what they considered superstitious practices. However, Chinese medicine was reintroduced and recognized as an important part of the state medical system in the 1960s. Currently, traditional Chinese medicine including acupuncture and herbs comprises approximately fifty percent of health care in China and is widely practiced in Europe and North America.

Notes

∽

Epigraph

1. *The Portable Nietzsche* (New York: Random House, 1954), p. 680.

Introduction

1. From the *Tao Teh Ching*, Chapter 21. The quotations from Lao Tzu that are
    used to introduce the concepts at the beginning of the chapters are based on
    verses of the *Tao Teh Ching* as translated by John Wu and Jonathan Star; this
    particular quotation is a combination of the two translations. In some cases,
    I have retranslated words in order to bring out a specific aspect of their
    meaning. Each of these introductory vignettes is rooted in original text. The
    specific chapter on which the vignette is based is indicated in the endnotes.

2. The actual word Lao Tzu uses in Chapter 21 of the *Tao Teh Ching* (John
    Wu's translation) as "what is within me" is *tz'u*, which in modern Chinese
    means "this." By examining the ancient etymology of the character, we dis-
    cover that it combines the radical *zhi*, meaning "stop" (a picture of the foot-
    print of a single left foot), with a picture of a man standing facing to the right
    (Wenlin CD Rom Version 2.1). The graphic communicates the character's
    original meaning: the place where a person's footsteps stop, right here, right
    now. The graphic opens us to Lao Tzu's crucial, and for his historical
    moment, radical insight. How do I know the world around me? I know the
    world from this very spot where my footsteps stop, the point where I stand
    at this place in space and time.

3. When I use the word "soul" in the pages of this book, I am not using it to mean
    the eternal spiritual entity often envisioned by the Judeo-Christian religions,
    which totally separates from the material body after death to reside with the
    angels in heaven above. I use the word "soul," for lack of a better term, to refer
    to a real yet extremely refined substance, sometimes referred to as the subtle

body. The soul or subtle body constellates through the intermingling of spirit and matter. It is the carrying medium of life, an ungraspable, immaterial substance that brings animation and vitality to living beings. The soul is the field of life where all spiritual growth and transformation occurs. It is the field of relationships, where opposites intermingle to form new possibilities. The soul is neither matter nor spirit, yet it contains qualities of both and cannot exist without the nourishing matrix of matter and the initiating fiery light of the divine. In human beings, the soul has a particular relationship to the heart, mind and emotions; it is the ephemeral substance that brings love, meaning and purpose to our lives. While most Eastern spiritual traditions are cautious about making definitive statements about the soul, they do not question the presence of a vitalizing breath that animates matter. This vitalizing breath is called *vata* in Vedic traditions, *ruach* in Hebrew and *qi* in Chinese. As we will see in Chapter Two, a reasonable correlation can be drawn between this vitalizing breath—i.e., *qi*—and the early Greek and Latin ideas about the *anima* or breath soul.

4. Thomas Cleary, *Twilight Goddess*, p. 59.
5. Soothill, *Dictionary of Buddhist Terms*.
6. Lao Tzu, *Tao Teh Ching*, Chapter 4, translated by John Wu.
7. Lao Tzu, *Tao Teh Ching*, Chapter 1, translated by Jonathan Star.
8. Translated by Thomas Cleary, *Practical Taoism*, p. 26.
9. Ted Kaptchuk uses this phrase as the title of his book *The Web That Has No Weaver*, one of the first popular texts on Chinese medicine to be published in North America.
10. Anthropologists and philosophers have used the term "mythical consciousness" to describe a non-linear way of organizing reality. The reader is referred to the work of Claude Levi-Strauss, *Structural Anthropology* and *The Savage Mind* as well as Jean Gebser's *Ever-Present Origin* for more detailed explorations of this topic.
11. Claude Larre and Elisabeth Rochat de la Vallée, *The Secret Treatise of the Spiritual Orchid*, p. 3.
12. Fritz Perls, *Ego, Hunger and Aggression*, p. 201.
13. In his book *The Time Falling Bodies Take to Light: Mythology, Sexuality and the Origins of Culture* (New York: St. Martin's Press, 1981), William Irwin Thompson offers a compelling argument that the Sumerian Descent Myth of Inanna, in addition to being a well-loved peasant's agricultural story and myth of woman's mysteries, is also a complex metaphysical description of the movement of the stars in the heavens, with each character representing the movement and nature of particular planets. He cites Professor Hertha von Dechend, who sees "myth as the technical language of a scientific and priestly elite" (p.173).

Part I: Introduction

1. Quoted without citation by Thomas Cleary, *Practical Taoism,* p. 28.

Chapter One: The Empty Center

1. Lao Tzu, *Tao Teh Ching,* Chapter 11, translated by Jonathan Star.
2. Giovanni Maciocia, *The Practice of Chinese Medicine,* p. 232.
3. In the terms of modern psychology, shamanic dancing induced states of "unity consciousness." Unity consciousness is accessed not only through ecstatic dance but also through various forms of meditation and dreams. It can also emerge spontaneously as a kind of grace during times of great crisis, love or overwhelming emotion. In this state of consciousness, boundaries dissolve, the individual "I" evaporates and all that is left is a sense of infinite connection with all of creation. There is an encounter with wu—the nothingness at the center of being. This experience is usually accompanied by a sense of divine presence, as if nothingness "makes room" for something other.
4. Quoted by Isabelle Robinet, *Taoism,* p. 84.
5. Claude Larre and Elisabeth Rochat de la Vallée, *The Secret Treatise of the Spiritual Orchid,* p. 19.
6. Marie-Louise von Franz, *Number and Time,* p. 121.
7. C. G. Jung, *Civilization in Transition,* Vol. X of the *Collected Works* (Princeton: Bollingen Foundation/Princeton University Press, 1953), p. 774. Cited in Marie-Louise von Franz, *Number and Time,* p. 121.
8. This explanation for the derivation of the character originates in Weiger and is pointed out by Larre and Rochat de la Vallée in their text *The Secret Treatise of the Spiritual Orchid,* p. 19.
9. Translated by Claude Larre and Elisabeth Rochat de la Vallée, *Rooted in Spirit,* and rendered into English by Sarah Stang.
10. Chad Hansen, "Language in the Heart-mind," in *Understanding the Chinese Mind: The Philosophical Roots,* edited by Robert Allinson.
11. Western ideas about the self derive from the tradition of the ancient Greek philosopher Plato, who proposed the idea that our physical form is based on an abstract structure that has an existence separate from the physical body. This abstract structure is an organizing principle that exists at the core of every human being. After the death of the physical body, this abstract entity maintains its integrity.
12. The teachings of the Golden Flower, the flower of transformation, are attributed to the Taoist alchemist Lu Tung Pin. Lu Tung Pin, also known as Lu Yan, lived in China during the tenth century. He is considered the founder of the Completely Real School of Taoism, which was started by his disciples in the eleventh century. The text of the *The Secret of the Golden Flower* is said to have been received "by direct transmission" from Lu Yan, many centuries

later. The Eastern concept of "transmission" refers to a kind of spiritual channeling where a living human receives wisdom from an enlightened being on another plane of existence. The text as we know it today was written and published during the mid-eighteenth century.

13. From C. G. Jung, "Commentary on *The Secret of the Golden Flower*," *Alchemical Studies*, p. 84.

14. C. G. Jung, "Commentary on *The Secret of the Golden Flower*," *Alchemical Studies*, p. 54.

15. Ibid., p. 21.

16. The term "backward-flowing path" is used extensively in both European and Taoist alchemy. It indicates a process in which a person decides to use the conscious will to stop the instinctual will from acting. Thus one is able to use the instinctual energies (that would otherwise have been used by nature for procreation) for inner growth and creativity. This backward path is discussed in more detail in Chapter 2.

17. Ken Wilber, *No Boundary*, p. 8.

18. Stephen Little, *Taoism and the Arts of China*, p.17.

19. A more detailed description of the experiential ground of ancient Chinese philosophy and culture is found in the anthology *Understanding the Chinese Mind*, edited by Robert Allinson.

20. C. G. Jung, Commentary on *The Secret of the Golden Flower*, translated by Richard Wilhelm, p. 95.

21. Ibid., p. 185.

22. From C. G. Jung, "Commentary on *The Secret of the Golden Flower*," *Alchemical Studies*, p. 37.

23. *The Secret of the Golden Flower*, translated by Richard Wilhelm, p. 36.

24. Post-Jungian depth psychologists recognize a similar kind of cataclysmic event as part of the individuation process that occurs during deep analytic work. It is the moment when the self has an actual encounter with something beyond itself. They refer to it as the moment when self encounters Self. This Self, intentionally written with a capital S to distinguish it from the knowable self of individual identity, is a reflection of cosmic wholeness. It is an unfathomable mystery that transcends the boundaries of self and not-self, I and cosmos. Dr. Nathan Schwartz-Salant, Jungian analyst and expert on European alchemy, is responsible for making this crucial distinction between the immanent, personal self that can be known by the ego and the Self that is a manifestation of the unbroken wholeness and mystery of the divine. He cites the theological concept of *homoousia*—the identity of the immanent and transcendent Self—as the Western version of the Taoist belief that a miniature version of Tao constellates at the center of the psyche.

25. From C. G. Jung's Commentary on *The Secret of the Golden Flower*, translated by Richard Wilhelm, p. 80.
26. Bach Flower Rescue Remedy is made by shining sunlight through the petals of several varieties of flowers and infusing purified water with this light. It is perfectly safe, has no side effects, and yet has a powerful calming effect on many people in states of acute shock and fright. I have also found it to be effective in the treatment of animals. It is available at most health food stores.
27. Pulse reading plays a role in healing traditions the world over and is an important part of Chinese medical diagnosis. A skilled acupuncturist can determine the severity, depth and organ location of disease by reading a patient's pulses. Sometimes it is even possible to determine how long a person has been sick and how soon he or she will recover.

    There are twelve different pulse positions located bilaterally on the wrist, just above the radial artery. However, unlike the Western doctor, the acupuncturist does not feel the actual blood pulse of the artery but rather the reflected vibration of the pulse in the body tissue. When I explain pulse taking to patients, I compare the radial pulse to a stone thrown in a pond. As an acupuncturist, I am not interested in the stone itself but in the waves that ripple outward from the splash. These ripples give me information about the movements of the qi, providing an inside view of the invisible dance of the life force.

    When an acupuncturist takes a patient's pulse, she or he places the fingers on the wrist just above the artery and "listens" to the ripples with the tips of the fingers. At first, students learning pulse diagnosis usually claim to feel nothing, but with time and practice, their sensitivity to sensation develops and a whole new world opens up at their fingertips. Over time, the pulses can be read and then "tuned" the way a master musician tunes the strings of a guitar. A single acupuncture needle well placed in a point is sometimes enough to change "off-key," twanging pulses into the harmonized chiming of a dozen golden bells.
28. Dr. J. R. Worsley was an English osteopath who went to China in the late 1960s and brought important traditional Chinese medical concepts, theories and techniques back to the West. He is known as the founder of European Five Element style acupuncture.
29. Translated from the *Lingshu*, Chapter 8, by Claude Larre and Elisabeth Rochat de la Vallée in *Rooted in Spirit*, p. 4.
30. *Rooted in Spirit*, p. xvii.

Chapter Two: Lead Into Gold
1. Lao Tzu, *Tao Teh Ching*, Chapter 15, translated by Jonathan Star.
2. Quoted by James Gleick in *Chaos: Making a New Science*, p. 68.

3. Nathan Schwartz-Salant, *Narcissism and Character Transformation*, p. 18.
4. Lao Tzu, *Tao Teh Ching*, Chapter 59, translated by Jonathan Star.
5. Zen master Eihei Dogen Zenji first presented the parable of the Zen cook or *tenzo* to his disciples in thirteenth-century Japan. The story was recorded by Master Dogen and finally completed by his students in 1237. It records the enlightenment experience that Dogen had in the company of a cook at a Chan Buddhist monastery in China. This story is presented again in modern form in Bernard Glassman's book *Instructions to the Cook: A Zen Master's Lessons in Living a Life That Matters*.
6. Quoted by James Gleick in *Chaos*, p. 307.
7. *Neijing Suwen*, translated by Ilza Veith, p. 97.
8. Ibid., p. 98.
9. I am grateful to Dr. Nathan Schwartz-Salant for inviting me to read his work-in-progress, *The Great Divide: The Emergence of the Modern Form of the Conservation of Energy*, which contributed to my understanding of the significance of entropy in ancient and modern healing systems.
10. Lao Tzu, *Tao Teh Ching*, Chapter 6, translated by Jonathan Star.
11. Lao Tzu, *Tao Teh Ching*, Chapter 15, translated by Jonathan Star.
12. Touching is an important part of Chinese diagnosis. Part of touching involves palpating certain acupuncture points and reflex zones to find areas of tenderness and temperature differences, but the most important part of touching is pulse taking. Pulse taking requires many years of training and experience, but once it is mastered it becomes an invaluable tool for the practitioner. The pulse can be felt at various places on the body but is generally read just above the radial artery. From the quality, speed and intensity of the pulse, the Chinese doctor can determine the state of the organs of the body as well as diagnose and locate areas of qi disturbance and imbalance. For example, from the pulse it is often possible to tell if a woman is pregnant, if the lungs are congested or if a patient has recently used drugs or alcohol. It is also possible to tell if a patient is tense or relaxed, where tension is located and how to best treat it. For more basic information on pulse taking, see Ted Kaptchuk's book *The Web That Has No Weaver*. For an in-depth study of this topic, see Shigehisa Kuriyama's *The Expressiveness of the Body*.
13. *The Secret of the Golden Flower*, translated by Richard Wilhelm, p. 55.
14. In the early 1990s, the "gate theory" was offered as an explanation for acupuncture's effectiveness, based on studies done on pain. According to this theory, acupuncture works to alleviate pain by inhibiting sensory nerve responses, closing the "gates" between various segments of the spinal cord. However, the theory did not bear out under scrutiny and was soon forgotten.
15. Moxibustion is an important part of Chinese medicine. It is a way to stimulate points through heat rather than needles. Moxa sticks are compressed

sticks of the herb *Artemisia vulgaris*. The sticks are lit and passed in circles an inch or two above the point or painful area.

Chapter Three: The Axle and the Wheel
1. Lao Tzu, *Tao Teh Ching*, Chapter 11, translated by John Wu.
2. Kiiko Matsumoto and Stephen Birch, *Five Elements and Ten Stems*, p. 1.
3. C. G. Jung, *The Archetypes of the Collective Unconscious*, p. 6.
4. *Neijing Suwen*, translated by Ilza Veith, p. 222.

Chapter Four: Tao Lost and Rediscovered
1. Lao Tzu, *Tao Teh Ching*, Chapter 29, translated by Jonathan Star.
2. Active imagination is a therapeutic process developed by C. G. Jung in which a person actively participates in a dialogue with images, fantasies and symbols drawn from the unconscious through dreams and meditation. I have found it to be a powerful adjunct to Alchemical Acupuncture treatment as it allows a patients to consciously integrate energetic shifts that occur at the unconscious somatic level. This leads to insights that often have a profound reorganizing effect on the self (for more on active imagination, see Glossary).

Chapter Five: The Mountain
1. Translated by Claude Larre and Elisabeth Rochat de la Vallée in *Rooted in Spirit*.
2. The phrase "mere dead weight" refers to Lao Tzu's *Tao Teh Ching*, Chapter 11, translated by Jonathan Star.
3. Quoted by W. Y. Evans-Wentz, in *Cuchama and Sacred Mountains*, p. xxx.
4. Stephen Little, *Taoism and the Arts of China*, p. 17.
5. *I Ching*, translated by Richard Wilhelm, p. 201.
6. C. G. Jung, *The Archetypes and the Collective Unconscious*, p. 19.

Part II: Introduction
1. From a translation of Shangqing texts quoted by Isabelle Robinet in *Taoism*, p. 131.

Chapter Six: Shen
1. Claude Larre and Elisabeth Rochat de la Vallée, *The Heart*, p. 42.
2. Anodea Judith, *Wheels of Life*, p. 216.
3. Claude Larre and Elisabeth Rochat de la Vallée, *The Heart*, p. 43.
4. Quoted by Claude Larre and Elisabeth Rochat de la Vallée in *The Seven Emotions*, p. 16.
5. Robert Aitken, *Mind of Clover*, p. 8.

Chapter Seven: Hun

1. *I Ching,* translated by Richard Wilhelm.
2. Claude Larre and Elisabeth Rochat de la Vallée, *The Heart,* p. 43.
3. This material is quoted from an unrevised transcript of a lecture on Chapter 8 of the *Neijing Suwen* given by Claude Larre and Elisabeth Rochat de la Vallée at a seminar in London in 1985.
4. Andrew Ellis, Nigel Wiseman, and Ken Boss, *Grasping the Wind,* p. 371.
5. *Neijing Suwen,* Chapter 8, as quoted by Larre and Rochat de la Vallée.
6. Nelson Foster and Jack Shoemaker, *The Roaring Stream,* p. 178.

Chapter Eight: Yi

1. Translated by John Wu.
2. Quoted by Claude Larre and Elisabeth Rochat de la Vallée in *Rooted in Spirit.*
3. Claude Larre and Elisabeth Rochat de la Vallée, *Rooted in Spirit,* p. 52.
4. Where there are ongoing problems with binging, bulimia, anorexia or sugar addiction, seek professional help. There is no way to truly nourish your intention and integrity until these physical-level issues have been dealt with. OA (Overeater's Anonymous) helps many people get in touch with the spiritual hunger that underlies erratic eating patterns. Or seek the help of a well-trained psychotherapist with experience in this area.
5. Herbal treatment for this patient consisted of low doses of *Gui Pi Tang* (Tonifying Spleen Decoction) in tincture form over several months. If her intermittent excess menstrual bleeding had not responded to this formula and the acupuncture treatment, I would have considered *Bu Zhong Yi Qi Tang* (Tonifying the Center and Benefiting Qi Decoction) as a next choice, but I have found that this second formula is more physical while the first affects the spirit more directly.
6. *The Secret of the Golden Flower,* translated by Richard Wilhelm, p. 50.

Chapter Nine: Po

1. Originally translated into German in 1929 and shortly afterward into English by Cary Baynes.
2. From C. G. Jung, "Commentary on *The Secret of the Golden Flower,*" *Alchemical Studies,* p. 39.
3. Giovanni Maciocia, *The Practice of Chinese Medicine,* p. 205.
4. Chuang Tzu, *Basic Writings,* from "Discussion on Making All Things Equal," p. 31.
5. *Ling Shu or The Spiritual Pivot,* Chapter 8.
6. Claude Larre and Elisabeth Rochat de la Vallée, *Rooted in Spirit,* p. 38.
7. Ibid., p. 38.

8. Lao Tzu, *Tao Teh Ching*, Chapter 10, compilation of translations by Jonathan Star and John Wu.

9. From a transcription of a talk on the *Secret Treatise of the Spiritual Orchid*, given at the Ricci Institute, published by the British Register of Oriental Medicine in 1985.

10. This information comes from a lecture given by Claude Larre and Elisabeth Rochat de la Vallée at the Traditional Acupuncture Institute in Columbia, Maryland in 1985.

11. Claude Larre and Elisabeth Rochat de la Vallée, *Rooted in Spirit*, p. 42.

12. For stubborn chronic pain, I have found that low doses of the blood-invigorating trauma formula *ShenTong Zhu-Yu Tang* (included as part of the Meridian Passage formula) is very effective not only in relieving pain but in helping to unlock emotions and uncover buried memories. It seems to soften the pain of psychological resistance and facilitate the process of uncovering buried emotions.

13. Claude Larre and Elisabeth Rochat de la Vallée, *Rooted in Spirit*, p. 41.

14. Quoted by C. G. Jung in *Alchemical Studies*, p. 103n.

Chapter Ten: Zhi

1. Translated by John Wu.

2. *I Ching*, translated by Richard Wilhelm, p. 16.

3. Lao Tzu, *Tao Teh Ching*, Chapter 21, translated by John Wu.

4. Chuang Tzu, *Basic Writings*, from "Mastering Life," p. 118.

5. Club drugs such as ecstasy (MDMA) and "special K" (Kaetamine) are a class of mostly illegal drugs that are popular with people who frequent all-night dance parties. These drugs are used to relax and energize as well as to help sustain a person's ability to dance for extended periods of time. Some users report enhanced sexual responses; however, the drugs often impair erectile and orgasmic function.

Part III: Introduction

1 Translated by Jonathan Star.

Chapter Eleven: Chaos

1. *I Ching*, translated by Richard Wilhelm, p. 17.

2. Chuang Tzu, *Basic Writings*, p. 127.

3. Lao Tzu, *Tao Teh Ching*, Chapter 6, translated by Jonathan Star.

4. From the Commentary of the *I Ching*, translated by Richard Wilhelm.

5. Isabelle Robinet, *Taoism*, page 134.

6. The joining together of the two souls brings life and their separation brings death. At each juncture, there is chaos. Perhaps this is why at the bottom of

death. At each juncture, there is chaos. Perhaps this is why at the bottom of the Chinese character *gui*, the graphic marker of two souls, we find the peculiar spiral of the whirlwind, the spiral Claude Larre speaks of as the "little whirling storm of dust that the ghosts leave behind them as they pass." (See figure 9.1 for a picture of the graphic for *gui*.)

7. Nathan Schwartz-Salant, *The Great Divide*, unpublished paper.

8. From James Gleick, *Chaos*, p. 308.

9. Ibid., p. 314.

10. Isabelle Robinet, *Taoism*, p. 735.

11. *The I Ching*, translated by James Legge. The Y'I King Text: Section I:III. www.sacred-texts.com/ich//ic03.htm.

12. The Chinese character for this clashing together of opposites is pronounced "chong," which sounds like two things hitting up against each other. The character is composed of two radicals. One is a picture of an arrow hitting the center of a target, thus penetrating the center of two opposites. The other radical is a picture of a wave of water. This wave of water is often found when there is a linguistic relationship to the concept of overflowing chaos. Thus the character reinforces our understanding that the sudden insight that arises spontaneously comes from the watery chaos of the unconscious.

13. Japanese Zen Buddhism, which has become relatively popular in the West, is based on even more ancient Taoist and Chinese Buddhist traditions. The great Zen master Eihei Dogen was a Japanese aristocrat who made the arduous journey to China in 1225 to study with teachers in the great Chinese monasteries. He became familiar with the practice of meditating on paradoxical questions that later became a central part of Zen practice.

14. *Neijing Suwen*, translated by Ilza Veith, p. 98.

15. Ibid.

16. This transcultural association tells us that the concept of "origin" is primal and universal and has its source in the archetypal imagination of human beings.

17. *Webster's Third New International Dictionary.*

18. In addition to the crucial work of Carl Jung, the idea of a core nature with a drive toward self-expression was explored in depth by Abraham Maslow, who is credited with being one of the founders of humanist psychology.

19. The Chinese character for "spontaneity" is *ziran,* which also means "nature." This word has a particular importance in Taoist thought, and a clue to its meaning can be discovered in the character that contains, as a radical, a picture of a phoenix roasting in the flames of a fire. The phoenix is the sacred bird of Xi Wang Mu, the Goddess of the Underworld, who lives deep in the labyrinths of the earth. She sits on a throne at the source of the Yellow Spring, whose gushing waters are the Waters of Life. Thus spontaneity is a

seminal quality of the natural world. It is the irrepressible energy of life, death and resurrection as symbolized by the phoenix, who roasts in the flames of the transformational fire of the underworld.

20. Quoted by Thomas Cleary in *The Secret of the Golden Flower,* p. 107.
21. Isabelle Robinet, *Taoism,* p. 237.
22. *The Secret of the Golden Flower,* translated by Thomas Cleary, p. 39.
23. Ibid., p. 107.
24. *The I Ching,* translated by Richard Wilhelm, p. 250.
25. This meditation is adapted from alchemical meditations described by Master Lu Tung Ping in *The Secret of the Golden Flower* as well as introductory Zen meditation practices. It is a wonderful practice for anyone involved in healing work for it helps us to get out of our own way and to be open and receptive to wisdom that comes from unconscious and transpersonal realms.
26. Lao Tzu, *Tao Teh Ching,* Chapter 4.

Chapter Twelve: Lead

1. Quoted by Fabricius in *Alchemy,* p. 98.
2. From *The Secret of the Golden Flower,* translated by Thomas Cleary, p.10.
3. Quoted by C. G. Jung in *Psychology and Alchemy,* p. 124.
4. A Gnostic text quoted by Nathan Schwartz-Salant in *Entropy, Negentropy and the Psyche,* p. 54.
5. Nathan Schwartz-Salant, *Entropy, Negentropy and the Psyche,* p. 55.
6. Lao Tzu, *Tao Teh Ching,* translated by John Wu, Chapter 8.
7. Ibid., Chapter 11.
8. Lao Tzu, *Tao Teh Ching,* translated by Jonathan Star, Chapter 6.
9. C. G. Jung, *Psychology and Alchemy,* p. 340.
10. Translated and quoted by Isabelle Robinet in *Taoism,* p. 239.
11. Ilza Veith translation.
12. *The Secret of the Golden Flower,* translated by Thomas Cleary, p. 108.
13. Ibid., p.19.
14. Richard Wilhelm reveals the secret, encrypted symbolism of the golden flower in his preface to his translation of *The Secret of the Golden Flower.*
15. Ted Kaptchuk, *The Web That Has No Weaver,* p. 4.
16. More information on focusing, including basic instructions for practice, can be found in Gene Gendlin's book *Focusing,* as well as online at www.focusing.org.

Chapter Thirteen: The Golden Flower

1. *Psychology and Alchemy,* p. 6.
2. Richard Wilhelm translation.
3. To the best of my understanding, it was the philosopher Jean Gebser who

first introduced the concept of integral consciousness to the world in his book *The Ever-Present Origin*. Today, most philosophers and even neuroscientists and explorers of consciousness recognize this term and use it to speak of a new, more expanded form of consciousness that has, as yet, manifested in only its first incipient form in such remarkable geniuses as Albert Einstein and Pablo Picasso. Yet integral consciousness has been a possibility for human beings for thousands of years, and we see hints of it in great mystic and spiritual teachers, such as Lao Tzu, Buddha and Jesus Christ.

4. Jean Gebser uses the phrase "ever-present origin" as the title of his book. For Gebser, the phrase reflects the play of change and constancy as human consciousness shifts through time.

5. I first discovered the concept of a "mutation of consciousness" in the work of Jean Gebser. For readers who wish to understand this concept more fully, Gebser offers a clear and elegant presentation in Chapter 3 of *The Ever-Present Origin*.

6. The *I Ching* or *Book of Changes*, Hexagram #3.

7. Claude Anshin Thomas, *At Hell's Gate*, p. 109.

8. Thich Nhat Hanh, *A Guide to Walking Meditation*.

Appendix

1. Archeological data from Cecilia Lindqvist, *China*, p. 46.

2. Lu Gwei-Djen and Joseph Needham, *Celestial Lancets*, p. 70.

Bibliography

∽

Modern Texts

Aitken, Robert. *The Mind of Clover: Essays in Zen Buddhist Ethics.* San Francisco: North Point Press, 1997.

Allinson, Robert, ed. *Understanding the Chinese Mind: The Philosophical Roots.* Oxford: Oxford University Press, 1991.

Aria, Barbara, and Russel Eng Gon. *The Spirit of the Chinese Character.* San Francisco: Chronicle Books, 1992.

Ballentine, Rudolph. *Radical Healing: Integrating the World's Great Therapeutic Traditions to Create a New Transformative Medicine.* New York: Harmony Books, 1999.

Cleary, Thomas. *Practical Taoism.* Boston: Shambhala Publications, 1996.

Cleary, Thomas, and Aziz Sartaz. *Twilight Goddess: Spiritual Feminism and Feminine Spirituality.* Boston: Shambhala Publications, 2000.

Connelly, Dianne. *Traditional Acupuncture: The Law of the Five Elements.* Columbia, Maryland: Traditional Acupuncture Institute, 1975.

Deadman, Peter, and Mazin Al-Khafaji. *A Manual of Acupuncture.* Hove, England: Journal of Chinese Medicine Publications, 1998.

Eckman, Peter. *In the Footsteps of the Yellow Emperor: Tracing the History of Traditional Acupuncture.* San Francisco: Cypress Book Company, 1996.

Edinger, Edward. *Ego and Archetype.* Boston: Shambhala Publications, 1992.

Ellis, Andrew, Nigel Wiseman and Ken Boss. *Grasping the Wind: An Exploration into the Meaning of Chinese Acupuncture Point Names.* Brookline, Massachusetts: Paradigm Publications, 1989.

Evans-Wentz, W. Y. *Cuchama and Sacred Mountains.* Athens, Ohio: Ohio University Press, 1981.

Fabricius, Johannes. *Alchemy: The Medieval Alchemists and Their Royal Art.* London: Diamond Books, 1976.

Foster, Nelson, and Jack Shoemaker. *The Roaring Stream: A New Zen Reader.* Hopewell, New Jersey: The Ecco Press, 1996.

Freud, Sigmund. *Introductory Lectures on Psycho-Analysis.* New York: W. W. Norton, 1966.

Frey-Rohn, Liliane. *From Freud to Jung.* New York: A Delta Book. 1974.

Gay, Peter, ed. *The Freud Reader.* New York: W. W. Norton, 1969.

Gebser, Jean. *The Ever-Present Origin*. Translated by Noel Barstad. Athens, Ohio: Ohio University Press, 1985.

Gendlin, Eugene. *Focusing*. New York: Bantam Books, 1982.

————. *Focusing-Oriented Psychotherapy*. New York: The Guilford Press, 1996.

Glassman, Bernard. *Instructions to the Cook: A Zen Master's Lessons in Living a Life That Matters*. New York: Bell Tower, 1996.

Gleick, James. *Chaos: Making a New Science*. New York: Penguin Books, 1987.

Grof, Stanislav. *Beyond the Brain*. Albany: SUNY Press, 1985.

Gwei-Djen, Lu, and Joseph Needham. *Celestial Lancets: A History and Rationale of Acupuncture and Moxa*. Cambridge; New York: Cambridge University Press, 1980.

Hall, Calvin. *A Primer of Freudian Psychology*. New York: New American Library, 1954.

Johnson, Robert. *Inner Work: Using Dreams and Active Imagination for Personal Growth*. San Francisco: HarperCollins, 1986.

Judith, Anodea. *Wheels of Life: A User's Guide to the Chakra System*. St. Paul, Minnesota: Llewellyn Publications, 1995.

Jung, C. G. *Aion: Researches into the Phenomenology of the Self*. Princeton: Bollingen Series, Princeton University Press, 1978.

————. *Alchemical Studies*. Princeton: Bollingen Series, Princeton University Press, 1983.

————. *The Archetypes and the Collective Unconscious*. Princeton: Bollingen Series, Princeton University Press, 1990.

————. *Psychology and Alchemy*. Princeton: Bollingen Series, Princeton University Press, 1980.

————. *Two Essays on Analytical Psychology*. Princeton: Bollingen Series, Princeton University Press, 1980.

Kanner, Allen D., Theodore Roszak and Mary E. Gomes, eds. *Ecopsychology: Restoring the Earth, Healing the Mind*. San Francisco: Sierra Club Books, 1995.

Kaptchuk, Ted. *The Web That Has No Weaver: Understanding Chinese Medicine*. Chicago: Congdon & Weed, 1983.

Kuryama, Shigehisa. *The Expressiveness of the Body*. New York: Zone Books, 1999.

Larre, Claude and Elisabeth Rochat de la Vallée. *The Heart: The Lingshu Chapter 8*. Cambridge: Monkey Press, 1996.

————. *Huang Di Nei Jing Su Wen: The Secret Treatise of the Spiritual Orchid*. Unrevised transcript of seminar presented at Ricci Institute, published by British Register of Oriental Medicine, 1985.

————. *Rooted in Spirit: The Heart of Chinese Medicine*. Translated by Sarah Stang. New York: Station Hill Press, 1995.

————. *The Seven Emotions*. Cambridge: Monkey Press, 1996.

Levine, Peter. *Waking the Tiger*. San Francisco: North Atlantic Books. 1997.

Lindqvist, Cecilia. *China: Empire of Living Symbols*. Reading, Massachusetts: Addison-Wesley Publishing, 1991.

Little, Steven. *Taoism and the Arts of China.* Chicago: The Art Institute of Chicago, 2000.

Maciocia, Giovanni. *The Practice of Chinese Medicine.* Edinburgh: Churchill Livingstone, 1994.

Matsumoto, Kiiko, and Stephen Birch. *Five Elements and Ten Stems.* Brookline, Massachusetts: Paradigm Publishers, 1983.

Neilson, William, Thomas Knot and Paul Carhart, eds. *Webster's International Dictionary of the English Language 2nd Edition Unabridged.* Springfield, Massachusetts: C. Merriam Company, 1950.

Perera, Sylvia. *Descent to the Goddess: A Way of Initiation for Women.* Toronto: Inner City Books, 1981.

Perls, F. S. *Ego, Hunger and Aggression.* New York: Vintage Books, 1969.

Perls, F. S., Robert Hefferline and Paul Goodman. *Gestalt Therapy: Excitement and Growth in the Human Personality.* Highland, New York: The Gestalt Journal Press, 1951.

Porkert, Manfred. *The Theoretical Foundations of Chinese Medicine.* Cambridge, Massachusetts: The MIT Press, 1978.

Powell, James. *The Tao of Symbols.* New York: Quill Press, 1982.

Nhat Hanh, Thich. *A Guide to Walking Meditation.* Nyack, New York: Fellowship of Reconciliation Publications, 1985.

Robinet, Isabelle. *Taoism: Growth of a Religion.* Translated by Phyllis Brooks. Stanford: Stanford University Press, 1997.

Schwartz-Salant, Nathan. *Narcissism and Character Transformation.* Toronto: Inner City Books, 1982.

———. *The Mystery of Human Relationship.* London and New York: Routledge Press, 1998.

———. *Entropy, Negentropy and the Psyche: An Inquiry into the Structure of Psychic Energy.* Unpublished thesis presented at the Jung Institute, Zurich, 1969.

———. *The Great Divide: The Emergence of the Modern Form of the Conservation of Energy.* Unpublished work in progress.

Sessions, George, ed. *Deep Ecology for the 21st Century.* Boston: Shambhala Publications, 1995.

Spretnek, Charlene, ed. *The Politics of Women's Spirituality.* Garden City, New York: Anchor Books, 1982.

Soulie de Morant, George. *Chinese Acupuncture.* Brookline, Massachusetts: Paradigm Publications, 1972.

Starhawk. *The Spiral Dance: A Rebirth of the Ancient Religion of the Great Goddess.* San Francisco: HarperCollins, 1989.

Thomas, Claude Anshin. *At Hell's Gate: A Soldier's Journey from War to Peace.* Boston: Shambhala Publications, 2004.

von Franz, Marie-Louise. *Alchemical Active Imagination.* Boston: Shambhala Publications, 1997.

———. *Archetypal Dimensions of the Psyche.* Boston: Shambhala Publications, 1997.

———. *Number and Time.* Evanston: Northwestern University Press, 1974.

Wenlin Institute. *Wenlin Software for Learning Chinese* (including ABC Dictionary by John DeFrancis). Version 2.0: www.wenlin.com, 1998.

Wieger, L. *Chinese Characters.* New York: Dover Publications, 1965.

Whitmont, Edward. *The Symbolic Quest: Basic Concepts of Analytical Psychology.* Princeton: Princeton University Press, 1969.

Wilber, Ken. *No Boundary: Eastern and Western Approaches to Personal Growth.* Boston: Shambhala Publications, 2001.

Wilmer, Harry, M.D. *Practical Jung: The Nuts and Bolts of Jungian Psychology.* Wilmette, Illinois: Chiron Publications, 1987.

Wong, Eva. *The Shambhala Guide to Taoism.* Boston: Shambhala Publications, 1997.

Translations of Classic Texts

Chuang Tzu. *Basic Writings.* Translated by Burton Watson. New York: Columbia University Press, 1996.

Hung Ti Nei Ching Su Wen: The Yellow Emperor's Classic of Internal Medicine. Translated by Ilza Veith. Berkeley: University of California Press, 1972.

I Ching. Translated by Rudolf Ritsema and Stephen Karcher. Dorset, England: Element Books, 1994.

The I Ching. Translated by Richard Wilhelm. Rendered into English by Cary Baynes. Princeton: Bollingen Series, Princeton University Press, 1950.

Lao Tzu. *Tao Te Ching: The Definitive Edition.* Translated by Jonathan Star. New York: Jeremy P. Tarcher/Putnam, 2001.

Lao Tzu. *Tao Teh Ching.* Translated by John C. H. Wu. Edited by Paul K. T. Sih. New York: St. John's University Press, 1961.

Ling Shu or The Spiritual Pivot. Translated by Wu Jing-Nuan. Washington, DC: Taoist Studies Series, 1993.

The Secret of the Golden Flower. Translated by Thomas Cleary. San Francisco: HarperSanFrancisco, 1991.

T'ai I Chin Hua Tsung Chih / The Secret of the Golden Flower. Translated by Richard Wilhelm. Rendered into English by Cary Baynes. London: Kegan Paul, Trench, Trubner & Co. Ltd., 1942.

The Yellow Emperor's Classic of Medicine: A New Translation of the Neijing Suwen *with Commentary.* Translated by Maoshing Ni. Boston: Shambhala Press, 1995.

Zen Master Dogen. *Instructions for the Zen Cook.* Translated by Thomas Wright. New York: Weatherhill Press, 1994.

Index

bodymind
    continuum, 17–18, 373
    spirit connection to, 19–20,
      62–63, 66, 73, 92,
      134–38, 249–50, 357
bones, 275
breath body
    ancient views about, xviii,
      23–24
    Five Spirits and, 23–24,
      146–48
    movement of, 147
    qi in, 135
breathing techniques, 131, 160
Brown's Pond, 353–54
bu land, 292
Bu Zhong Yi Qi Tang, 398n5
Buddhism, 4–5, 72–73, 400n13
bugs, 83, 85, 335
burning spaces, alchemical, 101

cancer, 347–52
Cauldrons of the Spirits, 321
causative factor, 104
caveat, xx–xxi
Celestial Pivot, 229–30
chakra system, xix, 22–23,
  147–48, 177, 199, 360
change
    in acupuncture practices, 3
    organic, 335–38
chaos. *See also huntun*
    during birth, 299–301
    definition of, 305
    leftover, 85–87, 333–35
    myth about, 85–87, 305
    resistance to, 330–33
    state, 141, 298
    symbols for, 303
    theory, 304–6
    transforming energies of,
      316–18
characters. *See* Chinese characters
chelidonium, 206
cheng shan, 325
ch'i. *See* qi

Ch'i Po, 75, 128, 336
child
    innocence of, 58, 355
    jing in, 81
    original nature of, 311
China
    ancient life in, 74–76
    history of, 385–86
    mountains of, 1, 150–52
    People's Republic of, 389
    religions of, 4
Chinese characters
    for alchemy, 99
    archetypes and, 14
    for elements, 118–20
    for Five Elements, 111
    guang, 344
    hun, 197
    huntun, 306
    jin hua, 344
    ling, 191
    for origin, 309
    origin of, 12–13
    po, 245
    qian, 333
    shen, 173–74
    structure of, xix–xx, 13–14
    tan, 99
    tao, 142
    tzu, 58
    understanding of, xvi
    weiji, 314
    wu, 37–39, 39–41
    xin, 42
    xing, 111–12
    yi, 218
    zhi, 276, 391n2
Chinese herbs, xxi, 80, 100–101,
  131, 206, 398n5, 399n12
Chinese Marxist philosophy, 327
Chinese medicine
    alchemical concepts in,
      69–70, 94–97, 310
    Five Spirits in, 144–46
    history of, 327, 371, 387–89
    psychology of, 15–17

skepticism of, 103
symbolic images in, 60–61,
    64
traditions of, xv, xvi–xvii,
    15–17, 31–33, 297, 327
wisdom of, 4, 140
Chinese medicine, traditional
    ancient texts of, xvi–xvii
    history of, 327
    psychology of, 15–17
    transformation with, xv, 297
Chinese Medicine, Traditional
    (TCM), xvii
Chinese mythology, 12, 51, 74,
    82, 261–62, 264, 349
Chuang Tzu, 178, 240, 284–85,
    301–2, 330, 367
cinnabar, 100–101, 151, 161
    field, 101–2, 182, 229,
        266–67, 382
circulatio, 367
civilization, ancient, 74–76, 82
Cleary, Thomas, 5, 316
cleaving strategy, 70
"cloud scrolls," 12
clouds, 193–94, 199
codependency, 225
collective unconscious, 45, 48,
    373–74
colon, 255, 257
color
    as element correspondence,
        114, 126
    as symbolic, 182, 244–45,
        315–16
Colorado Rocky Mountains, 322
communism, 16
compassion, 191
The Completely Real School of
    Taoism, 315, 393n12
conception, 78–79, 171, 275,
    303, 375
Conception Vessel, 148–49, 256,
    266
conflict, 84–85
Confucianism, 4, 5

coniunctio, 100
"conscious life," 53–54
consciousness. *See also* uncon-
    scious
    development of, 331–32
    dualistic, 357–58, 362, 374
    Five Spirits and, 166
    integrated, 359–62, 402n3
    logic and, 9–10
    modern, xv, 9–10, 50
    mythical, 9–10, 12
    symbols for, 166
    Taoist view of, 53–54
    transformation of, 19–20,
        23–24, 49, 65–66,
        341–42, 359–62
    unity, 393n3
    of Western culture, xv, 9–10,
        50, 355, 362
container, of life, 106
contra natura, 159
control, of elements, 114–16
correspondences, to elements,
    112–14
cosmic light, 172
cosmology, Taoist, 108–10,
    150–52, 297
cosmos
    alignment of, 26, 85
    connection to, 70
    emergence of, 307–8
    mountains and, 150–52
    reflection of, 51
creation
    origin of, 83–85, 305, 307–8,
        333–34
    patterns of, 9–10
    yin/yang in, 156–58, 277
creative process, 83–85
crisis
    identity, 250
    point, 313–16, 325–26,
        362–66
cycles/rhythms
    biorhythms, 134–35
    of Five Elements, 114–16

of Five Spirits, 114–16, 274,
342
of hun, 209–10
menstrual, 201, 204–5
in nature, 74–76, 108–11,
114–16
sheng/k'o, 114–16, 128, 274

dance, 58
rain, 191–92
shamanic, 37–39, 368,
393n3
dandelion, 206, 209
Dark Gate, 291–92, 301–2
dark goddess, 328, 337, 342
Dark Mother, 283–84, 290
Darling Island, 215
death, 81, 88
po and, 242, 252, 261, 266,
268
decisions, 197, 199, 201, 212–13
deities, 144, 146, 159, 173
demons, 61, 140, 197–98,
243–44, 262, 265, 375
depression, 144, 202, 232, 323,
346, 351
depth psychology, 53, 56, 68–69,
139, 250, 357, 373
desire, 288
destiny, 51, 80. See also Tao
hun and, 200–201
shen and, 174–75
spirit alignment and, 145–46
yi and, 216, 222
detoxification, of liver, 205–7,
209
devotion, 234–35
dharma, 5–6
diagnosis, pulse, 64, 90–91, 130,
379, 395n27, 396n12
diet, 103–4, 131, 206, 224–27, 233,
375. See also eating disorders
directed thought, 10–12
disease
heart, 184
manifestation of, 18, 144–45

spirit level problems,
144–46, 202, 231–32,
255, 278
diversity, of life, 6
divine
energies of, 24
inspiration from, 247
lifeless matter and, 328
Tao and, 5–6
Door of the Corporeal Soul, 257
Dove Tail, 256
dreams
images in, 130–31, 208, 318
organization of, 199
symbols in, 14, 48, 52
drugs, abuse of, 125–26, 144,
203, 205, 287, 289, 292,
399n5
dualism, 357–58, 362, 374

earth element, 103–4, 112–14,
120, 125, 217–18, 220–21,
346
eating disorders, 204, 226–27.
See also diet; nourishment
ego
awareness of, 20, 52–53,
313, 318
identity and, 47–48, 308–9
electromagnetic energy, 77
electromagnetic fields, 40, 98–99
elements. See also Five elements;
specific elements
Chinese characters for,
118–20
color for, 114, 126
control of, 114–16
correspondences of, 112–14
function of, 114
in nature, 118–21
organ systems with, 114
seasons of, 114, 118–20
sound and, 114, 126
spirits of, 114, 167–68
embryo, 56–57, 60
emergence, 280–82

emotions
    awareness of, 25–26
    balanced, 196–97
    blocked, 124–25
    in body, 271–72
    experience of, overwhelming,
        204
    Five Elements and, 121–23
    heart and, 177–80
    imbalanced, 126–28,
        144–45, 196, 219,
        317–18
    movement of, 123, 240
    organ systems and, 123
    origin of, 240–41
    po and, 240–41
    qi and, 241
    strain of, 62, 86
    as symptoms, 317–18
    wind and, 240, 248–49
emotum, 123
emperor
    heart like, 41–42, 175
    yellow, 151
empress, 78, 175
emptiness, 37–39, 53, 377
enantiodromia, 102, 277, 374
endocrine system, 130–33, 275
energy
    aggressive, 64
    bipolar spectrum of, 87–89
    chaotic, 316–18
    electromagnetic, 77
    female, 8–9, 51, 71, 356
    huntun, 305–6
    male, 8–9
    negentropic, 73–74, 78, 147,
        190, 275, 328, 336
    polarities of, 77–78, 83–85
    psychic, 88–89
    sexual, 288
    systems, 76–81, 83–85
enlightenment, 49. *See also*
    immortality
entropy, 68, 73, 76–81, 85, 91,
    96–97, 114–15, 235, 262, 298,
    304, 328, 330, 374

essences
    flower, xxi, 63–64, 182,
        395n26
    of jing, 374–75
    po and, 239–40
Essences of Anterior Heaven, 375
Essences of Posterior Heaven, 375
essential nature, 11
European alchemy, 303, 328,
    332, 357–58, 389
exercise, 223, 293
eyes, 62, 199

Fabricius, Johannes, 372
fatigue, chronic, 231–32, 352
fear, 105, 122, 132, 283–85, 319,
    324, 346
fertility, of yin, 71–72
fire
    element, 112–14, 119, 125,
        184–87
    excess, 186
    spirits and, 101–2, 175
five
    as center, 112
    as symbol, 39–41
Five Elements. *See also specific*
    element
    archetypes of, 117–21
    in balance, 143–44, 289
    Chinese character for, 111
    correspondences of, 112–14
    cycles of, 114–16
    emotions and, 121–23
    law of, 111–12, 335–38
    origin of, 108–10
    qi movement through, 336
    soul and, 121
Five Spirits. *See also specific spirits*
    archetypes and, 23–24
    breath body and, 23–24,
        146–48
    in Chinese medicine, 144–46
    consciousness and, 166
    cycles of, 114–16, 274, 342
    descent of, 156–58
    modern views of, 23

in pneumatic system, 147
soma as, 249–51
symptoms associated with,
246–47, 252–53
yin and, 147, 246, 252
possession, 257
poetry
discussion of, 185
of language, 59–60
Polaris. *See* North Star
polarities
of energy, 77–78, 83–85
of yin/yang, 40, 74–75, 88,
98, 134–36, 145, 383
Pole Star, 152. *See also* North
Star
practitioner
relationships of, 92, 128, 139
vision of, 65–66
prana, 378
present, staying in, 210
prima materia, 86–87, 328,
332–33, 335, 378–79
psyche, xviii, xix, 379
psyche, modern human
alchemical view of, 87–89
archetype of, 45–46, 61
gui and, 265–66
mind/body splits in, 20–21,
52–53, 134–38
torments of, 263–64
unity in, 24, 52n20
psychic energy, 88–89
psychological function, 145
psychology
Freudian, 382
modern depth, 53, 56,
68–69, 139, 250, 357,
373
Taoism and, xviii, 23–24, 60,
150
of traditional Chinese medicine, 15–17
psychosomatic illness, 16, 20,
281, 317
psychosomatic pain, 247, 252–53

pulse diagnosis, 64, 90–91, 130,
379, 395n27, 396n12

qi
balance of, 17–18, 44, 64
blocked, 95–97, 124–25,
223, 356
in breath body, 135
chaotic, 62
emotions and, 241
Five Spirits and, 22–23,
108–10, 144, 149, 336
jing, 241–42
life experiences and, 16
liver, 205, 209
movement of, 336
nature of, 7–8, 379, 392n3
needling of, 326, 369–70
sheng/k'o cycles of, 114–16,
128, 274
soul and, 11–12
Tao and, 26, 134–36, 311
touch and, xx, 396n12
qian, 96, 327–30, 332–33
qing, 241
Quan Yin, 191
quinta essentia, 39n6

radical, xx, 379–80
rebirth, 55, 58, 156–58, 268,
277, 342–44, 349–50
regression, 364
relationships
of elements, 114–16
to elements, 121
intimate, 184, 186
patient/practitioner, 92, 128,
139
repolarization, of yin/yang, 98
reproductive organ system,
71–72, 79, 275, 292
Rescue Remedy. *See* Bach Flower
Rescue Remedy
restorative acupuncture, 89–91
rhythm, of hun, 209–10
ri, xix, 13

self and, 56, 355
Tao and, 5–6, 46, 56–58,
    62–63
Wilber, Ken, 49
Wilhelm, Richard, 45
will
    disharmonies of, 285–86
    individual, 47, 79–81, 317
    instinctual, 316, 321–22
    zhi and, 275, 280–82
willpower, 275
wind
    chaos and, 303
    emotions and, 240, 248–49
winter, 114, 119, 354
wisdom, 4, 81, 133, 140, 320–22
woman. *See also* Mysterious
    Feminine
    body of, symbolic, 71–72,
        78, 265–66
    cancer of, 347–52
    hun spirit in, 204–5
    male connection to, 366
    original nature of, 311
    yin energy as characteristics
        of, 8–9, 51, 71, 356
wood element, 103, 112–14, 119,
124
    hun and, 195–96, 199, 211
    vision in, 196, 257–58
"the Word," 219
words, 14–15
World Trade Center, 63
worry, 222–25
Worsely, Dr. J.R., 64, 395n28
wu
    Chinese character for, 37–39,
        39–41
    as emptiness, 37–39, 53, 377
    experience of, 53, 55–56
    importance of, 36
    as number five, 39–41
    self and, 36, 43
    spirits and, 38–39
    tradition of, 3–4, 35
wushen, xviii, 32, 138, 144, 165

wuwei, 32, 61, 71–72, 176–77,
    316–18, 322, 324, 326, 352
wuxing, 32, 111–13

Xi Wang Mu, 79, 150, 159, 161,
    268–69, 297, 305, 310, 349,
    383, 400n19
    zhi and, 274–75, 277, 280,
        283
xin
    Chinese character for, 42
    experience and, 12, 41
    heart and, xvi, 42–43
    translation of, xvi
xing, 111–12
xue, 36

yang
    balance of, 17–18, 40,
        74–75, 80–81, 288
    creation/rebirth and, 156–58,
        277
    hun and, 147
    nature of, 8–9, 71
    in original nature, 310
    polar, 40, 74–75, 88, 98,
        134–36, 145, 383
    repolarization of, 98
    shen and, 170–73
    sulfide and, 100
    in Taoist cosmology, 108–10
Yellow Emperor, 151, 376, 378,
    388
*The Yellow Emperor's Classic of
    Internal Medicine*, xvi–xvii,
    74–75, 378. *See also* Neijing
    Suwen
Yellow River, 12, 26
yi
    balanced, 228, 230
    Chinese character for, 218
    correlations with, 220
    cultivation of, 225–28
    destiny and, 216, 222
    disturbances of, 222–25
    heart and, 218–19

heart and, 218–19
  as heavenly pivot, 221–22
  nature of, 145, 216–18
  organs associated with,
    220–21
  surrender to, 317
  zhi and, 277
yi she, 233
yin, 8–9
  balance of, 17–18, 40,
    74–75, 80–81, 288
  creation/rebirth and, 156–58,
    277
  as female energy, 8–9, 51,
    71, 356
  fertility of, 71–72
  mercury and, 100
  Mysterious Feminine and,
    6–7, 51, 158, 161
  in original nature, 310
  po and, 147, 246, 252
  polar, 40, 74–75, 88, 98,
    134–36, 145, 383
  recognition of, 330–31
  repolarization of, 98
  spirits, 159
  in Taoist cosmology, 108–10
yoga, 324–25
you men, 291
Yu Yuwu, 9
yuan, 309
yun, 197

zangfu, 123, 383
Zen Buddhism, 4–5, 72–73,
  400n13
Zen cook, 72–73, 86, 334, 396n5
Zen koan, 308–9
zhi
  associations with, 278
  balanced, 293
  Chinese character for, 276,
    391n2
  cultivation of, 292–93
  disturbances of, 279
  dual nature of, 279–80

healing stages of, 280–85
heart and, 277, 283
identity and, 285
imbalanced symptoms of,
  278–79, 281, 286
nature of, 145, 149, 274–76
underworld and, 274–76
will and, 275, 280–82
Xi Wang Mu and, 274–75,
  277, 280, 283
yi and, 277
zi, 44, 141
ziran, 382, 400n19